The Craving Cure

ALSO BY JULIA ROSS

The Diet Cure
The Mood Cure

The Craving Cure

IDENTIFY YOUR CRAVING TYPE TO ACTIVATE YOUR NATURAL APPETITE CONTROL

Julia Ross

FLATIRON
BOOKS
NEW YORK

This book contains the opinions and ideas of its author. It is intended to provide helpful general information on the subjects that it addresses. It is not in any way a substitute for the advice of the reader's own physician(s) or other medical professionals based on the reader's own individual conditions, symptoms, or concerns. If the reader needs personal medical, health, dietary, exercise, or other assistance or advice, the reader should consult a competent physician and/or other qualified health care professionals. The author and publisher specifically disclaim all responsibility for injury, damage, or loss that the reader may incur as a direct or indirect consequence of following any directions or suggestions given in the book or participating in any programs described in the book.

The fact that a physician, medical professional, organization, or web site is mentioned in this book, as a potential source of information or treatments, does not mean that the author or the publisher endorses any particular physician or medical professional, or the information they may provide, or the medications, equipment, products, or courses of treatment they may have used or recommended.

To Prayer

Contents

Part IV. Craving-Free Eating | 199

Part V. Vital Resources | 265

Introducing the Craving Cure

LIKE MOST AMERICANS, YOU'RE PROBABLY looking for answers to three of the most desperately asked questions of our time: "Why can't I stop eating the wrong food?," "Why is my weight still out of control?," and "Is there any safe and permanent solution?" *The Craving Cure* gives you definitive, complete answers to these questions and shows you, step by step, how to end the struggle, take charge of your own appetite, and stop unnatural weight gain. But first, let's dispose of some of the wrong answers:

- It's not in your mind. You're not an uncontrollable emotional mess who should just get it together. *Most of us* now find it impossible to consistently eat well, feel well, or look our best.

- It's not your willpower. More than 70 percent of Americans (230 million adults) are now *un*willingly overweight, despite their repeated and heroic attempts to change the way they eat.

- It's not a character flaw and you aren't lazy. In fact, you've probably been trying *anything* that might work for years.

Since the onset of the weight-gain epidemic more than fifty years ago, thousands of experts have dispensed advice, some of it very good, about how to eat, think, feel, exercise, or meditate to cope with what has now become a worldwide public health crisis. Yet the increasingly frantic public has found that, year after year, the new approaches never quite solve the problem. Why? Because *none of these approaches has ever addressed it.*

The problem is not that we're misinformed, mindless, or undisciplined. The problem is that we belong to a nation of cravers—*involuntary* consumers of the most addictive substances ever known. Only if our cravings for these substances are silenced can we return to our former eating habits—the ones that, until just a few decades ago, had kept us fit throughout human history.

How would I know? I've been a specialist in eating disorders, addiction, and nutrition for more than thirty years, directing programs specifically for food cravers in the San Francisco Bay Area since 1983 and training health practitioners from around the world since 2004.

The Principles of the Craving Cure

The elimination of cravings is the critical missing key in our struggle to free ourselves from the wrong food, the wrong weight, and the wrong health. *The Craving Cure* provides that key, forged from everything I've learned in the last thirty years through research into neuronutrition and from the real-life experiences of the thousands of clients who have come through the programs at my clinics. Here are its essential elements:

- Healthy eating and healthy weight are our birthright. They were a given throughout human history until the 1970s.

- In the 1970s, several dietary changes, unprecedented in all of human history, radically altered our relationship to food and to our bodies.

- Commercially designed food-like substances are turning us into helpless cravers and overconsumers of the most caloric and least nutritious diet ever known; a diet that nature never intended us to eat.

- Our brain's five primary appetite-control forces, including powerful neurotransmitters like serotonin and endorphin, are being hijacked by our new eating habits and need an emergency rescue operation.

- Each of us has a unique food craving profile determined by the functioning or malfunctioning of our brains' five appetite-control forces.

- Special, brain-targeted nutrient supplements called amino acids can be used to form an immediate line of defense against cravings by directly supporting any of those forces that have been compromised.

- A twenty-first-century eating strategy that restores the ancient nutritional fundamentals can build in permanent protection from modern dietary dangers, once the amino acids have done their work.

THERE IS AN EXPLANATION—AND A SOLUTION

Food cravings come in all sizes and strengths, from the vision of chocolate that lingers for hours until we finally succumb to the unstoppable drive-to-the-store-and-eat-it-all-in-the-car variety. Cravings have nothing to do with real hunger or the need for nourishment. They are blind, brain-triggered drives for a chemical "fix" that only carefully constructed, high-calorie, drug-like brain-bombs can temporarily supply.

Cravings were not our problem until just a few decades ago. Then, in the 1970s, we made three reckless dietary shifts that have since catapulted us into an international weight-gain spiral and set in motion the greatest nutritional crisis of all time. This crisis is propelled by an endless procession of increasingly sophisticated confections. All of them are scrumptious, but they are not foods. They are specifically formulated to create explosive cravings at the expense of our health and weight. Not understanding the distinction between real foods and drug foods will certainly keep you from losing unneeded weight. It could also kill you. The rates of diabetes and other diet-related diseases are rising in direct parallel with our intake of food-like products that are simply unsafe for human consumption—but impossible to pass up.

Part I of *The Craving Cure* explains how and why most of us have become overweight, sick, and riddled with cravings. But its value is limited if all you can think about is a Snickers. That's why Part II takes you right to the actual site of the problem. That problem is not located at your waistline or in your taste buds. That problem is in your brain. This powerful organ, which is supposed to be controlling your appetite, has been turned against you. Time to call in a neurologist? Not at all. The repair work needed to get your brain back in gear is a do-it-yourself project. By taking the Craving-Type Questionnaire that follows this introduction (see page 12), you will quickly discover which of the five types of brain-generated cravings you have. Then you'll read the chapters in Part II that apply to any of the Craving Types specific to you. In Part III, you will learn how to make simple but potent nutritional repairs tailored to your own brain's needs. Once you've started taking the amino acid supplements that are indicated for your Craving Type, you'll start experiencing life without cravings, overeating, or weight gain, *on the first day.*

Our clients, thousands of them over the past thirty years, typically call in with the same report after their first day on their brain-targeted nutrients: "Amazing! My cravings have disappeared." It soon becomes evident that their weight gain is disappearing, too, often as much as ten pounds in the first two weeks, and after that at a steady, sustainable clip. Without cravings, Part IV's Craving-Free Eating options (including one specifically for diabetics) are easy to implement. You have very little to lose but everything to gain. Except weight and disease.

What Are Amino Acids?

An amino acid is a protein. There are twenty of them. We get lots from high protein foods like steak and eggs and some, but fewer, from nuts, beans, and grains. Junk foods contain almost none. Amino acids are called "the building blocks of protein" because they are used alone or in thousands of combinations, like multicolored bricks, to build every structure in the body, including the brain cells that control our appetites.

None of our brain's appetite-regulating cells can function well without a good supply of at least five of the twenty aminos. The better the amino supply, the more satisfied we feel. The more depleted the amino supply, the more we crave. Most of the five key aminos are readily available as inexpensive individual supplements that start working in minutes.

WHY TRUST ME?

This may all sound very intriguing, but after so many diet experts have made you promises they could not keep, why should you believe me?

I have been directing programs in the eating disorder and addiction fields since 1980. From the beginning, my programs provided all of the best conventional recovery strategies. But, much to the disappointment of all of us in these fields, they most often failed. That is why I began experimenting with *nutritional* strategies. Over 4,000 overeater and bulimic clients have since come to my clinic and benefited dramatically from these strategies. As a result, I am now one of a small group of world experts in the field of applied neuronutrition; the care and feeding of the powerful brain neurotransmitters that control how we feel emotionally as well as what we crave. At this point, after all my experiences with the clients in my clinic and the successful case reports of hundreds of health practitioners who've gone through my trainings, I can honestly say that the strategies in this book are virtually fail-proof.

Although I'd begun to be beware of the new research on addiction and the brain when it first emerged in the early 1980s, it wasn't till 1985 that I was introduced to several studies authored by Kenneth Blum, Ph.D., one of the leaders among the neuroscientists focusing on addiction research. He had documented a brain-targeted nutrient treatment process that seemed to be able to heal the addicted brain using a few individual amino acids from which the brain could make its powerful appetite- and pleasure-generating neurotransmitters. When the targeted brain sites were supplied with supplements of these particular amino acids, his study subjects, all addicted to either alcohol or cocaine, consistently experienced relief of the cravings and negative moods that had always led them back into their addictions.

I asked the nutritionist at my clinic to implement a pilot study of Dr. Blum's amino acid approach and we found it to be just as effective as we had hoped. So we began to try it in our new program for overeaters and bulimics. The results were nothing short of miraculous. Eventually, we started trialing the amino acids during our very first sessions with these clients—and saw their food cravings disappear *even before they walked out the door.* Their supplements had helped eradicate their cravings even before they had made any dietary changes. In fact, we don't *let* our clients change their diets until their cravings, the ones that have defeated their every prior attempt, are gone.

But wait. You've been told that quick fixes, silver bullets, and easy answers don't exist. Only hard work, mindfulness, constant vigilance, portion control, calorie control, fat control, carbohydrate control, or meat control will solve the greatest dietary crisis of all time, right? Wrong.

ANTI-CRAVING FOODS

Millions of people have been working hard to "get their eating habits on the right track"—yet those same millions fail, again and again. The reality is that no system of dietary restriction yet devised has been able to combat our drive to consume our favorite treats. In fact, it turns out that dietary restriction is often a biochemical boomerang that sets off rebound cravings and weight gain by disrupting genetic, metabolic, and hormonal regulation, as you'll see in Chapter 4, The Weight-Gain Pandemic: Uncovering True Causes and How *The Craving Cure* Can Help.

It is true, of course, that you will have to change your eating habits. But after just twenty-four hours on the right amino supplements, you'll *want* to. You won't be craving junk foods, so not eating them will be easy. You *will* be eating more protein (which is composed of amino acids) and more traditional saturated fats (which, happy surprise, *are not* weight-promoting or heart threatening, as you'll learn in Chapter 3) as well as traditional carbohydrates (depending on your tolerance). You'll also be eating more calories than you would imagine. In other words, you'll be eating the diet of normal-weight people everywhere before 1970.

Though undeniably amazing, the amino acids are intended only to make us feel satisfied with the traditional foods that our normal-weight ancestors enjoyed for so long. Typically, after two to twelve months, our clients can dispense with the amino supplements altogether. By then they're relying solely on the aminos they get from their anti-craving foods, bolstered by the secret wisdom of the "three squares" and other nearly extinct but essential traditional eating practices. The recipes and menus section will come in handy here. What you will *not* find in *The Craving Cure* is a low-calorie, low-fat, or low-protein diet.

OPEN THE DOOR

Every chapter of this book is aimed at helping you to eliminate highly addictive, industrially designed edibles from your life. But don't expect to live with feelings of deprivation. It would never work! Once on your program of amino acids and anti-craving foods, you'll feel fine without the old treats. Without them, the rich supply of nutrients in your now consistently wholesome cuisine will work to restore your health and allow your body to reveal its true weight.

The Craving Cure is the key that can return you to your birthright: your natural appetite, your natural health, and your natural shape. I hope that you'll turn this key in the lock and come home.

Take the first step by turning the page and then filling out the Craving-Type Questionnaire that will open the way to your craving-free life.

Are You a Craver?
The Craving-Type Questionnaire

MORE THAN FOUR THOUSAND PEOPLE have come to my clinics since 1988. Almost 100 percent of them have been food cravers, but many of them didn't know it. You may be wondering about this, too. Like our clients do at first, you may be asking yourself right now:

"What does she mean by craving? I don't think I crave."

"I only crave a few things and only some of the time."

"Sure I've got cravings, but everyone does and I'm not sure it's the problem."

"I don't know why I keep eating stuff that I know will keep me fat. I hope I am a craver and that she can help me, but it sounds too easy."

COMMON MISUNDERSTANDINGS

Some of our clients are outright convinced that craving is not their problem. They're desperate to eat better, but they have their own theories about why they haven't been able to. Like them, you probably think it's your own fault—that you're either too lazy, too emotional, too tired, or too busy. Or maybe you're convinced that you "just have some bad eating habits" or that you "just aren't exercising enough." So, before you take the questionnaire, let's get some common misunderstandings out of the way.

Is It Lack of Motivation?

Like so many of our clients, you're probably convinced that you're not trying hard enough. Is this you? "I'm just undisciplined, I guess. Making pasta is easy and the pre-made garlic bread is really good. I buy veggies, but they just rot in the refrigerator." Our clinic staff points out to the self-described weak-willed that they don't seem to slack in other areas of their lives. It's obvious to us that, like *230 million* other Americans who can't control their eating or their weight, their lack of control has nothing to do with willpower and is certainly not their fault. Our inborn ability to control our own food intake was stolen from us when our brains were exposed to a force more powerful than any amount of self-control could ever overcome—the force of modern food technology.

Is It All Emotional?

Remember that I'm an experienced psychotherapist. When I meet with a new client, I'm better prepared than most to deal with the emotional-eating hypothesis: "I think it's really because I haven't gotten past the pain of my childhood (and my life now is pretty stressful, too). I've been in therapy for quite a while and I don't feel as bad as I used to, but I still need that comfort food because I still feel sad, lonely, and stressed a lot."

To those clients I say, "We've found that emotional eating is most often the result of specific (and reversible!) deficits in the parts of the brain that should be regulating both our moods and our appetite, deficits caused by the non-foods in the modern diet. Your psychotherapy was probably effective, but you won't be able to experience all of its benefits until your brain gets some *nutritional* therapy."

Is It Lack of Energy or Time?

Does this sound like you? "I'm too tired to cook when I get home." Or, "I don't have time to eat well in the mornings, plus I don't feel like it because I ate junk late the night before and I'm feeling guilty, as usual." If so, you'd get the following response from us: "Junk foods can make you too tired to cook, night or morning, and skipping real-food meals makes you crave. Please don't feel guilty. Your snack foods have been tampered with and secretly drugged, which makes you an innocent victim. You never really chose to overeat junk food in the first place. You started out eating it for fun and only later discovered that you'd been hooked and couldn't stop. The labels did not read 'highly addictive' or 'potentially disfiguring and lethal.'"

Just a Bad Habit?

"I always eat cereal and drink orange juice for breakfast and I always get out the ice cream and cookies at night." A "habit" is a term commonly used by hard drug users to describe their addictions. As an addiction specialist, I point out that no minor "habit" distorts body shape or has a negative impact on mood, energy, health, and self-respect. Minor habits are fairly easy to break. You are eating against your own best interest and your most primal feeding instincts. This can only be forced on you by the same brain-generated imperatives that hard drug users struggle against.

Not Enough Exercise?

Are you one of the "I just need to exercise more" group? I agree that exercise is important for health but, surprisingly, the research about exercise and weight loss is quite weak. Permanent weight changes require permanent dietary changes, which can't be made without permanent craving eradication.

No Clue?

Many of our clients have run out of theories. They've been burned too often and are almost defeated. They say, "You're my last hope and I don't expect much. But after all the things I've tried that have failed, I don't know what else to do." To them, my staff and I say, "That's understandable! But you'll know by tomorrow whether this is for real or not. Please hang in just a bit longer."

I hope that you're more like the clients who immediately see the light as soon as they hear the word "craving." Like them, you know that you're a craver, that you have become a biochemical prisoner in your own body. Like quite a few of them, you may also be very angry about it. "You mean all this time hating my belly and fighting to stay on a diet every day, and feeling like a stupid failure most days, even though I spin the rest of my life like a top, was so that those responsible could make more money? And they knew all along what their stuff would do to us?" To those angry ones we say, "Your anger is beautiful and healthy, but get back to it later when you're in condition to take on Big Food. Your battle right now is to get completely free and recovered from the dietary ordeal you've been subjected to."

WHAT TYPE OF CRAVING DO YOU HAVE? USE THE CRAVING-TYPE QUESTIONNAIRE TO IDENTIFY THE REAL CAUSE OF YOUR FRUSTRATION

The first step in your Craving Cure is to understand the nature of your own struggle. The Craving-Type Questionnaire, which I've developed and refined over more than thirty years, has proven to be the key to this discovery process. It takes the guesswork, the theories, and the blame out of the equation and pinpoints the true source of the problem, the exact food-brain disconnect that needs attention. The Questionnaire is a two-part affair. It allows you to both check off your symptoms and rate the severity of those symptoms

THE SYMPTOM CHECKOFF

The questionnaire is divided into five sections, one for each Craving Type. Each section contains a set of very distinctive symptoms. These symptoms, identified through years of neuroscientific study, are known to indicate deficiency in one of the brain's key appetite-regulating functions. In Part II, a whole chapter is devoted to each of the five Craving Types, the biochemical origins of their symptoms, and how specific nutrients called amino acids work to quickly eliminate these symptoms.

Over the years, we've refined the questionnaire as we've learned more about each of the Craving Types. My clinic staff has verified each symptom by watching the results of more than twenty thousand amino acid trials. How? By confirming that the deficiency symptoms of each one of the five Craving Types has been consistently eliminated by an amino well known to be the unique nutrient from which only *a particular one* of them can be produced.

THE SEVERITY SCALE

This part of the questionnaire allows you to identify not how many symptoms of a particular Craving Type you have, but *how intense* those symptoms are. The 0-to-10 scoring reveals important individual differences in craving. Some people have mild cases of Type 1 craving while others have severe cases. Occasionally clients have checked off only a few symptoms of a particular Craving Type, but their severity ratings have been high. Those clients have trialed the amino acid indicated and benefitted. When a rare client checks off many symptoms, but has very low severity ratings, he or she has usually either underreported and needs to rescore or needs to explore other Craving Types with higher severity ratings.

Some craving clients have been such underreporters that all of their severity ratings are on the low end and we have had to ask them to have family members fill out the questionnaire with them. (Men have been apt to be underreporters more often than women.) It is not uncommon for clients to not realize how often they seem irritable or sad or tired. If you're not sure about your own rating, don't hesitate to ask someone close to you for an opinion.

The Severity Scale will make it possible for you to closely monitor the changes in your craving and other symptoms as your Cure progresses. Initially, like our clients, you'll *rescore* your questionnaire weekly (using a shorter mini-version) to make sure that your severity scores start dropping rapidly. If any score stops dropping, the unchanged score will alert you to the need to increase your doses of the indicated amino supplement.

You're about to learn how to get your cravings put to rest—and to get them to stay put. So, let's get you started!

The Craving-Type Questionnaire

WHAT IS YOUR CRAVING STATUS TODAY?

Directions:

Fill out the Questionnaire and Profile here, at the end of the book on page 272 (in Tracking and Testing Tools), or at cravingcure.com/trackingtools.

<u>Step 1.</u> To determine your *symptom score,* check off each symptom statement that accurately describes you on a typical day. Each check mark equals a score of one. When you finish a section, add up the number of checks to see if your total symptom score indicates that you have that Craving Type. Then move on to the next section.

<u>Step 2.</u> To determine your *severity rating* on a scale of 0 to 10, rate the *strength* of each symptom statement on the blank line next to any box you've checked off. A rating of 1 is rare and/or quite weak; a 10 is daily and powerful.

<u>Step 3.</u> Enter your symptom score totals on the Profile Graph that follows the questionnaire on page 19. This will give you a quick visual perspective: How many Craving Types do you have? How high above the cutoff are your scores? How do you compare with the profile of one of our clients (on page 18)?

TYPE 1. THE DEPRESSED CRAVER

Are your cravings caused by a deficiency of serotonin, your brain's inner sunshine?

To determine if you are a Depressed Craver: Check off the box next to each symptom statement that applies to you. Next, rate each *checked* statement on the Severity Scale of 0–10 (0 none, 10 frequent and severe) by placing your number on the blank line next to any checked-off box.

_____ ☐ Your cravings are strongest toward the end of the day—in the afternoon or evening.

_____ ☐ You eat to get to, or get back to, sleep.

_____ ☐ You wake up in the night and head for the fridge.

_____ ☐ You crave more (and perhaps gain more) in fall and winter. Your mood is worse in winter, too.

_____ ☐ You tend to be negative, depressed, or pessimistic.

_____ ☐ You frequently worry or feel anxious.

_____ ☐ You have frequent feelings of low self-esteem, guilt, or shame.

_____ ☐ You are obsessed with certain thoughts or behaviors (e.g., your body, your weight, biting your nails, pulling your eyelashes out).

_____ ☐ You are a perfectionist or a neat freak. You tend to be controlling with others.

_____ ☐ You are subject to irritability or anger.

_____ ☐ You have panic attacks.

_____ ☐ You have phobias: fear of heights, small spaces, crowds, snakes, etc.

_____ ☐ You are hyperactive.

_____ ☐ You often have a nervous stomach (knots, butterflies).

_____ ☐ You are a night owl or have middle of the night insomnia.

_____ ☐ You suffer pain from headaches, TMJ, or fibromyalgia.

_____ ☐ You are using or have used an SSRI antidepressant drug (like Zoloft, Lexapro, or Prozac) with some benefit.

Your symptom total: _____ **(Each check mark equals a score of one.)**

If your symptom score is over 7, especially if most of your severity ratings are over 3, you are a Type 1 Depressed Craver.

TYPE 2. THE CRASHED CRAVER

Are your cravings caused by blood sugar deficits?

To determine if you are a Crashed Craver: Check off the box next to each symptom statement that applies to you. Next, rate each *checked* statement on the Severity Scale of 0–10 (0 none, 10 frequent and severe) by placing your number on the blank line next to any checked-off box.

_____ ☐ Your cravings for sugar or starch are stronger when you have skipped or delayed a meal.

_____ ☐ You tend to skip breakfast and/or other meals.

_____ ☐ Your cravings spike later in the day if you've skipped any earlier meals.

_____ ☐ You suspect you have (or you have been diagnosed with) hypoglycemia.

_____ ☐ You are diabetic or prediabetic. (Your blood sugar levels rise too high, but drop too low at times, as well.)

_____ ☐ You get dizzy, shaky, or headachy if you go too long between meals.

_____ ☐ You find it harder to concentrate when you go too long without healthy meals.

_____ ☐ You can get irritable, or blow up, if you go too long without full meals.

_____ ☐ You feel more stressed the fewer regular meals you eat.

_____ ☐ Hypoglycemia, diabetes, or alcoholism run in your family.

_____ ☐ You are drawn to alcohol on a regular basis.

Your symptom total: _____ **(Each check mark equals a score of one.)**

If your score is over 4, especially if your severity ratings are mostly over 3, you are a Type 2 Crashed Craver.

TYPE 3. THE COMFORT CRAVER

Are your cravings caused by a deficiency of pleasuring endorphin?

To determine if you are a Comfort Craver: Check off the box next to each symptom statement that applies to you. Next, rate each *checked* statement on the Severity Scale of 0–10 (0 none, 10 frequent and severe) by placing your number on the blank line next to any checked-off box.

_____ ☐ You crave—no, love—certain foods. They are treats that give you feelings of pleasure, enjoyment, or reward and taste "sooo goood."

_____ ☐ You think of your comfort foods as your best friends.

_____ ☐ Chocolate is particularly beloved.

_____ ☐ You get extra pleasure if you read, watch TV, or play with the computer, tablet, or phone while you eat.

_____ ☐ You are very sensitive to emotional or physical pain.

_____ ☐ You often feel sad, lonely, or hurt.

_____ ☐ You tear up or cry easily; even at TV commercials.

_____ ☐ You adore animals and need their loving company.

_____ ☐ You get a high from bulimic bingeing or purging or from restricting calories.

_____ ☐ You have a history of chronic physical pain from back or other injuries, or have chronic emotional pain from unresolved trauma or protracted personal ordeals.

_____ ☐ You are a dough lover—bread, cookies, and pasta are at the top of your list. You have trouble eating even whole wheat products moderately.

_____ ☐ Cheese, ice cream, frozen yogurt, butter, and even milk are irresistible.

_____ ☐ Dough and milk *combined* are your top treats: crackers and cheese, pizza, macaroni and cheese or the ultimate, dough and milk with chocolate—chocolate cheesecake, and cookie dough ice cream.

_____ ☐ You may also crave certain other substances or activities that give you similar feelings: painkillers, pot, or alcohol; serious aerobic exercise, porn, or self-harm.

Your symptom total: _____ **(Each check mark equals a score of one.)**

If your symptom score is over 6, especially if most of your severity ratings are over 3, you are a Type 3 Comfort Craver.

TYPE 4. THE STRESSED CRAVER

Do you crave because your brain's levels of calming GABA are too low?

To determine if you are a Stressed Craver: Check off the box next to each symptom statement that applies to you. Next, rate each *checked* statement on the Severity Scale of 0–10 (0 none, 10 frequent and severe) by placing your number on the blank line next to any checked-off box.

_____ ☐ You are overstressed or burnt out.

_____ ☐ You reach for snack food to counteract stress.

_____ ☐ You are unable to relax and loosen up easily.

_____ ☐ You have stiff, tense, or painful muscles.

_____ ☐ Your mind is cluttered and it's hard to focus.

_____ ☐ It's hard to meditate, pray, or be mindful, still, or at peace.

_____ ☐ You feel easily overwhelmed.

_____ ☐ You can feel close to panic.

_____ ☐ You don't get away on regular vacations to relax, rest, and regenerate.

_____ ☐ It is hard to get to sleep (or stay asleep) at times because of the above symptoms.

Your symptom total: _____ **(Each check mark equals a score of one.)**

If your symptom score is over 4, especially if most of severity ratings are over 4, you are a Type 4 Stressed Craver.

TYPE 5. THE FATIGUED CRAVER

Do you crave an energy boost because you're deficient in naturally stimulating catecholamines?

To determine if you are a Fatigued Craver: Check off the box next to each symptom statement that applies to you. Next, rate each *checked* statement on the Severity Scale of 0–10 (0 none, 10 frequent and severe) by placing a number on the blank line next to any checked-off box.

_____ ☐ You gravitate toward the stimulant effect of caffeine, coffees, sodas (including artificially sweetened ones), iced teas, energy drinks, or anything chocolate.

_____ ☐ Your energy is on the low side.

_____ ☐ You frequently feel the need to be more alert and focused.

_____ ☐ You are low in drive and motivation.

_____ ☐ Sweets give you a "pick-me-up."

_____ ☐ You have trouble concentrating, or have attention problems.

_____ ☐ You are easily bored and feel the need for some excitement.

_____ ☐ You have tried, and liked, stimulant drugs like Ritalin, Adderall, diet pills, methamphetamine, cocaine.

Your symptom total: _____*(Each check mark equals a score of one.)*

If your symptom score is over 4, especially if most of your severity ratings are over 3, you are a Type 5 Fatigued Craver.

THE PROFILE GRAPH

On the blank graph on the next page, transfer your total symptom score for each Craving Type to the corresponding Profile columns. Draw a line across the column where your score falls. See if your score is above the cutoff score and by how much. Shade in the space below your score, as shown in the example graph on the following page. Any score above the cutoff verifies that you have that particular Craving Type. The higher the score above the cutoff line, the more certain it is that you have that particular type of craving, particularly if the severity ratings tend to be over 3.

YOUR PROFILE GRAPH

	TYPE 1 Depressed Craver	TYPE 2 Crashed Craver	TYPE 3 Comfort Craver	TYPE 4 Stressed Craver	TYPE 5 Fatigued Craver
Max. Possible Score	17	11	15	9	8
	16	10	14	8	7
	15		13		
	14	9	12	7	6
	13	8	11		
	12	7	10	6	5
	11		9		
	10	6	8	5	
	9	5	7		
	8				4
Cutoff Score	7	4	6	4	
	6	3	5		
	5		4	3	3
	4	2	3	2	
	3	1	2		2
	2		1	1	
	1				1
Total Symptom Score					

THE EXAMPLE PROFILE OF ONE OF OUR CLIENTS,
A CRAVER WITH TYPES 1 AND 2

	TYPE I Depressed Craver	TYPE 2 Crashed Craver	TYPE 3 Comfort Craver	TYPE 4 Stressed Craver	TYPE 5 Fatigued Craver
Max. Possible Score	17	11	15	9	8
	16	(10)	14		
	15	9	13	8	7
	14		12		
	13	8	11	7	6
	(12)	7	10		
	11		9	6	
	10	6	8		5
	9	5		5	
	8		7		
Cutoff Score	7	4	6	4	4
	6	3	(5)		
	5		4	(3)	3
	4	2	3		
	3		2	2	
	2	1	1		2
	1			1	
					1
Total Symptom Score	12	10	5	3	0

Next Stop: Your Complete Craving Cure

Once you've scored your Questionnaire, which is the real key to this book, you'll have three more jobs to do. The first is to become aware of how we've been transformed from a people who'd always loved healthy food into compulsive consumers of industrial chemicals. Part I will help you with that. Parts II and III will train you to perform the second and more thrilling task: freeing your brain's battered appetite-control squad from the clutches of food science with a few amino acids. Your last job, laid out in Part IV, will be to craving-proof your diet by returning to the traditional eating habits of your healthy and shapely forbears.

A *complete* Craving Cure will then be yours.

PART I

How We Got Here

1

Your Favorite Carbohydrates: Twice as Addictive as Cocaine

A NUTRITIONAL CRIME HAS BEEN COMMITTED. An ancient and healthful nutrient has been transformed into the most harmful substance ever known. It is now the main ingredient in the American diet. What is the violated substance in question? Carbohydrate.

Carbohydrate is one of only three kinds of food available for our consumption here on earth. The other two are protein and fat. We have been thriving on these three elemental fuels in various forms and proportions since the beginning of human time. Tragically, all three have been subjected to damage and defamation in recent decades. But carbohydrate, grotesquely deformed by commercial processing into sweet and starchy weapons of mass destruction, is having its revenge. It is igniting cravings that we cannot resist and destroying us as we succumb.

WHAT IS A CARBOHYDRATE?

Most people think that a carbohydrate is a starchy food like bread, pasta, rice, beans, or potatoes—and they're right. But carbohydrate also comes in sweet forms; as apples, grapes, sodas, and gum drops. Most foods contain some carbohydrate, but any food that is *primarily* either sweet *or* starchy is officially called a carbohydrate.

Why are these two types of carbohydrate lumped together under one name when their flavors is so different? These sweet and starchy sisters are composed of almost identical chemical elements. They're also identical in that both can *very* quickly be converted into our bodies' primary energy source; its gas. (More on this miraculous process shortly.)

Carbohydrate-containing foods in their original, undamaged forms are rich in nutrients and include the world's most beautiful and colorful edibles. Vegetables and fruits, which were originally our only sources of carbohydrate (as well as fiber) gave us all the reds, purples, yellows, and, of course, greens in our diet. They gave us myriad sweet and subtle flavors and many health benefits. Those of us who are still eating several vegetables and fruits a day have been found to be healthier (our cancer rate is lower, for example)[1] and happier (our depression rate is lower).[2] Unfortunately, we're now eating less than half the fresh produce that we traditionally ate before 1970.[3] And I think it's fair to say that we're less than half as healthy and happy.

The foods highest in carbohydrate—fruits, roots, beans, grains, and, of course, sugarcane—also contain valuable nutrients. But it's their naturally high content of nature's sugars and starches that has made them the primary victims of modern nutritional crime.

THE CARBOHYDRATE-ENERGY MIRACLE—AND ITS DEMISE

Many of carbohydrate's natural properties are health- and pleasure-enhancing, but I have hardly begun to tout their most vital function. All sweets and starches contain, or can be instantly transformed into, the life-sustaining, cell-ready fuel called "glucose." Glucose absorption begins right in your mouth and continues in your digestive tract. The glucose released can be burned immediately or stored as backup energy.

Almost all sweet-tasting high carbohydrate foods like oranges and yams contain not only glucose, but lots of another natural sugar called fructose, as well. Glucose converts into energy immediately. Fructose is absorbed more slowly (you'll hear all about that process soon), but most of it eventually converts into glucose. High-carbohydrate foods like potatoes and pasta contain a starch called amylose, some of which is converted into glucose by the saliva in the mouth in milliseconds, the rest in the gut soon after.

Why all this focus on glucose? Glucose is your body's primary energy source; it is the vital fuel that keeps every cell in your body running. You can't build body *parts* out of it, though, any more than you can build a car out of gas. All of your body's structures, not just your muscles, but also your bones, organs, and everything else, are made from protein, fat, and water. But the miracle of carbo-hydrate provides the glucose that brings it all to life.

Our bodies require glucose twenty-four hours a day. Our cells can't ever turn off. Even when we're sleeping, they're still at work. But the precious glucose sup-plies we need are no longer consistently available to us. Despite the fact that our diet is higher in sugar and starch than at any other time in human history, these days, *we can't count on the availability of glucose.* That's because the unnatural, processed, carbohydrate *concentrates* we're now consuming so often can only fuel us with big, initially pleasurable, but short, bursts of glucose. In between bursts, we drop too low in glucose. We drop too low because excess insulin, stimulated by any high-carbohydrate foods, removes both any excess glucose *and* much of the *needed* glucose as well. The result: the low blood sugar crash called hypo-glycemia. How do we know if we've become hypoglycemic? We crave carbohy-drate.

Our *hyper*-carbohydrate diet has made us a nation of carb-craving hypogly-cemics. Since so many of us now typically skip meals and often go without eat-ing anything but sweet or starchy treats for long periods, glucose crashes just keep alternating with glucose overdoses. This roller coaster puts a strain on the entire body, distorts the body's natural hunger signals, and leads directly to the over-eating of carbohyrates that ends up in fat storage. (That's where insulin disposes of all that excess glucose.)

THE CARBOHYDRATE-CRAVING CONNECTION

Do you crave garbanzo beans, blueberries, or acorn squash? Nope. Why? Because these ancient, healthful carbohydrates are only mildly pleasurable. As a result, they have helped fuel human life since the beginning of time *without unnatural weight gain or disease.*

Since a moderate serving of these carbohydrates does not produce blood glucose bombs, these whole, naturally occurring foods don't stimulate insulin rushes. That means our blood sugar levels tend to rise a little and then steady-up till we eat again in a few hours. Our traditional meals used to give us a balance of complex carbohydrates, proteins, and fats. These latter two foods could pinch-hit if the glucose supply from the carbohydrate in the meal didn't last long enough. That's because the body can burn them when needed, by transforming them into glucose substitutes like ketones and lactate. In fact, it does this very smoothly while we sleep at night.

Nice design. Too bad we've wrecked it.

How did we do it? We took the foods that are naturally the highest in carbohydrate—sugarcane, sugar beet, corn, wheat, fruit, and cactus—and savagely processed them into white sugar, high-fructose syrups, and white flour. This "de-naturing" of our ancient sweets and starches, and the adding of their concentrated remains to the food supply, is the felony that's being committed wherever today's commercial foods are made. Almost every processed food product and restaurant item includes these felonious substances, everything from baby formula to "health" bars and frozen dinners. Here's why:

Very few substances in their original, whole forms can force the brain to set off the potentially fatal attraction called craving. But some whole foods contain chemicals within them that, when extracted and concentrated, become so powerful that we call them irresistible and divine. We can't get enough of them.

Think about it. What turns a leaf into crack? What turns a poppy into heroin? Most people addicted to cocaine would not chew coca leaves for long and heroin users would certainly not binge on poppies. No bread lover would settle for a wheat berry and no candy craver would settle for a piece of sugarcane. But when sugar is extracted from the cane and concentrated, it becomes hundreds of times sweeter,[4] hence the sugar rush provided by countless candies and soft drinks.

Highly refined sweets and starches are two of the most potent drugs ever extracted from plants. Like poppies and coca leaves, sugarcane, sugar beets, wheat, and corn can now be quickly and cheaply transformed into ultrapotent white powders and colorless syrups. Like all drug substances, they are designed to impact the brain neurotransmitters that produce enjoyable sensations. First they amplify these sensations tremendously, then, when the impact wears off, those same neurotransmitters start broadcasting powerful craving messages; messages that guarantee quick new sales. (There will be much more on the brain and our cravings in Part II, Understanding Your Craving Type.)

Naming the Enemy: Techno-Karbz

Some people call them Franken-Carbs, most people call them junk foods, but from now on I'm going to refer to these industrial-strength carbohydrates as "Techno-Karbz."

These "doctored" sweets and starches are no longer foods. They are neither fruit, bean, vegetable, nor grain. They are cold cereal, juice, ice cream, cookies, and chips. They are the bun on the burger, the batter on the chicken, the crust on the pizza, and the wrap on the burrito. The beef, chicken, tomatoes, and cheese in the latter products are real foods. When artificially created sugars and flours outweigh these real foods in a product, a Techno-Karb is created. More and more, the real food is being left out altogether. It has been determined that 60 percent of our diet is now composed of stripped sugars and starches with some flavoring and damaging fat thrown in (we'll get to the wronged fats in Chapter 3). This means that about 60 percent of our diet contains *none* of the nutrients required to keep us fit, healthy, and happy.[5] No wonder we aren't.

Sugar and starch concentrates are the world's top-selling and, as we'll see, the world's top-killing designer drugs. As such, they need to be given a warning label. It's imperative that we start making the distinction between Techno-Karbz and whole, natural carbohydrates. It's worth our lives. We must find a way to see through the familiar, cute, and misleading images; the pet names, the funny voice-overs, and the darling graphics. Or, almost worse, the ones that convince us that they're good for us and our children.

Techno-Karbz are actually just narcotics dressed up in skirts. Adorably packaged and sublime tasting, these substances are designed to pass as foods. But they have much more in common with hard drugs. Actually, as you'll see, your favorite goodies are more potent than heroin and cocaine *combined*.

SCIENCE EXPOSES THE FOOD INDUSTRY'S CRAVING STRATEGY

Up until very recently, the food industry has been able to get away with saying, "It's the consumer's choice. We don't *force* anyone to eat our products." But this stance is now slipping under concerted scientific scrutiny.

In 2010, the ultimate food industry insider, former FDA chief, David Kessler, Ph.D., blew the whistle. In his book, *The End of Overeating*, Kessler quoted food industry leaders who acknowledged that their products were destroying our health because we could not limit our intake of them due to their inflated "palatability" (read: addictiveness), achieved through careful and increasingly sophisticated food technology. This was news to the general public, but not to addiction scientists. Three years earlier, in 2007, at the University of Bordeaux, a study using the same methods that had originally certified cocaine as the most addictive drug ever known, had found table sugar, alone, to be *more than twice as addictive*.[6]

Animal studies comparing the effects of sugar to those of street drugs had first started to trickle in after 1980. That trickle has since become a torrent. The French study is now only one of hundreds of scientific papers that continue to be published on this topic. These studies have found the effects of Techno-Karbz on the brain to be comparable to the effects of not just cocaine, but drugs like heroin, Ecstasy, and Xanax, as well. Researchers have documented that foods containing highly refined sugars and starches can have an impact *on all* of the same pleasure centers in the brain that hard drugs do. The director of the National Institute on Drug Abuse (NIDA), neuroscientist Nora Volkow, Ph.D., has repeatedly made it clear that some foods, like certain drugs, set off powerfully addictive brain chemistry processes that leave millions devastated, and that no pharmaceutical solutions are yet in sight, despite her agency's years of committed research.[7]

Research and the Craving Cure

I disagree in this book with a number of opinions that have been held firmly for a long time. But I've only done so after years of experience with thousands of clients, years of digging through the research, and years of discussion with experts in the field of health and nutrition. Even so, I do not want you to just take my word. That's why I've included fifty pages of jewel-like references in the Notes section. I strongly encourage you to scan them and locate the studies that interest you on the Internet. Just type the first five words of any study into the search bar of your favorite search engine to find the study itself (not the blog posts *about* it).

IF OUR FOOD IS NOW SO ADDICTIVE, HAVE WE BECOME A NATION OF FOOD ADDICTS?

I've just explained that our diet has come to consist largely of addictive drugs in disguise and that our cravings for them are involuntary and harmful, so I don't think that you'll be surprised when I say that you are very likely to have become addicted. How could you *not* have? Craving is the primary symptom of any addiction. Most of us have been led all the way into a full-blown addiction trap by cravings that have been building since childhood, when we were first exposed to these shrewdly designed and mercilessly marketed substances.

You have likely been trying to escape that trap for years. No matter the strength of your own cravings, the methods you'll find in Part III, The Amino Breakthrough, will free you. But I don't want to minimize what's at stake here. You now know, from scoring your Craving Profile, how many Craving Types you have and how severe their symptoms are. You could have as many as five separate brain-generated forces propelling you toward the Techno-Karbz. This internal pressure is formidable. But, on top of it, you are faced with massive *external* pressures. Big Food's entire advertising industry is arrayed against you. And Techno-Karbz are everywhere, always a big part of "having fun." It's an addictive gang-up. Yet, most people, probably including you, still think that it's "all my own fault"; that it's about lack of motivation or poor self-discipline. That's what you're supposed to think. It really is a conspiracy!

HOW MANY OF US ARE FOOD ADDICTED?

Scientific interest in what constitutes addicted eating has been aroused by the helpless struggle with food and weight that most Americans are now engaged in. What have they concluded about how foods compare to drug and alcohol addiction? There are 28 million[8] drug and alcohol addicts in the United States. NIDA chief Volkow[9] and the influential Yale Food Addiction Study estimate that, in contrast, between 70 and 200 million Americans are addicted to foods. That's 20 to 60 percent[10] of the U.S. population. In a speech given in 2012, Volkow said that "20 percent of drug users become addicted and behave in health-risking ways because of their use. By this standard, food could actually be considered several times more addictive than crack."[11] Her estimate and that of the Yale study factor in the fact that over 70 percent of the U.S. population is now either obese or overweight and that the majority are suffering serious health and other consequences. They also take into account that those who are overweight and obese are *not all* food addicted, and that some of those at normal weight, like most of our bulimics, *are*.

The Most Addictive Foods

The international team associated with the Yale Food Addiction Study conducted research, published in 2014, that identified the top most addictive foods. Pizza and chocolate-flavored baked desserts topped the list, with chips, cookies, fries, and ice cream close behind.[12]

How did wholesome natural carbohydrates score? Bananas, strawberries, and apples were near the bottom of the list. Carrots and cucumbers were at the rock bottom.

Most important, the team found that *over 90 percent* of the cross section of 500 people they'd surveyed "had a persistent desire to, or repeatedly made unsuccessful attempts to, quit eating" those foods.

THE SIGNS OF TECHNO-KARBZ ADDICTION:
SIZING UP YOUR OWN EATING HABIT

The essential criteria for a diagnosis of chemical dependency, first developed in the alcohol and drug addiction recovery field, are now being applied to food addiction. There are many signs and degrees of addiction and the negative consequences of it, but the simple definition is *"continued use despite adverse consequences."* For you, is it four squares of chocolate every afternoon that you have to have? A pint of ice cream most nights and a constant struggle with fifteen pounds? Or daily binges, type 2 diabetes, and obesity? Can you stay away from your particular favorites? How often have you tried and "failed" despite the guilt, shame, expense, weight gain, and hangovers; despite the comments of friends, a spouse, your personal trainer, or your doctor?

Another common feature of addiction that you may have experienced is increased tolerance. Any addictive substance can become more addictive if we are exposed to greater amounts of it. Remember that in the 1980s, portion sizes *doubled* in the fast food and chain restaurant outlets[13] and we began to frequent them about twice as often. Soda sizes in particular really started to jump; Big Gulp is now ten times larger than the original Gulp. This is a good example of the fact that being addicted is not a voluntary activity. *You* didn't decide to raise portion sizes. As I said earlier, it takes a gang-up to hook one person, let alone a whole country-full. The *gang* decided that it was time to bump up the addictiveness of its foods by increasing our access to them, on top of the gang's continuing efforts to further "enhance the palatability" of their products.

In spite of all this, if you had come to my addiction recovery clinic before 1983, I wouldn't have known how to help you. If you had complained to me of cravings for foods, I would just have assumed that you were emotionally troubled; I would not have imagined that you were addicted. Even as a seven-year veteran in the drug and alcohol addiction field, when I first encountered food cravers, I didn't recognize them. And then one day Cathy, one of the top counselors at my first outpatient addiction recovery clinic in San Francisco, came to talk to me privately and told me her own story.

Cathy's Story

Cathy came from a long line of pretty, blond, blue-eyed, stocky German women. Always popular and lively, she was a cheerleader in high school, during the '50s, and the star of every dance party. In college, in the '60s, on high-

carbohydrate dorm food, she suddenly put on the freshman fifteen. She had a new boyfriend who loved his "nice armful," but she'd started to hate her own "thick" legs and waist because being thin had recently become the only look that counted, according to fashion magazines and advertisements. Cathy started drinking diet sodas, went low fat, and launched into her first "serious" diet: grapefruit and hard-boiled eggs. Without carbohydrates, including beer, she lost twenty pounds and felt better about herself, though she never again felt proud of her body's naturally full shape. Then she was back to parties and the typical '70s high-carbohydrate, low-fat fare. When she'd regained fifteen pounds, she dieted again.

This became the story of her life, except that after four low-calorie diets she began regaining more weight than she lost—despite becoming a Jane Fonda home workout fanatic—as her appetite for carbohydrates increased. Her diets got shorter as the cravings got stronger. After her second child was born, she could not lose all forty pounds of baby weight. She couldn't face another diet because she couldn't give up the cookies, crackers, chips, cheese, and ice cream. Instead, like so many young women in the '70s (and so many women and girls since), she started throwing up. After several years of almost daily bulimia, the shame, guilt, malnutrition, dental damage, and her husband's disgust drove Cathy to look for help.

Cathy had already been seeing a psychotherapist, and she herself had become a professional counselor by then, but she was experiencing little success. Realizing that she was a lot like the clients in our alcohol and drug program, she decided to try Overeaters Anonymous (O.A.). There she became convinced that she really was the victim of a full-blown addiction, and that helped a lot. She was still struggling with her cravings and her weight, but she was making some headway. She had been able to cut back on the bingeing and stopped all of the purging by the time she told me her story. She was hoping that we could help women like her, who were in the O.A. 12-Step program, but had no addiction-savvy counselors or nutritionists to support them.

Cathy asked me to attend some Overeaters Anonymous meetings with her. I did, but, even so, it took me months to recognize all the familiar signs of the unwilling, agonized struggle we call addiction. I just couldn't see it. Partly because I was older than Cathy and had grown up on a more nutritious diet, closer to the traditional diet of my ancestors, in my mind, food was still synonymous with safety, nurturance, health, and strength.

And, unlike cocaine or alcohol, we cannot live without food, so how could we ask people to abstain from it? But two things became was very clear to me when I attended those Overeaters Anonymous meetings: I saw people who were suffering in exactly the same way as the drug addicts at my clinic were. I also saw that they had all identified the same two specific foods as the triggers for most of their overwhelming cravings. Those foods were sugar and flour, in other words, Techno-Karbz. When I learned that mostly just these two foods were operating like drugs in their brains, I realized that "abstinence" was not only necessary but feasible. No one would starve to death by cutting those two substances out of their diets.

At that time, the list of fifteen questions that O.A. asked all prospective members to check off to determine if they really were food-addicted seemed extreme, unusual, and even bizarre. But now, most of them seem to me to apply to most women in this country. *See what you think:*

1) Do I eat when I'm not hungry, or not eat when my body needs nourishment? Yes/No

2) Do I go on eating binges for no apparent reason, sometimes eating until I'm stuffed or even feel sick? Yes/No

3) Do I have feelings of guilt, shame, or embarrassment about my weight or the way I eat? Yes/No

4) Do I eat sensibly in front of others and then make up for it when I am alone? Yes/No

5) Is my eating affecting my health or the way I live my life? Yes/No

6) When my emotions are intense—whether positive or negative—do I find myself reaching for food? Yes/No

7) Do my eating behaviors make me or others unhappy? Yes/No

8) Have I ever used laxatives, vomiting, diuretics, excessive exercise, diet pills, shots, or other medical interventions (including surgery) to try to control my weight? Yes/No

9) Do I fast or severely restrict my food intake to control my weight? Yes/No

10) Do I fantasize about how much better life would be if I were a different size or weight? Yes/No

11) Do I need to chew or have something in my mouth all the time: food, gum, mints, candies, or beverages? Yes/No

12) Have I ever eaten food that is burned, frozen, or spoiled; from containers in the grocery store; or out of the garbage? Yes/No

13) Are there certain foods I can't stop eating after having the first bite? Yes/No

14) Have I lost weight with a diet or "period of control" only to be followed by bouts of uncontrolled eating and/or weight gain? Yes/No

15) Do I spend too much time thinking about food, arguing with myself about whether or what to eat, planning the next diet or exercise cure, or counting calories? Yes/No[14]

Within a year of attending that first O.A. meeting, I had started the first treatment program for food addicts in Northern California. I experimented, with the help of some of the first holistic dieticians in the area, to find a safe and effective anti-craving food plan (which I'll tell you all about in Part IV, Craving-Free Eating). By dint of intensive addiction-focused counseling and O.A. support, together with a food plan that included adequate calories and eliminated all Techno-Karbz, all grains, fruits, and any other foods that were addictive for particular individuals, we were able to help most of our clients overcome most of their cravings. It took eight to twelve weeks of headaches, mood problems, and other withdrawal symptoms, including ongoing (but diminishing) cravings. But once past those difficult twelve weeks, our clients felt mentally terrific and lost their premenstrual syndrome (PMS), chronic bloat, and considerable weight. The trouble was that their cravings were not entirely gone. In fact, we didn't expect them to be. At best, addiction recovery seemed to be a constant struggle to stay abstinent alternating with inevitable periods of relapse.

A two-year follow-up of clients showed that 70 percent had relapsed but, because they had all found our anti-craving diet to be the best they'd ever tried, 70 percent of them had gotten back on it whenever they could, for as long as they could hold out against their residual cravings. Fortunately, a few frustrating years later, we learned about the brain-food connection and the amino acid supplements that would be more than a match for the addictive technology of the food industry.

THE TECHNO-KARBZ INDUSTRY PRODUCES
THE WORLD'S GREATEST HEALTH CRISIS

Almost two decades ago, shortly after the publication of my first book, *The Diet Cure,* I got a call from a representative of one of the world's largest breakfast cereal manufacturers. He started the conversation by volunteering the following information: To create all the cute cereal shapes, his company had to process their grain-based starches so heavily that there was no food value left in them. They used poor-quality fats. They regularly increased the amount of sugar in their products. They aggressively marketed their products to children.

When, astonished by his frankness, I asked why he'd called me, his response was: "I have just one question for you: Do you think that, in addition to the problems I've just admitted to, our products are also *physically addictive*?" Of course I replied, "Yes, your products are hard drugs and I'd be glad to show you more of the science that proves it. And let me try to help you to fill your boxes with something healthy so that you can become the children's true champion." (He wasn't interested.)

Since that conversation, more than fifteen years ago, this corporation has gained millions of new customers for products that have continued to inflict the same damaged starches and fats and even higher doses of sugar on us. It has been verified that most cold cereals started out with sugar contents of about 20 percent,[15] but, in 2015, for example, Kellogg's Honey Smacks were 60 percent sugar[16] and Lieber's Cocoa Frosted Flakes were 88 percent sugar.[17] (Chillingly, children's cereals typically contain much more sugar than "adult" cereals do.[18]) These progressively more addictive and harmful "breakfast foods" are still marketed to children who are easily persuaded to continue to consume these products lifelong.

Clearly, creating a nation of Techno-Karbz addicts has been a great business concept. How has it worked as a health concept?

All substance addictions have direct health consequences: smokers' lung cancer, alcoholics' cirrhosis, and meth users' stroke, to name a few. Techno-Karb users suffer similar consequences and many others besides such as pre-diabetes, and type 2 diabetes, food-related cancers, non-alcoholic liver disease, and obesity. These conditions have made ordeals like stomach surgery and kidney dialysis commonplace in the United States and around the world today.

Most of our clients know that their chronic health problems are caused by the foods they can't stop eating. Of course, they suffer from inappropriate weight gain and regular food hangovers, but in addition, they frequently report anxiety, depression, insomnia, aching joints, fatigue, reflux, and irritable bowel syndrome (IBS). They also report the pain of seeing their children develop many of the same problems.

The adverse health effects of Techno-Karbz are now known to be legion, and new reports are published every week. They include the crippling of even our most basic functions, with most children now unable to run and young men and women in their prime no longer able to pass the physical to enter the armed forces. But there are worse consequences that you may not be aware of. Consequences that will likely overtake anyone who cannot find a craving cure.

Alyssa, a young mother, came to us with a bad pizza, pasta, and ice cream habit. She took the Craving-Type Questionnaire and identified as a Depressed (Type 1), Crashed (Type 2), and Comfort (Type 3) Craver. She also had chronic digestive problems that had her doubled up with pain on a regular basis. Once on her three aminos (one for each of her Craving Types) she was quickly able to go off of her cheesy, creamy, doughy treats and her chronic digestive distress disappeared.

A few months later she brought in her temperamental eleven-year-old daughter who had constant tummy aches and distressing weight gain. The Type 1 Depressed Craver's amino was all she needed to mellow out, and she did so so much that a week later she agreed to give up her daily doses of pizza and mac and cheese. She was suddenly happy to sit down with her mom for healthy breakfasts and dinners and willingly took a lunch from home that her mom packed. The Craving Cure worked for this mother and daughter, giving each of them a new future, one without pain, illness, or unnatural weight gain.

TECHNO-KARBZ AND DIABETES

Our rate of diabetes, now the most widely disabling of all food-related illnesses, was less than 1 percent in 1960. In 2016, it was 50 percent.[19] And it is still rising. This number includes the category of *pre*diabetes. Those millions now diagnosed with this condition often become full-fledged diabetics within six to ten years after their initial diagnoses.[20] Five percent of children[21] and 20 percent of teens[22] are contracting "adult onset" diabetes, as well, often a more virulent form of it.

A diagnosis of diabetes is often a death sentence, and the progression of the disease is a slow and torturous one. Diabetes is associated with high rates of often fatal forms of heart, kidney, and liver disease.[23] Diabetics also have increased risks of *almost all cancers*[24] and Alzheimer's disease is now being called diabetes III.[25] And then there are blindness, impotence, and amputation.

What is the method by which refined sugars in particular are wreaking this devastation? We know that they chronically elevate glucose and insulin levels and that this is an essential factor in the development of diabetes. In fact, several studies have found the amount of sugar consumed to be the specific factor that correlates worldwide with the incidence of diabetes.[26]

No sugar, no diabetes.

But sugar plays a second role.

GLYCATION: THE SILENT ENEMY

Excess sugars, both glucose and fructose, have been circulating freely, as never before, in the American bloodstream since the 1970s and quietly damaging cells throughout our bodies *on contact*. This phenomenon of unregulated "free sugars" roaming throughout the brain and body and injuring us in innumerable searing collisions is called *glycation*. Although excess glucose glycates our cells, glycation by excess fructose is now an even greater problem because it is *ten times* more damaging.[27] You may never have heard about this direct means by which sugars lead to diabetes (and other degenerative diseases), but it is well known in medical science. There, glycated cells are referred to as AGEs, or *advanced glycation end products*. The acronym speaks for itself; prematurely aging cells, body-wide.

There are actually two types of glycation. One occurs in human tissues, as I've just described. The other comes from foods we eat that are themselves glycated; foods exposed to excessive heat—like our favorite seared barbecue, the crust on the fried chicken and the crunch of breakfast cereals, crackers, chips, and cookies. This is also called the browning or Maillard reaction. We could get away with traditionally glycated foods like our breakfast toast and bacon before 1970, but now we're eating a diet *mostly composed* of toasted foods and the sugars that toast our cells.

Glycation is a primary cause of diabetes.[28] Among the many kinds of glycated cells throughout the bodies of diabetics are their red blood cells (their hemoglobin). The blood test that measures levels of *glycated* hemoglobin (HbA1c) is used to identify if someone is prediabetic (with a score of 5–7 percent) or diabetic (with a score over 7 percent). This number can drop if dietary first aid is administered early enough and is sustained. (Which it can be with the use of the aminos.) Glycation is also a big contributor to heart disease and stroke,[29] to our increasing number of diet-related cancers,[30] and to many other degenerative conditions. The only cure for glycation is being able to stay away from the Techno-Karbz that cause it. In fact, scientist and glycation expert Helen Vlassara, Ph.D., whose studies and books I recommend to you, assures us that cutting glycated food consumption by just 50 percent can result in decreased AGEs and normalized blood levels, within just a few months.[31] On the aminos, we can easily cut 50 percent and still enjoy some bacon. *Note:* If you are already diabetic or suffering from other degenerative diseases associated with glycation, I urge you to go to the diabetic eaters' section at the end of Chapter 14 and cut out *more* than 50 percent of AGE-promoting foods. Also try the anti-glycation supplements I discuss in Chapter 7 on page 124.

TECHNO-KARBZ AND THE AMERICAN HEART

Techno-Karbz have destructive effects on all of our organs, including our hearts, largely by fueling diabetes and glycation. But Techno-Karbz (as well as the hydrogenated fats that are still in our food supply as of 2017) are also prime sources of heart-harmful (LDL) cholesterol. In addition, the glucose glut that follows the overconsumption of sweet and starchy foods stimulates the overproduction of *triglycerides* in the liver. Triglycerides are essential storage fuels made up of one fat and three sugar molecules. When amounts are excessive, they can certainly raise our risk of heart disease.[32] The cardiovascular problems caused by sugar-triggered excesses of LDL cholesterol and triglycerides were recognized in the 1960s, but the information was suppressed, despite solid research by reputable scientists. This suppression was accomplished with the help of the sugar industry which, we learned in 2016, had paid scientists from Harvard and elsewhere to blame saturated fat, instead of sugar, for our by then epidemic rates of heart disease.[33] That same year the conservative American Heart Association (AHA) broke ranks and published a chilling scientific report in the journal *Circulation* warning of heart damage *starting in infancy* as a direct result of sugar consumption. (For example, there is virtually no brand of baby formula that is sugar-free.) It recommended *zero* sugar for children under the age of two, and very little after that.[34]

The intentional mass addiction of infants and children to substances known to be deadly is one of the most shocking acts of all time.

Soda and Our Health

Studies have shown that drinking two high-fructose corn syrup–sweetened sodas a day for two weeks triples the risk of death by heart attack and raises diabetes markers and insulin resistance by 17 percent.[35, 36] One soda a day can increase liver fat by close to 150 percent. Although the effective campaign against soda, led by Robert Lustig, M.D., Michael Goran, M.D., and other heroes, has reduced the consumption of it, soda is still one of the nation's top-selling products. That's because it is one of the *top-addicting* products (you'll discover why in Chapter 2).

DEATH AND THE TECHNO-KARBZ

Addiction is always considered to be a potentially terminal condition, shortening lives through diseases like hepatitis and cirrhosis, not to mention overdose. More than 150,000 drug and alcohol addicts die in the United States every year because of their addictions.[37] Techno-Karbz addiction is no exception, *except that it harms and kills so many more by so many more means.* When we compare Techno-Karbz ingestion to the ingestion of another addictive substance, tobacco, we see the true extent of our peril. Among deadly drugs, tobacco is known as the great killer. Worldwide, almost 5 million smokers are killed by their tobacco use every year.[38] Sugar, however, has now far surpassed tobacco in deadliness. Sugar is now strongly implicated in diseases such as heart disease, cancer, and diabetes, which contribute to *35 million deaths* worldwide annually. Indeed, now that we have exported diabetes to the rest of the world, along with our Techno-Karbz, the International Diabetes Federation has estimated that it is killing one person every six seconds.[39]

The U.S. food industry has perfected its addictive and deadly technology and the world, up to this point, has been helpless before it. That's why *The Craving Cure* is so important now. The next two chapters explain how addictive food technology has "advanced" over the past 3,000 years and how three abrupt changes in our dietary habits, starting in the 1970s, have allowed this technology to perpetuate mass cravings for the toxic foods that are now destroying us.

2

The Invasion of the Techno-Karbz: 3,000 Years of Bliss-Point Technology

WHETHER CRUNCHY OR CREAMY, SOLID or liquid, highly processed sweet and starchy Techno-Karbz are the central ingredients in today's diet. That's because they are so intoxicating to the brain. But, as addictive as they are, they almost always come carefully "enhanced" by a bevy of alluring add-ons. Chocolate, cheese, and other co-addictors significantly boost the total brain impact. With this bevy on board, you literally can't say no.

The lightbulb went off for Belinda when we broke down her cinnamon-churro-and-latte habit into its basic chemical components. That habit had, over the last year, gone from a weekend treat to a daily necessity. Churros are composed of two kinds of highly processed white flour and three kinds of sugar, plus frying oil, salt, and "flavorings." As for the latte, it combined milk and coffee with a powdered mix containing beet syrup, corn syrup, and chocolate. For Belinda, each one of these components lit up a different pleasure center in her brain, adding up to a blast of bliss.

In this chapter, we'll examine each of the most addictive ingredients in today's industrial concoctions, starting with the stars: the sugars and the starches. Then we'll look at the supporting cast: salt, fat, milk products, chocolate, caffeine, and the most recent addition, cannabis. This tour will reveal how your own favorite flavors and textures are nothing other than chemical constructs. Seeing them this way, from the vantage point of a food scientist, will make it easier for you to turn your back on your deliberately "loaded" favorites.

We'll start at the top, with the most addictive substances on earth, the sugars.

THE SAGA OF SUCROSE: THE ORIGINAL SUGAR

The first plant to be industrially processed or "technoed," if you will, was the sugarcane. From ancient times, sugarcane was famed for its beauty and its usefulness as a medicinal plant, a dense source of carbohydrates, and as a building material. In 500 BCE, it began to be systematically subjected to the sugar extraction process, very similar to that still used today: squeeze out the syrupy contents and boil until the white sugar crystals separate from the brown molasses. What resulted was a crystalline concentrate *800 percent sweeter* than nature ever intended.[1] We call it "sucrose," based on the Latin word for "sweet."

Sucrose is actually made up of two sugars bound together. Fifty percent of it is glucose and 50 percent of it is fructose, just as it is in the cane. These two component sugars are quite different in the way they impact us, particularly in the way they impact our appetite chemistry. As you'll see in the following section on the new high-fructose sugars, the ratio between the two component sugars seems to be one of the most critical factors in today's diet, weight, and health crises.

Sucrose was first mass-produced in India and then in Asia and the Middle East, where it was highly prized and worth its weight in silver. At that time, sugar was valued, not as a new food, but as a new *pharmaceutical*. For almost seventeen centuries it was handled only through apothecaries, the world's original druggists.

The list of sucrose's early pharmaceutical uses, in India, Arabia, Greece, Rome, and the rest of Europe, is long: it was used to treat everything from heart problems to blindness.[2] The French used a popular expression for centuries to describe someone experiencing a loss: "he was like an apothecary without sugar."[3] In England, in as late as the 1880s, it was still considered a "powerful antiseptic and preservative, but not capable of supporting human life as a food."[4]

After 1400, sucrose became a street drug, as so many pharmaceuticals have since. The aristocrats, who could afford this luxury, got it, loved it, and abused it. Their sumptuous meals were replete with sucrose-infused confections like bonbons and meringues. Sucrose's reputation for pleasure spread and the demand for it increased. Sales of honey, the ancient and much cheaper product of the bee industry, suddenly went into a decline.

When supplies of sucrose ran low, it was "cut" with other white powders to maintain profits. Eventually, the slave trade was hugely expanded to carry out the harsh processes required to make sucrose affordable for and available to a broader market. Europe, and later America, took to eating it by the pound. In the 1900s, sucrose began to be extracted in the United States from locally grown sugar beets as well as from imported cane; intake in the United States increased rapidly from 6 pounds per person per year in 1822 to 97 pounds per person per year in 1950.[5] By the 1970s, the average American was consuming 122 pounds per year.[6]

Any negative consequences of our sucrose addiction (except to our teeth) up to that point had gone unremarked upon, partly because most people could afford to consume so little of it until after World War II, and because, even when our consumption rose more steeply, our weight and health seemed to remain normal. By the 1930s, though, heart disease had begun to be a concern for the first time ever. In the 1960s, we decided it was because of our saturated fat consumption. That was partly because the sucrose industry began fighting to protect an image of safety in the 1960s by paying scientists to point the finger at saturated fat thereby discrediting the reputable scientists who were starting to call sucrose to account.[7] (More on this in Chapter 3.) We now know that it's the sweet and starchy Techno-Karbz (still starring sucrose), not the saturated fats, that raise "bad" LDL cholesterol levels. The sucrose-generated triglycerides (that excess sugar is converted into on its way to being stored as fat) have also certainly contributed significantly to the development of our continuing heart disease problems. But the recent surge in heart disease is a consequence of the diabetes pandemic; though that is clearly a sugar-related phenomenon, it is *not* a sucrose-related one. The diabetes surge occurred after the consumption of sucrose had given way to high-fructose corn syrup (HFCS) consumption in the 1970s. According to the USDA, sucrose use has actually been cut in half since 1970, when the cheaper and more addictive HFCS was introduced (more on this in a few lines).[8] The sucrose industry has been fighting for its life against the corn industry in the courts and trying to make an advertising comeback as the innocent, "old-fashioned" or "pure organic" option. As for sucrose's drug impact on the appetite-regulating systems in the brain and body: Sucrose can briefly set off all five Craving Types at once by raising serotonin levels, glucose levels, natural opiate (endorphin) levels, levels of soothing GABA, and those of energizing and rewarding dopamine. Much recent scientific inquiry, including several studies conducted at NIDA (the National Institute on Drug Abuse), has confirmed this, as I'll detail in Chapter 5, Your Brain, Craving Control Central.

THE SECOND TECHNO-SUGAR: HIGH-FRUCTOSE SYRUPS

Almost two millennia after sucrose was invented and the sugarcane and sugar beet industries rose to power, a different sweet drug was created from corn, agave cactus, and fruit. Starting in the 1970s, the new Techno-Sugar that was cheaper, twice as sweet, and much more addictive than sucrose bounded into the marketplace. Food engineers had discovered that they could manipulate the fructose content of corn syrup, and therefore increase the addictive potential of most commercial foods. They started by replacing sucrose with high-fructose corn syrup in sodas, and produced the most popular beverages of all time.

HIGH-FRUCTOSE CORN SYRUP

What exactly is the difference between the new high-fructose corn syrup and the "old" sucrose? That's the critical question. Sucrose contains glucose and fructose bound together in the equal, one-to-one ratio found naturally in the cane, the beet, and in other fruits and vegetables. Despite the elaborate processing required to make HFCS (ironically, corn naturally contains only glucose which has to be heavily processed to be converted into fructose), it is still much less expensive to produce than sucrose. Then the two sugars are combined in various ratios. The HFCS in foods and beverages can contain anywhere from 42 to 90 percent fructose.[9] As labels have not been required to reveal the exact amount of fructose, we're only now learning exactly how much we've actually been exposed to.

Because of the unique properties of fructose, this new sugar has broken through our bodies' protective barriers, snapping the leash that we'd previously been able to keep on our consumption of sucrose-sweetened foods. Our bodies have always been familiar with both glucose and fructose, in both their bound and free forms, in the modest amounts that most fruits and sweet vegetables contain. We do not respond well to excessive amounts of glucose, but our bodies know what to do with it (activate insulin to store it, largely as fat). When the sugar we consumed was primarily sucrose, the 50:50 sugar, eaten in increasing but more controlled amounts, we were suffering galloping rates of heart disease but not of weight gain or diabetes. After 1970, though, the ratio of fructose to glucose began to rise. The extra fructose now contained in HFCS-sweetened sodas, for example, is undisputed. Anything HFCS-sweetened is sweeter and more addictive than anything sucrose-sweetened. As a result, the amounts of the sweet substances we're consuming have skyrocketed. Between 1970 and 1999, our sweets intake overall went from 120 pounds of sugar a year to 160 pounds a year—and high-fructose corn syrup accounted for more than half of that overall intake.[10]

FRUCTOSE ADDICTION

Of all of the effects of fructose on our bodies, one of the most extraordinary is its ability to increase our sweet cravings. Fructose impacts all of our five brain-centered craving functions. But it goes beyond that. It also disrupts many other ancient signal systems that the body uses to protect itself from too many sweets or starches. Glucose actually turns these productive systems *on* so that we can stop short of poisoning ourselves. Fructose turns them *off*.

The body doesn't know how to react to a fructose overdose. In fact, our bodies don't even recognize that a fructose overdose is in progress because fructose disables the body's alarm systems. Because it blocks the warning signals, we literally can't protect ourselves; we *can't* say no. There are at least ten built-in hormonal appetite guardians that are disabled by fructose. For each guardian that no longer functions, our cravings are magnified exponentially. Perhaps the most important of them are the hormones ghrelin, leptin, and insulin:[11]

Ghrelin: This hormone makes us hungry. When we eat, this hormone gets turned off, signaling the body that we are no longer hungry. Fructose, apparently not recognized as a food by the body, does not turn it off. So we keep eating.

Leptin: This powerful hormone lets us know when we're satiated. Again, the body does not recognize fructose as food, so when we ingest fructose, leptin is not released and we continue to eat.

Insulin: When levels of this hormone rise in response to an ingestion of too much glucose, our appetites drop. But fructose does not raise the insulin alarm as glucose does. Its stealthy entry goes unrecognized—and we keep eating. Eventually fructose does convert into glucose and insulin levels do rise, but it's too late by then to curb our intake.

Now are you beginning to see how modern sugar has become something that you simply cannot contend with? And I'm just getting started!

A REFRESHING SCIENTIFIC EXPOSÉ OF THE FRUCTOSE
CONTENTS OF SODAS AND "FRUIT JUICE DRINKS"

While scientists have suspected that fructose dominance is the prime cause of our current weight and health crisis—they've had no proof of exactly how much fructose we're actually being exposed to. Could a 5 to 10 percent higher ratio of fructose to glucose in sweet beverages and foods be responsible for the greatest health crisis in history? Possibly. In the last few years, Michael Goran, Ph.D., a professor and researcher at the University of Southern California, and his team decided to find out by analyzing the contents of specific brands of sodas and fruit juice drinks and documenting the exact amounts of fructose contained in them.

Goran's research proved that most sodas actually contain much higher amounts of fructose than the soda manufacturers have admitted to: close to 60 percent of the sugar in these drinks is fructose and only 40 percent is glucose.[12]

Dr. Goran's team has also discovered that some beverage labels contain other grossly misleading information. On some labels, sucrose was listed as an ingredient although none was present in the beverage, and on others high-fructose corn syrup was not listed even though it was present in high concentrations in the beverage.

"Excess Free Fructose" (EFF) is now known to pose a well-defined and serious national health threat. The fact that it is so addictive ensures that we'll keep consuming it and keep suffering the consequences—unless we limit our access to it by arming ourselves with anti-craving amino acids.

WHAT ABOUT THE "NATURAL" FRUCTOSE IN
FRUIT SYRUP, AGAVE SYRUP, AND WHOLE FRUIT?

While HFCS sales are reportedly dropping because of scientific, media, and parental pressure, *agave (along with fruit syrup) use is rising*. Ninety percent of the highly concentrated syrup from the agave cactus is fructose![13] Like fruit juice syrup, it is marketed as a "healthier option" and used in massive quantities. Agave is a highly processed substance about which there has been much controversy.

Fresh and dried fruits contain a combination of glucose and fructose in three forms: sucrose, the 50:50 bonded fructose-glucose combo; free glucose; and free fructose (the kind of fructose found in HFCS). The amounts of each form vary quite a bit. Apples and pears contain by far the most free fructose. Soda sales are now dropping, but sales of fruit drinks are rising, so again, Dr. Goran started analyzing and found that fruit juice beverages contained even *more* fructose than sodas did! Additional studies have found that apple juice alone contains 67 percent fructose and just 33 percent glucose. This is an enormous departure from the 50:50 content of sucrose.[14] The ratio is the same in the natural juice, but the others often add sugar to it. Any juice made from concentrate is similar to a sugar-sweetened juice. The natural doses of free fructose we consume in one serving of nutrient- and fiber-packed fresh fruit does not strain the body. But the free fructose in fruit, in excess, can create problems. Two dried figs contain more fructose than a twelve-ounce Coke, but are also loaded with the vitamins, minerals, and fiber that partly compensate for their high-fructose content. In Part IV of this book, I tell a story about one of our clients who became prediabetic by eating too much fruit.

DAMAGE BY EXCESS FRUCTOSE

The excessive amounts of *unopposed,* or "free," fructose in high-fructose corn syrup that we've now been exposed to for decades is associated not just with diabetes, glycation, and heart disease, but also with our increased rates of the *often fatal fatty liver disease* that is now suffered by 30 percent of the general population and 70 percent of diabetics.[15] High-fructose corn syrup is also a major cause of the *degradation of the microbiome*, the coexisting body of bacteria in our gut that has regulating effects on our weight, our metabolism, and our overall health.[16]

In addition, excess free fructose (EFF) is the specific cause of an entirely new kind of illness. It's called *fructose malabsorption* and it has resulted in new types of arthritic, digestive, respiratory, and depressive conditions whose incidences have much increased since the 1970s. As much as 30 percent of the population is affected.[17] In the next chapter, you'll get a look at how fructose has been freed so that it can do this kind of damage.

What About Kombucha?

My observation is that this fermented beverage can be addictive and its popularity may be due at least as much to the power of sugars, caffeine, and alcohol as to its probiotic power. Its sugar content is 2–24 grams per 8-ounce serving depending on how long it ferments and what sweeteners are added. Check the labels. It's not included among the beverages in *The Craving Cure* (though you can reintroduce it, as per Chapter 15, after the first month and see what *you* think about it then).

THE SUGARLESS TECHNO-SWEETENERS

We're just starting to understand that these popular calorie-free chemical sweeteners can be addictive and harmful, whether consumed in sodas, candies, gums, or other foods. How could they *not* have adverse effects? No matter which type or brand, these are almost all bizarre chemicals, hundreds of times sweeter than sugar, that were mostly discovered as the result of lab accidents![18]

You may keep cases of diet soda in the garage. Do you drink it for energy? Probably so if you're a Type 5 Fatigued Craver. Artificially sweetened sodas contain as much synthetic caffeine as sweetened sodas do, and like energy drinks, they have been associated with a heightened risk of stroke.[19] Like coffee, caffeinated sodas blunt our appetite for real food—and when we skip meals, we end up hungrier for Techno-Karbz later. If you also crave soda for its sweet flavor (and its icy fizziness), you're likely to be a Type 3 Comfort Craver. Regardless, you probably drink "diet" soda to avoid the weight gain and the risk of diabetes you know are associated with caloric sugar consumption. Unfortunately, through their effects on your taste buds, your gut bacteria, and other functions, diet sugars can promote cravings, raise blood sugar and insulin levels, and are clearly associated with weight gain and type 2 diabetes.[20]

The French study that found sugar to be more than twice as addictive as cocaine, found that saccharin, one of the first and still a primary zero-calorie sweetener (the pink one) was just as addictive![21] One study showed a 7 percent increase in BMI for diet sugar users versus those who use caloric sugar![22] All artificial sweeteners, including highly processed Stevia, have *zero nutritional value;* therefore, they prevent the normal growth of helpful gut bacteria (which require a variety of nutrients, notably fiber from whole carbohydrate). A disrupted microbiome is known to promote weight gain and diabetes (among many other misfortunes).[23]

TECHNO-STARCH: THE ALLURE OF DOUGH

The fact that high-starch foods can create pleasurable highs and insatiable cravings is common knowledge, but the particular starch that we now consume *most* insatiably was quite unknown for most of human history. As hunter-gatherers, we ate starchy vegetables like yams, potatoes, and fruit. But about 10,000 years ago we learned how to convert inedible grass into plump, tasty grain. The chief result of this experiment is now called wheat. Wheat had several invaluable properties: It was a high-calorie food that also contained more protein than other grains and it could be safely stored for long periods. These unique attributes eventually made it Egypt's primary crop and the source of its empire's extraordinary wealth.

When the Egyptians learned to make bread out of it, wheat also became the core of a radical new high-carbohydrate diet. Egyptian soldiers, for example, were provided with five pounds of bread a day. Thousands of Egyptian mummies have since been analyzed to determine the health of these ancient wheat-eaters. The results: the essentially vegetarian Egyptians died grossly overweight, with clogged arteries, and with teeth worn down to diseased gums.[24]

What the Egyptians didn't know was that their new grain, like its grassy forbear, was in many ways *still inedible*. Wheat contains over one hundred proteins—mostly in forms with no biological value. Wheat's primary "usable" protein is an elastic substance with exceptionally irritating and addictive properties called gluten, from the Latin word for "glue"! In addition, like all seeds (grains are seeds), wheat contains phytates that prevent us from absorbing the minerals it contains and can only be neutralized by lengthy sprouting or fermenting processes (that are now rarely employed in Westernized countries). Gradually, many adjustments have been made in how wheat is grown, processed, and consumed, which have made it a still more damaging and addictive substance. Over the millennia, much of the world adapted to various versions of wheat as a dietary staple. But most peoples, unlike the Egyptians, tended to consume it along with animal protein as only one *part* of their diet. This seems to have minimized its negative health impacts, until now.

MAKING WHEAT MORE ADDICTIVE

There's a reason you feel you can't live without bread.

First, we mastered the art of grinding wheat into flour. Then we figured out how to bake it with a variety of leavenings to make it rise. Later, we made it rise even higher when we learned how to separate out and discard the two most nutritious parts of the grain: the bran and the germ. We found that the fiber in the bran made it heavy and that the fat in the germ got rancid and spoiled the flavor, so we engineered a way to remove those two parts of the full grain. What was left? Eighty percent of what remained was white powdered carbohydrate: the first Techno-Starch. Almost instantly, while it is still in your mouth, starchy flour starts converting into glucose, delivering pleasure through the stimulation of all five brain reward functions.

But that's not the full story. There's another pleasurable, drug-like effect that results when you sink your teeth into warm bread or slurp up some pasta. That delight is delivered by the glue! Twenty percent of wheat flour is actually a protein called gliadin. Gliadin gives baked wheat its elastic, puffy, sensually thrilling texture and its addictive impact on the brain.

Does today's wheat actually contain *more* gliadin? This is a very hot topic and nutritional science has been strangely slow to answer the question (we asked researchers on three continents). What we do know is that we are eating thirty-five pounds more wheat flour products a year than we did in the early '70s.[25] This is partly due to the now common practice of mixing a *gliadin concentrate* called "vital gluten" into most baked goods and many other foods, like canned soups, to "improve" their texture and taste, (and to increase our cravings!).[26] Modern baked goods, especially the sweetened ones, have, not surprisingly, now become the top comfort foods of all time. Dough is king—whether as pizza or pasta, bagels or cinnamon rolls. Dough combined with sugar and vegetable oil in cookies, cakes, pies, and doughnuts top any other food ever known in "palatability."

Most relevant to dough cravers, gliadin has a brain effect much like that of morphine. As it does with morphine, our brain mistakes gliadin for our body's own painkilling, pleasure-promoting chemicals, the *endorphins*. In fact, because of this unique property, gliadin is officially called gluteomorphin. Knowing about gliadin's drug-like properties helps explain the potent pleasure-enhancement and emotional pain-relief that thousands of our clients have reported experiencing in dough's arms. And, of course, dough's refined flour delivers a glucose bomb almost as quickly as sugar does, which stimulates all five Craving Types.

All of this means that we can easily fall in love with one of the least nutritious and most indigestible foods on earth. At our clinic, we've seen (and cured) thousands of sufferers of gas, bloat, reflux, fatigue, chronic constipation, and dozens of other ailments, from anxiety to depression, by helping them detach from the glue. Gliadin has a much-researched capacity to cause a variety of health problems, from irritable bowel syndrome to psoriasis. The incidence of celiac disease and nonceliac gluten/gliadin sensitivity conditions has increased since 1970. (In the UK, the incidence has tripled.[27]) Since the '70s we've altered the nature of the wheat plant. It now produces three times more wheat, and in its many "modified" forms it has been added to so many products that we have been eating much more of it than we realized (thirty-five pounds more to be exact!).

Let's take licorice whips, a client favorite, as an example.

Two handsome, intelligent, health-obsessed brothers in their sixties came to my clinic for a consult. They both loved the licorice whips by Panda, whose package states, in large print, ALL NATURAL! The brothers ate these whips frequently by the large bagful, even though one had a severe case of type 2 diabetes and both were seriously constipated and considerably overweight. Neither could give up sweets, but they thought that they were at least "off gluten." They were depressed and sheepish when I asked them to read that third entry on the ingredients list.

WHAT ABOUT WHOLE WHEAT AND "GLUTEN-FREE" STARCH?

Whole wheat products are not exempt from the chemical facts. In fact, to make them lighter, more wheat gluten concentrate is often added. Completely whole wheat and organic products (hard to find) produce a lesser glucose and insulin impact because their greater protein, fat, and fiber contents blunt blood sugar spikes. But be warned: an opioid kick is still present. However, if you are not addicted to and/or sickened by gluten, this is the way to go.

Gluten-free, refined white starches made from hulled and de-germed corn, rice, other grains, or potatoes also raise glucose levels, insulin levels, and weight. These are some of the documented concerns about the current popularity of gluten-free foods.[28] They can manipulate neurotransmitter levels as quickly as white wheat flour does (and almost as quickly as sugar does). So if you decide to see how you might feel off of gluten-containing products, please don't substitute these starchy junk food products (with added sugar, typically). Look for whole-grain substitutes or take the opportunity to try life without any dough, as I advise in Chapter 14.

CULINARY SPEEDBALLS: COMBINING SUGAR AND STARCH WITH EIGHT OTHER ADDICTIVE SUBSTANCES

For those of you not familiar with drug jargon, a speedball is a combination of heroin and cocaine. It's considered by many to be the ultimate high. I've already made the point that Techno-Sugars and Techno-Starches are as addictive as, or more addictive than, street drugs. But even the most hard-core food cravers would not sit down with a bowl of granulated sugar, a glass of high-fructose corn syrup, or a bag of flour. The truth is that these substances must be carefully *combined* for the most addictive results. Addictive potency multiplies when the two Techno-Karbz are combined, and multiplies exponentially with each additional addictive substance added. Commercial food producers know that they can notch up the feeding frenzy by applying this speedball principle. The performance of the sweet or starchy Techno-Karbz "stars" is strongly supported by the addition of a cast of substances with their own distinctive addictive properties. These supporting roles are played by milk products, fat, salt, chocolate, caffeine, and cannabis. (And then there are the lesser lights: nuts and flavorings like pepper, cinnamon, vinegar, vanilla, and licorice.) The concoctions that result are *the complete Techno-Karb,* filled with damaged carbohydrates and laced with the co-addicting substances I'm about to describe.

THE CREAMY CO-ADDICTORS: CHEESE AND OTHER MILK PRODUCTS

Cheese, milk, cream, butter, and yogurt are complete, natural, traditional foods full of nourishing vitamins, minerals, proteins, and fats. They also come mildly sweetened with their own natural sugar, lactose. So what is it about milk products that makes them so excessively yummy to so many of us? It's the morphine! Seriously, the problem is that modern milk products, especially cheese, contain a unique type of protein called *casein.* Like the *gluteomorphin* in wheat, this milk protein can function so much like the opiate drug, morphine, that it's often referred to formally as *casomorphin.* Its impact can be very enjoyable for Type 3 Cravers. But when it's *combined* with wheat and/or sugar, look out. Though milk products can be addictive all by themselves, they most often serve as powerful components of the most effective speedballs of all. Think chocolate-chip-cookie-dough ice cream, mac and cheese, crème brûlée, and, of course, pizza.

Our butter and cheese addicts prefer their casomorphin on crackers, bread, rolls, or muffins. They laugh and say that they eat bread just to have something to put on their butter. Of course, we help them to see that the bread's gluteomorphin can't help but amplify the effect.

One of our clients was heavily addicted to cheese, which contains concentrated amounts of casein. She was so addicted that she named her three dogs Swiss, Feta, and Cheddar. Like so many others, she preferred to combine her cheese with dough, so she named her cat Pizza. She was a pure Type 3 Comfort Craver. On her Type 3 endorphin-building aminos and big servings of protein at every meal, she was able to leave the cheese (and the pizza dough) behind with ease.

Nonfat and low-fat milk products have more concentrated milk sugar (lactose) and casomorphin contents than full-fat versions, plus, typically, lots of added sugar to help exert addictive influence to offset the absence of luscious fat. Low fat became popular in the 1970s and many of us still insist on buying low-fat products—but because they offer a false sense of safety, it's easy to overeat them.

Many people crave butter and plain yogurt and other unsweetened milk products too. We've even had a number of adult clients who were drinking quarts of milk a day with no idea that they were addicted to it. If milk products are a trigger for you (or if they give you any of the respiratory, bowel, or other troubles listed in Chapter 14), the aminos will help you live easily without them. (Honestly!)

The casomorphin story has one more twist: Not all milk contains this unique protein. Casomorphin is a characteristic feature of the milk of Holstein cows, who produce much more milk than any other breed and are therefore preferred by most dairy farmers. Now, though, we can have access to pre-modern milk with none of the Holstein's A1 beta-casein content. It's being distributed as A2 Milk at major markets through the United States. This may be better tolerated and less addictive. For example, it may be associated with less severe symptoms of autism and schizophrenia.[29] More on this in Chapter 15.

THE ESSENTIAL CO-ADDICTORS: FAT AND SALT

Fat and salt are essential to life! They also have the potential to become at least moderately addictive, although, again, no one would sit down with a bowl of salt or swallow a bottle of olive oil. But without salt and fat, even sugar and starch can lose their allure. We have always known that these two ingredients made food more delectable. On the other hand, we can fairly easily adapt to moderate or even low amounts of either. The salt and fat scares have taught us that. But the food industry has been increasing both the fat and the salt contents of our prepared and packaged food right along with its sugar and starch contents for decades. Prime example: aisles and aisles of fat and salt, combined with a little corn or potato, attest to the concerted power of *the irresistible chip*.

Fat

When fat is combined with starch or sugar, it spells entrapment for lots of us. Especially if fried. French fries and battered chicken or shrimp are always near the top of food popularity lists. Without the fat, the starchy potatoes and flour would be dry mush, not moist crunch. It's the combining of these ingredients that makes the end products so irresistible. The addictive effects of the fat added to crackers, cookies, and other baked products are less intense, but the added richness of flavor and crispy or creamy texture is definitely registered by the brain's pleasure centers. The appeal of the frozen fat-and-sugar speedball called ice cream never flags because it registers on *all five* of the brain's pleasure centers and double-registers on Type 3 endorphin-triggered cravings.

Then there are the nutty fats in either creamy or crunchy textures that always keep Reese's and Snickers among the top five candies sold in America. Unfortunately, whatever fats we eat will always *feel* good going down, and because of industrial processing, they will almost always smell and taste fine. The brain can't help us distinguish between a safe, traditional, relatively unprocessed fat—such as extra-virgin olive oil or butter—and an unsafe modern one—like hydrogenated margarine and some of the "salad" oils that you'll read more about in the next chapter.

Fortunately, it will not be hard for you to moderate your own fat consumption without resorting to low-fat foods. In spite of all the years of fingers pointing at the "fatty" content of junk foods, it's actually the sugar and starch content that's the greater addiction problem. Fat is simply not as chemically addictive.[30] Although it always rings the pleasure bells of the brain's Type 3 Craving opioid (endorphin) system, fat typically does nothing for the other four Craving Types. Armed with naturally endorphin-promoting amino acids, you'll be able to ignore damaged fats and enjoy the generous amounts of safe traditional fats we'll discuss in Part IV, Craving-Free Eating.

Salt

No less an expert than Mark Gold, M.D., famous for his leading work in cocaine addiction and, more recently, food addiction, has published several studies documenting the drug-like effects of salt. He and others have found that salt has moderate effects on our pleasure- and reward-generating neurotransmitters endorphin and dopamine.[31] Other scientists have also confirmed salt's addictiveness, especially when added in careful ratios to starch, fat, and sugar. These golden combinations have been much studied by food chemists to determine the exact line between flavor-enhancement—that is, addiction-enhancement—and oversalting.

Like fat, salt has real nutritive value. We need the minerals it is composed of—both its sodium and its chloride contents are essential to life. But they must be balanced in a ratio of 1 to 4 with the potassium and magnesium in vegetables and fruits to prevent the sodium excess that leads to high blood pressure.[32] On a high Techno-Karbz diet, no one is eating fresh produce. This is a big part of the reason for our high-blood-pressure epidemic. With the help of the aminos, though, we can avoid salt-saturated processed foods, eat more produce, and get into the safe zone.

Note: Severe salt cravings don't usually suggest the need to cut back. They often indicate problems in the crucial balance between sodium and potassium and warrant a visit to a doctor.

THE CO-ADDICTING DRUGS: CHOCOLATE, COFFEE, TEA, SYNTHETIC CAFFEINE, AND CANNABIS

We'll complete our tour of addictive ingredients with four well-recognized psychoactive drugs that are often added to foods. We've been combining drugs with food since the 1800s, when Coca-Cola was formulated by pharmacists to actually contain cocaine, and morphine and alcohol were common additives in many elixirs. Two of the drugs that are currently added to foods and beverages have become so familiar that we've forgotten that they actually *are* psychoactive substances. But coffee and chocolate are not known as "bliss" and "food of the gods," respectively, for nothing. They are addictive stars on their own, but add them to sugar, starch, fat, or cream and you have a galactic effect. These two ancient and exotic plants were introduced along with tea, sucrose, and tobacco, and developed the same kind of international mass appeal at about the same time, five hundred years ago. Combining the bitter drugs with the sweet one increased their mutual addictiveness many-fold as coffee, tea, and chocolate came to be consumed together and tobacco came to be cured with sugar.

CHOCOLATE

The pleasuring and stimulating powers of *chocolate* are legendary and sales are ever-rising. Chocolate is loaded with drug compounds including some with opiate properties (that account for its attraction for Type 3 Cravers) and several different kinds of energizing properties (that appeal to Type 5 Cravers). Unsweetened (dark) chocolate contains three times more caffeine and other stimulants than sweetened chocolate does. Combining it with milk, sugar, coffee, butter, flour, nuts, and various flavors creates a collective increase in its attraction for Craving Types 3 and 5.

COFFEE, TEA, AND SYNTHETIC CAFFEINE

Coffee is the number one drug consumed worldwide. Like chocolate, it is loaded with many compounds. Its stimulant effects are most attractive to Type 5 Fatigued Cravers. But coffee also has pleasure-promoting properties, triggering endorphin effects in Type 3 Comfort Cravers.[33] The sugared, creamed, and flavored blends have become our morning and afternoon cocktails of choice, and are often a necessary part of after-dinner pleasures.

Even moderate coffee drinking (say, one or two cups a day) can constitute a real problem for a food craver. Why? Because it *suppresses the appetite for real food,* and *raises and drops blood glucose levels* so that we turn to quick Techno-Karbz fixes instead of to regular meals. With our clinic clients we insist that coffee, if consumed at all, be consumed only *after* meals. (Since we can typically use the aminos to provide natural energy and pleasure, it's rarely a struggle for our Type 3 and 5 clients to give up.)

THE OTHER CAFFEINATED BEVERAGES

Because *tea* contains caffeine (and many other complex and pleasant-tasting chemicals), hot and sweetened iced tea are still popular beverages, whether the sweetener is HFCS or a calorie-free version. But tea's caffeine content isn't strong enough for most Americans. In fact, even coffee isn't enough anymore for many of us.

Sugared and sugar-free *colas* are also loaded with synthetic caffeine and high-fructose corn syrup. Our consumption of pop doubled in the '80s. While that consumption has been dropping, it's still common to see people lugging giant cups or bottles of soda around.

And then there are the *"energy drinks"* (more like sweetened methamphetamine than coffee). One of our clients, at age thirty-six, sustained three strokes after his habit reached nine per day. I will have more to say about colas and energy drinks in Chapter 9, when I talk about the special issues for the Type 5 Fatigued Cravers, who are the most vulnerable to them. I'll talk there, too, about how easy it can be to walk away from caffeine using naturally stimulating aminos.

THE NEW CO-ADDICTOR: CANNABIS

Several states in the United States have decided to add a new drug to food, one that has well-established addictive effects: the glorified hemp plant called lots of things, but now mostly cannabis.

A fourteen-year-old-boy with a big sweet tooth could not stay away from "pot" either—though he was already in legal, academic, health, and family trouble because of it. He was able to escape detection for a long time because, after he'd started coughing blood from smoking high THC "Dabs" with an acetylene torch, he'd found a source, through a local pot club member, of what he called "heaven." This came in the form of chocolate fudge cookies baked with lots of high-THC cannabis. The package said that one quarter of a cookie was a serving. But it was so sweet and yummy that he could never stop there. His addiction to cannabis and sugar was so fierce that we had to refer him to a residential treatment program where we arranged for him to be given several aminos and a wholesome diet that, together, made it possible for him to be comfortable in his own skin and eliminate his cannabis cravings. After that, he was able to benefit even more from the group and family counseling and the Marijuana Anonymous meetings he attended.

Cannabis is legendary for setting off the exaggerated enjoyment of food called the munchies. So it's a boon for the Techno-Karbz industry. Where cannabis has been legalized, its addictive, psychoactive properties have been added to everything from candy to ketchup. When cannabis is cooked in foods, its psychoactive effects are much amplified, but they come on slowly. This makes some imbibers, impatient for the high, start smoking too and end up much more intoxicated than they'd planned or wanted to be. Especially now that the drug's THC content has increased so much.

THC, cannabis's primary pleasure- and addiction-promoting component has been increasing in potency since the 1960s, when hybridization became a major focus for the growers of what has become one of the most lucrative crops ever known. THC contents have now increased from .5 percent to levels as high as 90 percent in "dabs," "wax," and other super-concentrated and toxic preparations.[34]

THC's effects on the brain are complex, and as its levels have increased, its unusual tendency to be stored for long periods in the brain has been amplified. This may not extend the high, but can also contribute to long-term personality and other changes. (Fortunately, they are reversible if the drug is avoided, as stored THC will slowly but eventually leach from the brain.) We have found that this plant can impact any or all of the brain's five Craving Types, amplifying the naturally mellowing effects of brain neurotransmitters like serotonin, endorphin, and GABA for some, but also able to trigger energizing dopaminergic[35] symptoms in others. In addition, THC stimulates the cannabinoid one neurotransmitter, which further magnifies the pleasurable, addictive, and other effects it adds to the wide variety of foods it's being legally combined with now. The new potencies are having many disturbing consequences such as a doubling of ER visits for psychotic symptoms.[36]

As an addiction professional, I have seen cannabis's negative effects on mind and body up close. I am afraid of the consequences of our making it so readily available in the most potent drugged-foods of all. For those increasing numbers who find themselves seriously addicted to this drug, the aminos have been found to be very helpful. (See the cannabis page on the Alliance for Addiction Solutions website for more on this.)

I hope I've just put a dent in some of the romance and the mystery of your love of certain foods and other substances. The mission of this book is to set you free. Knowing more about the mechanisms of craving can help. Of course, you won't waltz out of the Techno-Karbz trap until you've started your aminos and begun eating anti-craving foods, but this chapter's perspectives should make it easier for you to head for the exit. So should the revelations in the next chapter.

3

The Craving Generations: Reshaped by Three Dietary Trends of the 1970s

DO YOU ASSUME THAT IT'S always been this way—that as a nation we've always struggled with our diet, our weight, and our health? No, you were just born at the wrong time. If you'd grown up in any period of world history before 1970, you would have worried about *losing* too much weight, not about *gaining* too much. You might not have had enough food, but most of that food would have been wholesome. When food was generally plentiful, you would have had no particular interest in eating more than you needed and you would never even have heard of obesity or diabetes. In short, you would have been an average human eater who looked fine and felt well.

But the 1970s changed all that. In spite of our long, relatively trouble-free eating and weight history, starting in what I call the disaster decade, we suddenly made three radical changes in the way we had been eating for thousands of years. What possessed us to make these changes *then*, when we were in such good shape? And why, in the face of the disastrous consequences, are we still pursuing them?

This chapter identifies the three dietary missteps that have lined the path to food addiction, unnatural weight gain, and diet-related illness. My plan is to take you backtracking through those missteps to uncover our culinary roots and reclaim the nutritional treasures that we've left behind. Let's start with a brief look back at what our eating habits were like right *before* it went so wrong, when we were enjoying a more traditional diet, more traditional weight, and more traditional health.

PRE-1970S USA

In the years prior to 1970, we tended to follow the collective wisdom handed down to us about when, what, and how much to eat. We generally enjoyed our meals. We certainly never felt guilty about eating them. In fact, we rarely worried about eating or weight at all. We had no reason to. We had plenty to eat and we were vital and attractive people. How do I know? I was there. I grew up in the '50s and '60s.

Here's what I know from my firsthand experience and from the historical record: Americans were typically fit and healthy until the 1970s. Although there were signs of erosion in the '60s after our sugar intake went up another big notch and we began Twiggy-inspired fad dieting, most of our weights were ideal for our genetic body types. Less than a third of us were overweight and less than 2 percent of us had type 2 diabetes. Let me remind you that now, 70 percent of us are overweight[1] and half of us are on the diabetic spectrum.[2]

Like almost every girl I knew, from grammar school to graduate school, I grew up with no self-consciousness about my weight. We considered "personality," not appearance to be the crucial factor in popularity. My friends and I—all growing up in middle- or working-class families—were in the healthy, average range, weight-wise. We knew that weight variations, just like variations in height and eye color, were to be expected and had to do with family heritage. Did we have any special dietary secrets? Eggs, bacon, toast with butter, and juice or whole milk (there was no other kind) for breakfast; a ham and cheese or leftover-meat sandwich with fruit and milk for lunch; meat loaf, veggies of some sort (salads were just starting to become popular), baked potatoes with butter and/or sour cream, and some homemade dessert with another glass of milk for dinner. We could always have "seconds" or thirds, if there was enough, and there was always more milk, bread, and butter if there wasn't. For after-school snacks, some of my school friends got sardines and crackers and shared them with me. We loved them. (That was before low-omega-3, high-mercury tuna replaced sardines as America's canned fish of choice.)

The 1950s diet was not perfectly nutritious. It could have been improved upon (as it was for a while in the '60s when we ate more whole wheat bread and discovered big salads). But whatever the imperfections, the way we ate before 1970 *worked* because we ate a fairly traditional balance of proteins, fats, and carbohydrates in foods that were fresh, largely unprocessed, and consumed regularly in adequate amounts. Our Depression-era parents used to call what we ate "good eats," "hearty grub," and "square meals." "What is a square meal?" I ask at my lectures and most people under fifty don't seem to know. One twentysomething once wondered if a "square meal" was "like, a nerdy meal?" He had no idea that I was talking about the hot, filling, homemade, and often tasty nourishment we expected to sit down to until the 1970s. Plenty of meat, saturated fat, and vegetables, fruit, beans, and grains. "Plenty" as in "the land of plenty," which is what the United States used to be. And can be again when the aminos give us back our desire for real food!

The most important thing about pre-1970s eating was what was *missing* from it: no skipped meals; no candy, no chips, no soda, no ice cream *except as special treats*, mostly when we went out. Very little pasta (just spaghetti with meat sauce or a tuna casserole once a week), no pizza, and no daily sugar-loaded cold cereal (it had not yet entirely ruined the great American breakfast).

Our mothers made sure that when we did eat sugar, most of it was consumed *after* a meal, saying, "That stuff ruins your appetite, so you can't have it until *after* dinner." Their homemade desserts were loaded with eggs, butter, cream, and nuts. Even when cake mixes became a fad in the '50s, our mothers doctored them up with real ingredients because "they didn't taste that good" without them.

How *often* did we have full meals? *Never less than three times a day.* Skipping meals was unthinkable. "What do you mean you're not hungry? Are you sick?" our mothers would say. "Well, if you're not sick, you must have been sneaking the cookies that I baked for dessert and you're in trouble!" (And they were always right!)

The same basic eating habits have worked everywhere in the world, and still do, where traditional diets are still in place. As long as our diets were mostly free of industrially processed food, overweight and diet-related diseases like diabetes were virtually unknown.[3,4]

THEN ALONG CAME THE '70S

As an eyewitness and an active participant in the happenings of the 1970s, I can tell you that, first and foremost, it was the decade of true believers. It was a time of cults, causes, and innovations of all kinds. Pull up a bandwagon and we'd jump on it. Think feminism and fitness, encounter groups and Eastern religion, a fascination with the brain, and an unprecedented interest in nutrition and health.

Ordinarily, making even *one permanent* change in an entire nation's entrenched eating habits would be an impossible task. For example, in the period between the World Wars, we were forced to eat processed food substitutes and we hated them: margarine and Spam instead of butter and ham! Saccharin instead of sugar! Outrage! As soon as we could, we went right back to "the real stuff."

In the revolutionary atmosphere of the '70s, though, we stepped up en masse and made *three* dietary pledges. We committed to dismantling all three of humanity's most fundamental eating practices. We made these pledges because we were convinced that they would save our lives, our looks, our souls, or the planet. With the best of intentions, we headed down the dead-end dietary trails that we continue to pursue today.

The Three Dietary Trends That Led Us from Moderate Eating and Ideal Weight to Craving and Obesity

1. *We made the Fat Switch:* we swore off traditional saturated fats and replaced them with damaged and inflammatory mystery oils.

2. *We went high carbohydrate:* we began to eat more of the new, higher-fructose sugars and the new wheat flour products.

3. *We went low protein:* we reduced our intake of animal protein, of red meat in particular.

THE FIRST TREND: THE FAT SWITCH

Despite the generally glowing health of Americans, there was one growing health concern: heart disease rates in the United States had been mysteriously rising since the 1930s. In the 1950s and 1960s they rose more steeply and we began to panic. The American Heart Association and the loudest voices in nutrition science assured us that cholesterol buildup was the cause. We were told that we needed to cut back on saturated fats like eggs, cheese, whole milk, and fatty meats, which contained some cholesterol. And we did! Whole milk consumption, for example, quickly dropped by 66 percent in the '70s and has never recovered.[5]

But saturated fat was an odd choice of villain. We'd been eating food full of it for millennia, *without* cardiovascular damage or weight gain. More oddly, we'd been eating *less* saturated fat since the '30s, because of butter shortages and a popular novel by Upton Sinclair Jr., which, by exposing the horrors of the meat-packing industry, reduced American meat consumption for years.[6] Despite all of this, in the '50s and '60s, famous and convincing scientists, notably nutrition expert Ancel Keys, insisted that the traditional saturated fats had somehow become the enemy.

With the saturated fats out of the way, sales of hydrogenated (artificially hardened) vegetable oil margarine and shortening took off. But thirty years later, in the 1990s, a flood of international research concluded that the hydrogenated fats, first introduced at about the same time that heart disease had started to become a problem in the United States, were causing a serious increase in "bad," heart-damaging LDL cholesterol. So, did that mean that *both* hydrogenated *and* saturated fats were causing heart disease? No. *The studies that condemned hydrogenated fat specifically vindicated saturated fat.*[7] This astonishing scientific about-face has been firmly supported by subsequent research. A definitive review of *all* the studies on fat and heart disease published up to 2010 found that *"saturated fat was not associated with increased risk of heart disease."*[8] Another exhaustive review, published in 2015, confirmed this yet again.[9] But did *you* ever hear about it?

No. You *did* hear about the first finding, that hydrogenated fats were dangerous, loud and clear. In fact, these "trans" fats will be entirely banned from our food supply as of the end of 2018.[10] But somehow the second finding, the one that exonerated the saturated fats, was universally ignored. Some light dawned as a result of the heroic journalism of Gary Taubes (and his subsequent books) starting early in the twenty-first century. But it wasn't until June of 2014 that a curl of butter would appear on the cover of *Time* magazine heralding an inside story exposing serious errors in the earlier scientific thinking about saturated fat. Even so, the rehabilitation of butter faced an uphill battle until the day in 2016 that a *JAMA Internal Medicine* study made the front page of the *New York Times*. Finally, and in one headline—"How the Sugar Industry Shifted Blame to Fat"—sixty years of nutritional obfuscation was exposed. Saturated fat had been made a decoy to protect the sugar industry from the responsibility for its major role in our heart disease epidemic (and in much of the ensuing weight and health disaster we now face).[11] It turns out that we've known since the '60s that it's been sugar, along with hydrogenated fat, *not saturated fat*, that have been the cardiovascular threats.

CLEARING UP THE SATURATED FAT FALLACY
AND THE CHOLESTEROL CONFUSION

With sugar's culpability along with that of hydrogenated fat now well established, we can take a new look at dear old butter and other saturated fats. Nina Teicholz's book, *The Big Fat Surprise: Why Butter, Meat and Cheese Belong in a Healthy Diet*, appeared not long after *Time* magazine's butter edition, and has been creating a stir ever since with its startlingly positive and densely documented facts on saturated fats. Let's take a peek at some of the treasures in her trove, starting with her report on the results of a thirty-year follow-up to the famous ongoing Framingham, Massachusetts Heart Study which included the following facts (are you seated?):

- The higher the amount of saturated fat eaten, the lower the body weight among the hundreds of carefully monitored subjects.

- Saturated fat consumption was *neither* associated with high cholesterol *nor* with heart disease.[15]

- For every percent *drop* in their cholesterol, the subjects experienced an 11 percent *increase* in coronary and other causes of death.[16]

Teicholz documents another, literally monumental failure of the low-fat diet. The U.S. Women's Health Initiative study's conclusion, after following 49,000 women on low-fat diets for ten years, was that a low-fat diet did *nothing* to prevent heart disease or weight gain![17] (Actually, it turns out that women are especially vulnerable to lowering their intake of saturated fats as it can drop their heart protective HDL levels by one-third![18]) Teicholz also unearthed an early study about Israel, which at the time boasted one of the world's lowest rates of saturated fat consumption and highest intakes of cholesterol-free vegetable oil but had one of Europe's highest rates of heart disease.[19]

This sort of solid evidence confirms historical common sense: saturated fat never did harm us and still doesn't. But does saturated fat do us any *good*? Let's consult the gorgeous African Masai, who have lived on their animals' milk and blood almost exclusively for millennia. Such a living testament to the health benefit of a high-saturated-fat diet encourages us to take seriously certain newly documented facts such as that milk fats are *specifically protective against type 2 diabetes*[20] and *heart disease*,[21] and that steady-burning saturated fat is not only the *preferred fuel of the heart* but *protective against stroke.*[22] American scientists have even dared recently to find that eggs are specifically protective against stroke.[23]

How about butter? Butter is packed with ten vitamins, ten minerals, eighteen amino acids, and eleven kinds of fat. It's loaded with vitamin A, which it helps deliver to our eyes (night vision is absolutely dependent on an adequate vitamin A supply). Vitamin A also regulates the female sex hormone progesterone, providing many mood, fertility, and other benefits. "A" also stands for "anti-tumor," and butter's saturated fats assist fat-soluble vitamin A absorption in this life-preserving function (which too many omega-6 fats from vegetable oil can block).[24] Butter is also rich in its namesake, butyrate, the fastest burning of all fats, used extensively in the brain and well known to protect us from colon cancer.[25] This is particularly true when butter is organic and grass-fed, because its omega-3 content is higher.

MORE ABOUT CHOLESTEROL

We know so much more about cholesterol now than we did when it was presented as the sole cause of heart disease in the '60s and '70s. It's a very complex matter and we're still learning about it. So far, studies have identified that there is "good," large, heart-protecting HDL and small "bad" HDL cholesterol, as well as large neutral (LDL) and small, "bad" (LDL) cholesterol. But what these types of cholesterol are good and bad for is still somewhat unclear.

With all the vilifying of cholesterol the past fifty years, we have certainly not heard much about its numerous *benefits.* High levels of bad cholesterol can contribute to health problems, but *low* levels of good cholesterol can pose an equally serious health risk. A 40-year study of 4,000 people in Hawaii found that *"the earlier that patients start to have lower cholesterol concentrations, the greater the risk of death."*[26] That is partly because cholesterol protects against cancer[27] and low cholesterol causes hemorrhagic stroke. Low cholesterol is linked with autism,[28] depression, anxiety, irritability, violence, suicide, and insomnia. Why? Partly because, in the brain, cholesterol is essential for the production of our natural antidepressant, serotonin,[29] and also because our adrenal glands can use *only cholesterol* to make the hormones that allow us to cope with stress (and reproduce). Precious vitamin D is also made from cholesterol.

THE OLD AND NEW FATS

Traditionally our fats have come from meats, eggs, and poultry; nuts and seeds; butter and cream; chicken fat, bacon fat, and lard (pork fat); and olive and coconut oils. *Before the 1930s, this fat consumption had resulted in neither weight gain nor heart disease.* Yet we were told to reduce our total fat as well as our saturated fat intake so radically that we would have had to drop dangerously low in overall calories to achieve it. That 10 percent loss (over 200 calories a day), for an already trim population, would have been experienced by the body as a threat to survival. We cannot tamper with such fundamental dietary requirements without penalty, as we are now learning. We did initially reduce the amount of fat we ate by the whopping 10 percent from the traditional 43 percent to 33 percent of our diet.[30] But we did not lower our overall caloric intake for long. To compensate for the sudden loss of calories from fat, we reached for calories elsewhere. We turned first to the new "fat-free" '70s inventions: the high sugar and starch, zero-fat Techno-Karbz. Fairly soon, though, the nonfat taste palled. No matter how much sugar or flour Entenmann's fat-free cakes contained, they just didn't have that deeper, yummier satisfaction that fat adds. Yet the food industry did not dare to restore saturated fat (even the previously popular tropical fats like coconut oil that contained *no* cholesterol). So it began to add more of the new, highly processed, inexpensive vegetable oils and hydrogenated margarine and shortening, all "cholesterol-free."

The actual "low-fat" period, though the concept lives on, was very brief. By 1980 our consumption of the new vegetable oil products was rising steeply and has continued to do so. In addition, we're eating more cheese. As a result, our fat intake, by 2011, was 850 calories a day, somewhat *higher* than it had been before we started to go "low fat."[31] To understand better what's happened in our mass fat-switch experiment, please pause for a quick fat lesson.

SOME FAT BASICS

Fat is complex and active. It's not an inert, greasy blob. It's made up of dozens of types of fatty acids, or lipids, all with very specific and active functions in the body.

The simplest distinctions between fats are that some are solid and some are liquid; some are natural and some are industrial.

The Firm, or Saturated, Fats

1. Naturally firm saturated fats (there are several kinds) from *animal sources* like butter, bacon fat, cheese, egg yolks, and chicken skin come along with varying amounts of what we now know is mostly helpful cholesterol. The safety of these fats has been scientifically verified since the 1990s.

2. Some naturally firm saturated fats come from tropical *plants* that contain no cholesterol, notably coconuts, whose oil is now famous for its health-promoting properties.

3. *Un-natural* saturated fat, industrially hardened by hydrogenation into margarine and shortening, is mostly made from what were, originally, unsaturated liquid plant oils. It has been known to be heart harmful since the 1990s.

The Liquid, or Unsaturated, Fats

All are cholesterol-free

1. Natural *omega-9* oils—the most stable liquid oils—are concentrated in olives, avocados, and macadamia nuts, but they also comprise up to one-third of animal fat (including bacon fat),[32] and smaller portions of peanut oil and other seed and nut oils.

2. Natural *omega-3* oils—are fragile, but essential. Their DHA and EPA contents are required by every cell in the body and are famously *anti*-inflammatory. "Essential" means that they can't be assembled by the body from other fats. We don't need lots of omega-3 fat, and that's a good thing because it's harder to come by than any other fat. It comes (in its most assimilated form) directly from fish and from the fat of grass-fed animals, which we don't eat much anymore. We're too busy eating Techno-Karbz. We're also, understandably, afraid that fish is contaminated by the mercury and other toxins that are now dumped so freely into our waterways, and we know that fish have their own contamination problems. They also contain less DHA and EPA and much more of the competing omega-6 fats.[33] The crude vegetable oil form of omega-3 (ALA) found in plants like flax and hemp is difficult for most animals, including humans, to convert into the essential and invaluable DHA/EPA forms. (Poultry can't convert well either, so "high omega-3 eggs" are not likely to be much help.) Even those humans who *can* make this conversion can only derive EPA, not DHA, from flax or other plant sources of ALA. DHA is the form of omega-3 fat most needed (in the brain, in particular). It can be converted into EPA but only with difficulty, as five enzymes are required to do the job. EPA cannot be converted to DHA at all. Fish oil provides both EPA and DHA. The United States is now among the lowest consumers of omega-3 fish oil in the world.[34]

3. Natural *omega-6* oils (there are several types) are fragile and essential, like the omega-3s, but they are mostly *inflammatory* oils. They are obtained traditionally from nuts and seeds. We do need these oils, but only in small amounts, consumed in a 1 to 1 ratio with the omega-3 fats.

4. *Unnatural, industrially extracted* omega-6 vegetable oils are damaged *and* inflammatory. We're eating so much of this oil now that we're losing what little benefit we're still getting from the tiny amount of omega-3 fats we're still consuming. *The ratio of omega-6 to omega-3 fat we consume is no longer the ideal 1 to 1; it is now closer to 20 to 1.*[35]

THE RISE OF THE TECHNO-FATS

We used to rely on saturated fats (in human breast milk, for example!) as well as some stable unsaturated omega-9 oils (like olive oil), a little omega-3 fish oil, and a little natural omega-6 oil from nuts or seeds. The hydrogenated fats and the heavily processed vegetable oils, both mostly composed of omega-6 fat, were never a human food before sophisticated equipment made their extraction and processing possible in the twentieth century. Whether liquid or hardened, these new vegetable oils have now become our primary source of fat. When we radically cut down on saturated fats, these mystery oils became the only game in town. As they contained no cholesterol, they were massively marketed as the "lite" oils in the 1970s, though their calorie content was as high as butter's and their other properties and effects had been little researched.

All fats trigger some pleasurable brain response, so without the guilt and fear that since the '70s accompanied any consumption of saturated fat, our intake of the seemingly innocent vegetable oils has predictably gone wild. Most of this intake has come, though, from commercially prepared foods (think *chips, fries, and mayo*) that comprise most of our diet now. Almost *everything* available on the supermarket and snack-shop shelves, as well as in any restaurant, includes or is cooked in cheap high-omega-6 fat (omega-9 olive oil is much more expensive) vegetable oil. This oily deluge has caused our total omega-6 fat intake to be higher by a third than it was *before* 1970. That's half a pound (about 225 calories) a day.[36]

What is the impact of all this unnatural fat? We know now, because of the research finally done on hydrogenated (solidified) vegetable oil in the '90s, that *it* is harmful. But what about the liquid vegetable oils? We're just starting to aggressively study their effects on humans. (Teicholz did find cancer resulting in studies which fed them to animals.[37]) More research is coming in fast, including one human study from the National Institutes of Health published in the *British Medical Journal* which found that the risk of death rose 22 percent for every unit of cholesterol reduced by a high–vegetable oil diet.[38]

The Omega-6 Oxidation Factor

For centuries, worldwide, a few traditional high-omega-6 vegetable oils, like flax oil, were pressed by hand, but were known to quickly become rancid and only to be safe to eat for a few days. These ultra-fragile, high-omega-6 oils are now squeezed from cheap, often GMO, cotton seeds, corn kernels, or soybeans, complete with pesticides.

All seeds are originally carefully protected by nature, wrapped in a brown coat of antioxidant vitamin E that keeps them stable. But this shield is stripped from them in processing. Once the naked oil is extracted, it is exposed to oxygen, heat, and light. Any one of the three is capable of damaging it further by oxidation (rancidity). Then it is processed *again* for deodorization, so that we won't smell the rancidity.[39] There are several kinds of omega-6 fat. The omega-6 fat now identified as our chief problem, LA (linoleic acid), so plentiful in soy, corn, canola, and most other "salad" oils (except olive), is known to be elevated in children with type 2 diabetes and in all those with potentially fatal *nonalcoholic fatty liver disease* (NAFLD), which afflicts 30 percent of the general population and 70 percent of diabetics.

Inflammation and Other Factors Even if these unstable oils arrived on our salads in pristine condition, they would still be harmful because they are also so inflammatory by nature. Linoleic acid (fat, like protein, is mildly acidic) breaks down into arachidonic acid, which has many known adverse effects in excess, including metabolic dysregulation. A little omega-6 fat is essential to our health if derived from a few fresh nuts or seeds a week. It facilitates menstruation and provides an initial localized inflammatory response to infection, injury, or allergies (the beesting swells and gets red and hot). Our bodies are now, though, vastly *overloaded* with omega-6 oils and our intake of counterbalancing, *anti*-inflammatory omega-3 fat is, as I said, among the lowest in the world. Much of the omega-6 oil we consume is taken into our cell walls—but only because we're so deficient in the omega-3 fats that those walls actually require. (This is particularly true of our brain cells.) Excess omega-6 fat is also stored in our adipose (fat) tissue because we consume so much more of this fat than we can burn off. But remember, our total calorie intake from fats is only a little higher than it was before 1970 when we had virtually no obesity. *It's only the type of fat that has changed.* It is becoming clear now that the more omega-6 fat we consume, particularly coupled with our now dangerously low consumption of counterbalancing and metabolism-enhancing omega-3 fat, the more metabolically impaired and overweight we become.[40] In several studies, lean subjects have tended to have lower omega-6 fat levels and higher omega-3 levels than obese subjects.[41]

WE NEED AN OMEGA-6 FLUSH-AND-BALANCE

We can and must stop consuming so much damaged and inflammatory mystery oil and stock up on safe *anti*-inflammatory omega-3-containing fish and grass-fed animal fats (as I detail in Chapter 13, page 204). Animal studies show that improving the current omega-6 to omega-3 ratio by adding in more omega-3 fat can reverse many of the adverse effects of a high omega-6 diet.[42] Introducing more fish oil into the diet, just enough to create not the perfect 1 (omega-3) to 1 (omega-6) ratio but a 1 to 8 (much better than the current 1 to 20 ratio) cured 100 percent of a Polish study's subjects of their non-alcoholic fatty liver disease and reduced their BMI, insulin, and other markers as well (despite their continuing on a high-Techno-Karbz diet)![43] There are also well-documented benefits to giving omega-3 oils to those with heart disease, brain injury, and learning problems. We can get even closer to the ideal ratios by cutting out high-omega-6-oil-infused commercial foods and eating a few nuts and seeds a few times a week instead. But to actually expel the excess omega-6 fats from the phospholipids that compose all of our cell linings, they must be replaced with more omega-3s from fish and from supplements of fish oil or oils from krill, cod liver, or algae oil. We can also make new phospholipids for the omega-3s to inhabit from organic egg yolks and liver to strengthen the flush process further. One study has shown that egg-derived phospholipids have positive effects on weight and blood pressure in patients with metabolic syndrome.[44] See more about eating fish in Chapter 13, page 209 and using omega supplements in Chapter 12, page 196.

THE SECOND TREND: GOING "HIGH-CARB"

Out of our extreme and, as you can see, mistaken fear of traditional saturated fats, in the '70s, we obediently adopted *low-fat and nonfat* products for the first time in history. However, we certainly didn't replace the lost fat calories with extra protein, fresh vegetables, fruit, beans, or whole grains. Instead, we immediately started replacing those calories with the new "fat-free" Techno-Karbz: more cereal, bread, pasta, bagels, pretzels, and sweetened dairy products than ever before. Then, in the 1980s, as I mentioned earlier, in fast-food and chain restaurant outlets, *portion sizes doubled*. So we were downing even more Techno-Karbz as half of our food was eaten "out" by then.[45] By this time, though, most of these refined carbs were no longer fat-free. They were laced with the hydrogenated fats and the damaged vegetable oils.

All this meant that the *quality* and safety of the food in our diets was dropping as the number of calories went up. A recent study has confirmed that fully 60 percent of our diet is now "pure" Techno-Food with *no* nutrient content other than calories.[46] *So we're starving and gaining weight at the same time.*

THE NEW SUGARS AND STARCHES

In the 1800s, our sugar intake went up from 6 pounds to 60 pounds of table sugar (sucrose) per year, but that sugar intake rose to 120 pounds a year in the 1960s.[47] This is when we first started to experience some weight gain. Some distinguished scientists at that time rightfully blamed sugar for our increasing incidences of weight gain and, more important, heart disease, but no alarm regarding sugar was sounded. All our attention was focused on saturated fat. As we know now, this obsession with saturated fat was partially orchestrated by the sugar industry, starting in the 1960s. High-starch breads and other "baked goods" also went under the radar almost entirely, though there was a boycott of Wonder Bread and a popularization of whole wheat products during the '60s "back to nature" period.

During the 1970s, our intake of brand-new forms of sugar and starch escalated. As I explained in Chapter 2, high-fructose corn syrup was introduced at that time, and so was the new "dwarf" wheat. Our consumption of the products containing them has doubled since then. We've been especially vulnerable to them because they came upon us just as we were embarking on the other two hazardous new dietary experiments at the same time: the *fat switch* you've just read about and the *protein drop* you'll read about next. As we saw it then, there was literally nothing left to eat but sugar and dough.

By 2000 we were consuming about *155 pounds of sugar per year, 35 pounds a year more than we'd been eating in 1970. More than half of it was high-fructose corn syrup.*[48] Our consumption of white flour went way up too—interestingly, by the same 35 pounds per year.[49] *Between the new sugars and the new starches, today, according to the USDA, we're eating, on average, over 500 more calories per day than we were eating before 1970.*[50]

Due to the addictive properties of the Techno-Karbz that comprise most of our current diet, we've almost entirely lost our taste for *nature's* highly nutritious carbohydrates. The new trends in commercial sweetness and starchiness have quite literally spoiled our appetites for the vegetables and fruits that, in the 1960s, still comprised 20 percent of our daily calories. Now they make up just 8 percent, mostly as tomato sauce and fried potatoes.[51]

CARBOHYDRATE-LOADING FOR FITNESS

In the '70s, before we knew all this, carbohydrates had developed a reputation as a fitness aid. Fitness was another new rage that ignited in the '70s. Based on the discovery that carbohydrates (in the form of glycogen) were stored in the muscles and the liver, and some very limited research with military recruits and mara-thoners, in the '70s, our athletes were told they should "carb-load" before every event. Since the new exercise craze had motivated *everyone* to become athletic, this meant Pop-Tarts before the kids' swim meets and pasta pig-outs before Daddy's and Mommy's runs. We assumed that we could easily "burn it all off" by participating in some form of "workout" (another concept first popularized in the 1970s). Because sweets and starches then were mostly low- or nonfat, "high-carb" actually became synonymous with fitness and health. Now we "carb-load" on a daily basis, despite our much reduced exercise level and the knowledge that these foods are seriously antifitness. Even those of us who are exercisers are unable to burn off all the Techno-Karbz they're overconsuming on a daily basis.

The result of our now involuntary Techno-Karb loading? Of 15,000 over-weight Dutch women, those who consumed the most refined carbohydrates were 80 percent more likely to have cardiovascular disease than those who consumed the fewest.[52] A similar study found a 50 percent greater incidence of diabetes among women who ate the most carbohydrates.[53]

THE THIRD TREND: WE WENT LOW PROTEIN

In our efforts, since the 1970s, to cut the fat, especially the saturated fat, out of our diets, and more recently, for ethical, religious, and other reasons, we've turned on the last of our three primal foods: animal protein. What turned us against the food we had most prized for the prior two million years? To begin with, we ob-jected to it because it contained saturated fat. Later we rejected it as we did *all* fatty foods, because it contained fat at all. *All* natural sources of protein (animal or vegetable) come inextricably combined with some sort of fat. The delicious fat in nuts and seeds, in the skins and muscle of meat and poultry, and in cheeses constitute as much as 50 percent of their total calories, or more. Even tofu's fat content is (not so lusciously) high. We didn't know then that the carbohydrates we were eating were much more weight-promoting than the saturated fat in meat. We didn't know that any excess was turned into fat in our bodies and stored.

We also rejected meat because of valid concerns about processed meat, but even fresh, lean meat was rejected for newly influential ethical and spiritual reasons, which I'll address shortly. *As a result, protein has gone from being our primary food source before 1970 to third place.* Sugar and starch are the new number one with fat (mostly high-omega-6 vegetable oil) in second place. Take eggs. We used to eat about ten per week[54] and called it "the perfect food." We're now down to five, even though the American Heart Association has acknowledged its earlier mistake and is encouraging us to add more.

The trouble is that everything in the body is made from protein, including our hair, bones, and, of course, our brain's anti-craving neurotransmitters. For most of our history on this planet, we have relied on the protein content of animal products to construct almost all of our body parts. Meat, poultry, fish, some cheeses, and yogurt concentrates (especially thick, Greek-style yogurt) have *two to four times more protein* per ounce than the equivalent amounts of plant proteins. And animal-derived protein is *complete*, meaning it contains all twenty of the amino acids required for brain and body maintenance, including *all nine of the "essential" ones*, which are the aminos our bodies can't manufacture themselves.

Each of the total twenty amino acids in protein is earmarked for very specific and unique construction and repair purposes in our bodies. The number of constituent aminos and total protein grams found in vegetables, beans, grains, nuts, and seeds are much lower per ounce than in animal protein, as I detail in Chapter 13.

As with traditional fats, traditional protein sources had always served us well. Remember, most of us in the United States were eating animal protein three times a day *long before* we developed any weight problems at all and long before heart disease became a problem.

Once they've started taking their aminos, our clients immediately begin to eat traditional amounts of animal protein and are aware of the difference right away. Later, if they start to eat too little protein again, their cravings quickly start to return (even if they're still using the aminos). This is due to the satiety power of protein, which is known to be greater than that of any other food.[55] This is why we tell clients that if they suddenly want a cookie, that's fine, as long as they eat a salmon steak or a lamb chop *first*.

Beef and lamb (especially when grass-fed) contain all the needed fats *and* can be converted into glucose-replacing, cell-fueling ketones. They also come with invaluable vitamins and minerals. Three of our most depleted micronutrients, vitamin B_{12} and the minerals zinc and iron, can only be derived in easily absorbable forms from animal protein; the latter two, only from red meat. This makes animal protein a true *superfood*.

VEGETARIANS AND VEGANS

Now you can see why we've depended on animal protein for two million years or so. We have only been eating so much carbohydrate for 12,000 years—since we started to grow grains, beans, and our own fruits. Our needs for proteins do vary. Some vegetarians seem to thrive on their all- or mostly plant diets. Some vegans even excel as athletes. But many others don't. I wish that we saw more physical, emotional, or spiritual health in our vegetarian or vegan clients, many of whom come to us weak, unhappy, and full of cravings for Techno-Karbz. We typically ask these understandably conflicted people to try some animal protein for a few days before they make a decision. Red meat in particular has been dramatically beneficial for many of them right away because of its uniquely strong and absorbable iron and zinc content, as well as its robust and complete protein content, high in two mental- and physical-energy-generating amino acids.

Cutting protein intake can be a particular problem for big veg exercisers whose muscles demand extra aminos to build and maintain size and strength. Young female athletes lose strength, stamina, their periods, and their ability to recover from injuries when amino supplies are limited by a high-carbohydrate, low–animal protein diet.[56]

A Vegan Story

A formerly vegan mother brought her currently vegan teenage daughter in to us because the girl's stamina was too limited to support her athletic talents. The young woman had lost her period and her athletic injuries were taking too long to heal. She was also living on Techno-Karbz, so her weight was climbing, despite all her physical exercise. Her coach insisted on a low-calorie diet, but we prevailed in our insistence on an increased-calorie, Techno-Karbz-free diet that included red meat. All of her complaints disappeared (though she found having regular periods again a nuisance).

Mom's own career as a college runner had almost fizzled for the same reasons. She, too, had been a vegan (raised as one by her own "hippy" mom). Her track coach had insisted she meet with a local sports M.D. who'd explained to her that red meat was by far the best source of iron and zinc—the former crucial for energy and stamina and the latter for optimal appetite, digestion, and wound healing. He prescribed a steak a day for a week, and at least two steaks a week thereafter, plus any other animal protein she liked, and lots of it. Within two weeks she was not only running much harder and longer, but she was bubbly and happy. (She hadn't realized until then that she was capable of feeling that good.) We saw the same personality transformation in her fifteen-year-old daughter in response to similar recommendations—except that we needed to add several aminos for her moods, including the Type 1 amino (she was a big

Type 1 Depressed [and obsessive] Craver, like most vegans) to help her relax her rigid thinking about her diet. This inner struggle was made harder for her because of all the current external pressure to be vegan that was not there when her mother was her age.

SPIRITUAL CONFLICTS

It's important to know that the vegan diet is *not* one of the traditional diets of mankind. For example, Buddhist communities worldwide are split in half between those who eat eggs and milk products and those who eat meat as well.[57] The Dalai Lama, the spiritual leader of the Tibetan Buddhists, explains in his autobiography that he made the decision to return to eating meat because of a serious health problem. The Buddha's own *nonvegan* diet, as detailed in scripture, included milk products and eggs. A similar "lacto-ovo" diet is followed by 40 percent of those in India, mostly for cultural, *not* religious or health, reasons.[58] Spiritual teachers from this tradition in India have been very influential in the United States, particularly since the 1970s, in spreading their esoteric dietary practices as well as yogic ones. The majority of Indian vegetarians are known to be low in iron or have frank anemia. Seventy percent[59] of the children in India are very low in iron. Low iron and B_{12} are serious and common deficiencies among Western vegans and vegetarians as well.[60, 61]

One of our spiritually motivated vegan clients unknowingly developed what could have become a serious and even fatal case of pernicious anemia (low vitamin B_{12}) not too long after becoming a vegan. But she happened to get a facial, which revealed the telltale yellow tone of her skin. Three B_{12} shots later and feeling perky again, she realized how tired she'd gradually became on her vegan diet and she came to see us for advice on alternatives. We told her, as we tell all of our spiritually conflicted vegan clients, that there are, and always have been, innumerable spiritually enlightened meat eaters all over the world. This client found that all of her faculties strengthened with the addition of animal protein (range-fed and organic) and she actually found that she became more spiritually in-tune after she stopped being a vegan!

Most of the vegetarians and vegans who have come to our clinics have found that their energy, mood, and cravings improve noticeably within forty-eight hours of their introducing meat, fish, or poultry. Some have noticed it *right after* their first red meat meal. One noticed that her brain started tingling *during* her first serving of steak. *The brain in particular requires very generous protein feedings.* In fact, the human brain only developed to begin with after we, as a species, began eating more meat. (More on this in Chapter 14, page 224.)

We've never worked with a vegan who was able to completely eliminate cravings or optimize energy or mood without adding some animal protein. We've always ended up asking our vegan clients to trial some "animal-medicine" and to decide, based on their own experience, what they should do. Many of them have had to bow to their own animal natures. We ask them to love themselves anyway, as much as they love their omnivore dogs and carnivore cats.

LEAVING ALL THREE TRENDS BEHIND

The runaway weight and health disaster that the trends of the 1970s have unleashed on us has prompted endless dietary debate. Since the 1970s, we have been barraged by ever-new dictums about what constitutes healthy and unhealthy eating. The *value of all our ancient food staples and food preparation traditions* have become suspect. In fact, we're being urged to change our minds about what we should or shouldn't eat every week! Some of this dialogue is constructive and new nutritional research helpful, but sorting through it is extraordinarily difficult because there is so much contradiction and passion involved. I hope that we can call a moratorium on newly invented diets and step back to see that our original diet gave us everything we need so badly now.

In the next chapter, you'll get my perspective on post-1970s weight gain, what has really caused it, and why our weight loss efforts up to now have failed. You'll also get a look at how the Craving Cure's approaches have worked for our clients in helping them unravel this as yet little understood problem.

4

The Weight-Gain Pandemic: Uncovering the True Causes and How the Craving Cure Can Help

MOST OF US BORN INTO the modern-dietary-disaster era are fighting for things we used to take for granted. Since the 1970s, we've been fighting for our beauty, our health, and even for our lives. The first sign of disaster broke out initially among American women, but it has since spread throughout the world, afflicting men, children, and infants as well. It was a plague of unnatural weight gain.

In the ethnic melting pot of the United States, some variation in weight had historically been regarded as healthy and normal. We considered weight to be a family trait, a genetic distinction, like height, that fell somewhere within the normal spectrum. For example, my father's side was slender, but not thin. My mother's side was curvy, but not overweight (though my grandfather and great-grandfather proudly described themselves in later years as "portly," modeling themselves on robust President Teddy Roosevelt). In fact, overweight in the United States had always been considered such an insignificant problem that no statistics were even collected on it until the 1960s. At that point there was just starting to be some concern about weight gain. Since then, over 70 percent of U.S. adults and 30 percent of children have become overweight,[1] more than half of them obese.[2]

As disturbing as it has been for us to endure this uncontrollable distortion of our appearance, modern weight gain has only been the visible evidence of what has actually been a *body-wide* calamity. It has certainly had nothing to do with weak willpower or poor food choices. We're no more or less disciplined or wise now than we were during the prior two million years. Modern weight gain has to do with much more formidable problems, like brain neurotransmitter dysfunction, appetite-hormone dysregulation, and genetic misprogramming. It is a much deeper, more complex, and more virulent phenomenon than we knew. *That's why we haven't been able to stop it.*

Up to now, our primary strategy for counteracting our loss of weight control has been extreme caloric restriction, but as you'll see, even the most highly structured and closely monitored diets actually make food cravings and weight problems worse.[3] Frequent low-calorie dieters, for example, are twelve times more likely to become bingers than nondieters.[4] The first part of this chapter focuses on exactly how low-calorie dieting harms us. Then you'll read about my clinics' alternative approaches to weight repair, including the exercise factor, and our client's responses. Finally, I'll describe some new developments in nutrient therapy aimed at correcting the genetic factors in weight gain.

Let's start with the calorie calamity. Ironically, just before we'd begun to eat the most weight-promoting diet of all time in the '70s, many American women had become obsessed with looking thinner than was genetically possible for most females over the age of twelve. This trend had started in the early '60s when the bizarrely thin (even for a model) Twiggy caught the national fancy. But it took a while for us to get seriously interested in looking scrawny. Looking like Marilyn Monroe was still plenty good enough for most of us at first, and most American women, with a few minor adjustments, could pull it off. In the innovative atmosphere of the '70s, though, game for anything new, more women of all ages and weights launched into what we assumed was a harmless competition to see who could lose the most weight. We thought that recreational dieting sounded like fun. We assumed that weight loss was just another "new look," like corseting our waists, binding our breasts, or perming our hair: a harmless fad, easily reversible when the style wore out.

Unfortunately, our commitment to this new "style" led us into what would turn out to be a fatal fascination with calorie restriction. The skinny ideal never did wear off and low-cal dieting got a stranglehold on us that has never let up. Instead of the radiant and voluptuous Marilyn, the sinewy Jane Fonda became our new role model. Jane has since publicly admitted that her obsession with the lean look turned her into a serious bulimic who badly neglected many important aspects of her life, including her children. Since then it has become commonplace for dieters to develop eating disorders.[5] In fact, low-calorie dieting has helped propel us into what has become a national *epidemic* of eating (and weight) disorders.

Ironically, in the 1980s, while our obsession with skinny was still in high gear, fast-food and chain restaurant portion sizes *doubled*.[6] That's when calorie overload, overeating, and overweight *really* took off. By the end of the '90s, the number of obese Americans began to exceed the number of overweight Americans. Desperation weight-loss efforts, including extended fasts and gastric surgery, started to become commonplace. Inexorably, though, our national weight disorder continued to spread. Eventually, it came to afflict most of the people we knew, including ourselves and our children.

In 2001, the Obesity Epidemic among adults in the United States was officially declared by the Centers for Disease Control (CDC). Not surprisingly, since children most often inherit abnormalities in appetite and weight from their parents,[7] in 2010, the U.S. Childhood Obesity Epidemic was announced with 15–20 percent of all children and teens qualifying.[8] Obesity is roughly defined as having a BMI (body mass index) greater than the "overweight" BMI, which is 25–30. There are now three categories of obesity, with BMIs ranging from 30 to 40. Between 1975 and 2014, rates of those in the third, most severe, category, called morbid obesity, rose from 1.6 to 13.3 percent: a 700 percent increase.[9] The United States now shares with China the highest obesity rate in the world.[10]

Fewer than one-third of us are at our genetically intended weight.

America has since exported its high-calorie, nutrient-empty diet to the rest of the world. In the twenty-first century, for the first time in history, the number of people who are overfed and overweight in the world outnumber the number of people who are underfed and underweight.[11] A new category of malnutrition, called *overnutrition*, defined as "an excess of sugar and fat in the diet," was identified and is now linked not just with weight gain, but with a myriad of other, far worse, health problems.

THE CALORIE-CUTTING SOLUTION REVISITED

The Twiggy-inspired experiment in voluntary mass starvation probably would have passed fairly quickly had it not coincided with the three radical new eating trends that emerged at the same time. We were not only increasing our consumption of calories from more addictive and weight-promoting new sugars, starches, and vegetable oils, we were also *decreasing* our consumption of calories from the traditional sources. We were eating less of the animal protein, saturated fat, vegetables, and fruit that had kept us in shape for so long. Did we reassess the new eating habits we'd adopted in the '70s? No. We got more serious about low-calorie dieting instead. Did it help? No. Low-calorie dieting has led, not to the land of the happy-at-weight-perfect, but to the land of the yo-yo syndrome, where, as so many dieters have learned, weight always rises, falls, and rises ever higher.

The fact that starving ourselves for weeks or months might be harmful should have been obvious. The human race had always dreaded food scarcity for very good reasons. So why were our daughters permitted to engage in starvation so casually, with no great medical or societal outcry? This was particularly puzzling as an exhaustive two-volume study of the alarming consequences of a single twelve-week, 1,500 calorie diet, "The Biology of Human Starvation," had fairly recently been published by the famous nutrition scientist Ancel Keys.[12] Keys continued to be a prominent leader in nutrition science for decades, but, ironically, in the 1970s he was busy leading the anti-fat crusade. This would eventually make him the single person most responsible for all the disastrous dietary blunders of our post-1970 era, including low-fat and low-calorie dieting.

It turns out that the body can mount insuperable survival responses when faced with inadequate calories: primary among them are the slowing down of the metabolic rate and the amplification of food cravings. Why? To keep us alive. The body can respond to food deprivation by ensuring that we hold onto whatever flesh we have. It can force us to eat and to gain. Then in 2016, the entire country was suddenly alerted to this previously unrecognized consequence of dieting.

"THE BIGGEST LOSER" STUDY EXPOSES THE SHOCKING RESULTS OF LOW-CALORIE DIETING

The television show *The Biggest Loser* was a great success and its winners became national celebrities. In a six-year follow-up study, published in 2016, however, it was discovered that the show's contestants had suffered a permanent reduction in their ability to burn calories. These celebrity dieters were *burning 500 fewer calories a day*, six years later, than they had been before the contest started. They were also suffering *much stronger and more constant food cravings*. As a result, most contestants had regained much of, all of, or more than the weight they'd worked so hard to lose.[13]

The study found that the contestants' increased food cravings and weight regain had been caused by their weight loss while in the program, which had altered the levels of several of their appetite-regulating *hormones*. We've known for decades that calorie reduction can lower the levels of one of our primary hormonal calorie-burning regulators, the thyroid hormone. The Biggest Loser Study confirmed this. But it also found decreased levels of the hormones leptin and increased levels of the hormone insulin. *Low levels of leptin and high levels of insulin are associated with constant cravings for food.* These hormonal changes were automatic responses to the program's weight-loss regimen, which was clearly considered by their bodies to constitute a dangerous threat. Though the contest formally recommended 1,500 calories a day, the contestants report that they were urged to eat far fewer calories by their trainers.[14] No one can be sure exactly how few or many calories each one actually consumed.

The news about the Biggest Losers spread throughout the country following the appearance of Gina Kolata's original story in the *New York Times*. The revelation was horrifying to millions of dieters, but it did blow open the implacable mystery of why we cannot keep the weight off. As grim as it was to discover that the Losers' seemingly "successful" dieting itself was the culprit, and that most of us were trapped in the aftermath of dozens or hundreds of similar diets, at least it was *no longer our fault*! The Biggest Losers themselves, after the terrible humiliation of their public weight regain, expressed particular relief.

Is there a specific number of calories consumed during a weight-loss effort that can cause such severe weight regain? The answer to this question was provided by an Australian study on the impact of a twelve-week *500-calorie-a-day* diet. This research found that this popular medically monitored fasting model of very low-calorie dieting can negatively alter dieters' appetite- and metabolism-regulating hormone levels even more seriously than the Biggest Loser regimen did. The function of *six additional hormones,* all also known to increase cravings and/or slow metabolism, were negatively impacted by the 500-calories-a-day allotment.[15] The patients, who actually pay for participating in this previously undocumented experiment, like the Biggest Losers, quickly regain their weight and more. This means that 500 calories a day is too few. What would a safe and effective number be?

We don't know. What we do know is that, according to the United Nations, the minimum number of calories considered adequate for sustaining human life is 1,800.[16] My clinic would rarely encourage a client to go even that low in calories. Keeping that in mind, we help our clients tailor their weight-loss efforts to their own unique needs, remembering that it's not only calories, but the *kind* of calories that makes so much difference. With the aminos, our clients can easily improve the *kind* of calories they eat as well as lose their desire for *excessive* calories. That automatically reduces the calories they consume without their having to go to what we've learned, from so many clients' experiences with low-calorie dieting, is a hazardous extreme.

The End of Yo-Yo Dieting

Ironically, the hormones that can be negatively altered by low-calorie diet-ing tend to be the same ones that are altered, with the same results, by the ex-cessive intake of *fructose* (see Chapter 3, page 68 for details). This means that, since the 1970s, on the standard American yo-yo diet, we have alternated between periods of high fructose consumption and periods of low-calorie dieting. This has created the perfect formula for permanently increasing food cravings and weight gain; *the perfect recipe for an obesity pandemic.* Fortunately, the now undisputed failure of the low-calorie approach may finally result in a new trend *away* from dieting programs and products. Already, by 2015, only 19 percent of people surveyed were on a diet. Some 77 percent of overweight Americans were instead trying to "eat healthy."[17] This non-dieting approach could be half of our answer. The other half is the elimination of our cravings for high-fructose sugar and other Techno-Karbz. For that I refer you to the possibilities you'll find laid out next.

THE CRAVING CURE'S APPROACH TO WEIGHT REPAIR

Too many Techno-Karbz and too many low-calorie diets have probably skewed your own weight-regulating mechanisms. Our clinic has developed eleven tech-niques that help to readjust those mechanisms. Here is a list of them followed by typical examples of how our clients have responded to them.

1. Brain-targeted amino acid supplements eliminate cravings for toxic, high-calorie, low-nutrient, weight-disturbing, craving-promoting foods.

2. These same aminos, teamed with a stabilizing diet, eliminate the negative moods and overstress that drive us to "emotional over-eating."

3. Regular exercise and calorie burning become possible and more productive with increases in high-protein foods (energizing iron-rich red meat in particular) combined with amino acids that restore the desire and capacity to be active.

4. Insomnia-targeted amino acids can provide the eight hours of sleep required for optimal weight loss.

5. Learning to establish a caloric intake in accordance with our own responses and needs can prevent, and reverse, the low-calorie weight-loss freeze.

6. Home food testing can identify hidden foods that contribute to cravings, weight retention, and ill health.

7. We can stabilize blood sugar levels and reduce insulin resistance in both hypoglycemics and diabetics with specific foods plus amino acids and other nutrient supplements.

8. We can stop PMS cravings with aminos and other nutrient or herbal supplements, plus a diet free of inflammatory fats and Techno-Karbz.

9. Loss of appetite for real food (especially in the morning) caused by zinc deficiency can be corrected with zinc supplementation, red meat consumption, or by identifying a genetic factor called pyroluria.

10. The slip prevention and recovery techniques developed at our clinic over the past thirty years further protect against relapse into cravings and overeating.

11. If weight loss and exercise efforts are impeded despite all of the above, we can identify whether an impaired thyroid or other trouble is contributing to metabolic shutdown and what can be done about it.

Six of these strategies are amino acid–based. You'll find them all in Parts II and III, Understanding Your Craving Type and The Amino Breakthrough. The eating strategies are described in Part IV, Craving-Free Eating. In case of exercise problems, PMS, poor appetite, minimal weight loss, or breakthrough cravings, go to Chapter 16, Dodging Slips and Shooting Trouble. My report on the exciting potential of nutritional strategies that target two big causes of weight gain, our malnutrition epidemic and diet-caused genetic dysfunction, is found here at the end of Chapter 4. Together, they comprise a multifaceted approach to weight repair that directly and safely addresses many of the newly recognized dimensions of the problem.

THE DIFFERING PATTERNS OF WEIGHT LOSS WE SEE

The Craving Cure skips the starvation and starts with permanent maintenance.

Most weight-loss diets automatically begin with radical food restriction. Whether called an induction period, a cleanse phase, or a detox, this punishing deprivation operates on the assumption (verified nowhere) that traumatic caloric reduction will somehow lead to the Holy Grail of weight loss, the Never-Never Land of "moderate eating" and "permanent maintenance." But since we now know that such calorie restriction is guaranteed *to prevent* lasting weight loss, we can understand why so few people ever arrive at maintenance and even fewer linger there.

When our clients cut out the Techno-Karbz, they typically drop hundreds of toxic calories, which alone constitutes a cleanse, without their having to cut the remaining *healthy* calories down to starvation levels.

With the amino acids—initially from supplements, but ultimately just from high-protein foods—our clients become immune from cravings for anything but the clean, healthful, maintenance-supporting foods they have been wanting to eat all along. And this blessed immunity can last for life!

THE EASY CLIENTS: LIGHT DIETERS, FOOD INTOLERANTS, CHRONIC UNDEREATERS, AND EMOTIONAL EATERS

Nobody responds to their Craving Cure in exactly the same way when it comes to weight loss. It is always a very individual matter. At our clinic, we're often surprised by which approaches work best for which clients. Here are some of the common weight changes we see:

The Light Dieters. The amount of metabolic battering caused by dieting seems to vary from person to person depending on how many diets they've attempted, how low in calories those diets have been, how long they've lasted, and their body's ability to rebound. Though we only rarely have a client who has *never* dieted, we have had many who'd long ago quit restricting calories. Instead, they'd just kept trying (and failing) to "eat healthy." They've also tended to have a history of easy weight loss when they have been able to avoid Techno-Karbz, but it's never lasted because of the power of their cravings. Once these clients begin the amino supplements, their cravings disappear and so does their excess weight.

Some of our clients really don't even care about their weight anymore. They have learned to value themselves, and to see that other people value them despite it. They say, "I have more important things to do than worry about my belly." They come to us *not* to lose weight, but because they want to stop being enslaved by the food industry or because they know they are headed toward illness and a slow death. Yet they sometimes lose more weight than other clients who, like our aspiring actors, obsess about their looks. Why? They are addicted to junk food, but they have *not* done much dieting. When we help them lose their cravings and quit eating Techno-Karbz, their less-suppressed metabolic rate allows them to burn calories faster than our chronic dieters, much to their surprise.

The Food Intolerants. When these clients cut out, in addition to the Techno-Karbz, certain otherwise healthy foods that, for them, seem to be metabolically unfavorable, they often find that they can then lose even more weight. They identify the possible culprits through the "food testing" process that I describe in Chapters 14 and 15. For example, one of our clients lost fifteen pounds when she quit junk food, lost another five pounds when she got off of whole wheat and other gluten-containing grains, and lost ten more pounds when she went off of all grains. (Yet she kept her daily calorie consumption between 2,100 and 2,500.)

Then there are the clients who always limit their daily calories to 1,500 or so but do *not* lose weight. These frustrated **undereaters** actually have to eat *more* calories (healthier, of course) to get any needed weight loss. This is also true for our **purgers**, who are often terrified of the weight gain they assume will follow if they consume and retain all the calories in our substantial regimens. They are all shocked when the scales show a loss. Even though they increase the number of calories, these new calories are *not weight-promoting.*

Losing Weight by Increasing Calories

We recently had a Skype intake session with a young woman who was on a creatively prepared diet consisting of good quality protein, fat, and carbohydrates three times a day. The problem? She was tired, irritable, and had started craving increasing amounts of chocolate every afternoon. She'd slipped out of "healthy" diets dozens of times before, so she knew the early signs and was determined not to "fail" again. We told her that her problem was that she was not eating enough of the good food. We told her we'd love to work with her if she'd be willing to eat more fat and protein. She said she'd try. Five days later, during her first formal session with her craving coach, before she'd trialed even one amino, she reported that her cravings, fatigue, and moodiness were 90 percent gone. She'd increased each meal's protein portion from three to four ounces and each meal's fat by one tablespoon, an increase of 500 calories per day with no weight gain. In fact, she'd lost the five pounds that the chocolate had put on. She still needed the aminos, for a time, to finish off her cravings, but the right foods had already done the lion's share of the job. This is not an isolated case. Myself and my trainers regularly see this with clients who habitually restrict calories.

The Emotional Eaters

My colleagues and I so enjoy watching as the aminos take effect during initial trialing sessions when our clients' negative moods drop away without high calorie assistance. And it lasts! This means that they have the opportunity to finally live without the comfort food. Of course, some emotions need additional attention, and typically the amino support makes psychotherapy more beneficial. I describe how we address our most emotionally impacted clients in Chapter 16, Dodging Slips and Shooting Trouble, on page 257.

THE DILEMMA OF THE FREQUENT DIETER

Our most impaired yo-yo dieting clients, because of their starvation-caused metabolic slow-down, have sometimes been gaining up to five pounds a week for some time before they get to us.

One of these clients had finally quit dieting because her cravings had become too strong to resist and because she was hardly losing any weight anymore, even on crash diets. She told us an interesting story we've now heard many times: "After one month with you, the scale showed a mere three-pound loss, but I'd actually lost fifteen pounds." What she meant was that she'd quit gaining the three pounds a week she'd been enduring for over a year (since her last low-calorie diet had turned off her long fading ability to burn calories). That added up to thirty pounds "lost" by the end of her second month. She'd actually lost a total of six pounds but had not gained the twenty-four pounds that she would have otherwise.

THE EXERCISE FACTOR

For many of our clients, being able to start or increase exercising is a major turning point. They may begin to feel energetic enough to exercise regularly because, on their relaxing aminos, they're getting enough sleep, or because they're using energizing aminos, or because they're gaining strength by eating more protein or calories—or they're able to cut screen or cell time on the aminos.

Whatever the case, many just start spontaneously stepping out more. After not exercising regularly in years, one day they come in and report having "just somehow" begun to be more active: walking longer or more briskly, biking, hiking, Jazzercising, or working out at the gym. They're enjoying it, too. Soon they report the expected benefits, including to their weight. No guilt or shame is motivating them. Their bodies are just coming back to life.

Others have to make sure that they're not getting *too much* exercise. We recommend they get any arduous exercise only on alternate days and caution them against burning themselves out by overdoing (which can so often turn into doing nothing again). Besides, they're just starting to get enough dietary amino acids to restore the brain and the rest of the body. Overusing muscles can siphon off the newly enhanced amino supply. How to keep this balance between activity level and protein intake? Increase protein intake on exercise days.

With increasing exercise (and protein) our clients steadily build muscle, and muscles burn fat for energy. We had one client who lost ten pounds, but went down *three* dress sizes because she was naturally athletic and her aminos plus more protein, minus Techno-Karbz, boosted both her energy and her muscle mass, which burned up more excess fat and rearranged her shape.

No matter how hard the workouts, though, trying to increase muscle mass, alone, without the amino acids and the diet changes, is an exercise in frustration.

A consultant to the nutrition and body-building industry told me that after he'd attended my weekend training, he'd been asked to consult with the frustrated coach of a hugely talented body builder who had developed the ultimate musculature, but was unable to get enough definition to even place in competitions. His inability to stay away from junk foods buried his contours. After just a few months on the aminos and a suddenly enjoyable Techno-Karbz-free diet, he was finally becoming a competition winner!

Many trainers have come to us for personal help with similar complaints and to get a new approach for their clients. Craving Techno-Karbz has been the big unsolved problem in the fitness industry for years, one that just hasn't responded to the standard diet-discipline-and-caffeine approach. Now you know why.

If our clients are not already pursuing much physical activity, we first suggest that they acquire a pedometer, a LifeTrak, or a Fitbit to track how many steps they are currently taking. We urge them to work toward getting between 10,000 steps known to promote health and prevent weight gain, and 14,000 steps known to assist with weight loss.[18] Cutting back on computer and phone time is often critical to making this happen.

If nothing gets clients moving, we've learned that it's not because of laziness. We always find that real health challenges are at work. See Chapter 16, Dodging Slips and Shooting Trouble, for how we identify and assist with those challenges.

THE WEIGHT-LOSS FRONTIER: FACING PROFOUND NUTRIENT DEFICIENCY AND GENETIC DYSREGULATION

How does our nutrient-empty diet promote weight gain? It's not just the useless sweet and starchy calories, although it's true that the caloric content of the current American diet is at an all-time high. Government statistics vary. Some estimate that we've increased our calorie intake since 1970 by 500 calories. Others estimate increases of over 1,500 calories. Whatever the exact number, 60 percent of those current calories are now known to be *completely devoid of nutrients.*[19] We are, as a result, grotesquely malnourished. Even whole foods today, unless they are organic, provide as much as 25 percent fewer nutrients than they did before 1970.[20] Consequently, we're consuming below the *minimum* amounts of almost half of the vitamins and minerals vital to human life. In addition, we're depleted in the essential amino acids and fatty acids we are not getting from our low-protein, high–vegetable oil diet. This new state is called *overnutrition.*

Intermittent low-calorie dieting has been the other great stripper of vital nutrients. Even high-quality food, *consumed in small quantities,* can drop nutrient levels (not to mention hormone levels) even below our already substandard levels. Take the adorably wholesome but stingy South Beach Diet. At 1,200 calories a day it could not only further lower the levels of our twelve already-depleted nutrients, it could deplete *nine additional* nutrients, making us deficient, not in twelve, but in *twenty-one* of the total of twenty-seven nutrients. This means that 75 percent of irreplaceable nutrients can drop below minimal levels on *any* comparable low-calorie diet.[21] (Not to mention the hormonal havoc that we now know such a diet can set in motion.)

What are the consequences of these two methods of starvation? Scientist have concluded that deficiencies of very specific nutrients are tightly associated with weight gain, obesity, and diabetes. They've also begun to study the possibility that these nutrients, *taken as supplements,* can help to reverse these problems.

Eating nutritious, preferably organic, wild and range-fed food, and taking amino acids and other nutrients as supplements can immediately start to counteract the ravages of twenty-first-century mega-malnutrition. Some supplemental nutrients do not absorb as well as nutrients from real foods, but at my clinic, we've found (of course) that amino acid concentrates absorb almost instantly and that a broad collection of vitamins and minerals mostly given in moderate amounts, can be very helpful as well. When, occasionally, the supply of our specially formulated multivitamin/mineral has been cut off, our clients have consistently reported not doing as well, even though they're still on the same aminos.

Some vitamins and minerals found to be particularly deficient among those who are most overweight (or diabetic) have been found to be helpful *when added as individual supplement concentrates.* They include *vitamin C, vitamin D, thiamine (vitamin B₁), and chromium.*[22] The multivitamin I recommend as the primary *support nutrient* includes a broad array of B-complex and other vitamins, notably vitamin B_1, plus extra chromium. It's accompanied by additional supplements of vitamins C and D (if testing shows deficiencies). (All of this is detailed in Chapter 12, on page 195.)

Other individual nutrients, not yet studied in humans as higher-dose concentrates, will certainly be found to be beneficial in the future. Our clinic will keep looking for promising new human study results, trial the potentially helpful nutrients with clients, and post the results on cravingcure.com/exploremore to share with you. We've actually been doing this for years. For example, before we added a higher dose of chromium to our multi, we trialed chromium at various doses by itself when it was just starting to be marketed as a supplement. Our clients' improved resistance to cravings and their improved relief from hypoglycemic symptoms was consistent and incontrovertible.

ADDRESSING THE GENETIC FACTORS IN WEIGHT GAIN AND LOSS

The twenty-first-century diet, alternating, as it does, between nutrient-empty Techno-Karbz and nutrient-depleting low-calorie diets, can't help but damage our health, including our genetic health. Yo-yo malnutrition can trigger thousands of genetic changes, which can negatively impact glucose tolerance, appetite, fat storage, calorie burning, and many other weight-related functions. How many? We have no complete genetic analysis yet of humans, but a thorough genetic analysis was done on young bulls who'd been subjected to a now common practice called Compensatory Growth. In this procedure, introduced in the 1970s (of course), bulls are starved for 90 days to accelerate weight gain later (at sale time). A before-and-after genetic analysis found that 2,600 abnormal genetic changes had been set off by this period of food restriction.[23]

We lack a complete genetic assessment of the effects of starvation on *humans,* but we do have some information. For example, we know that children exposed through their forbears to under- or overnutrition are known to have increased risks of obesity in adulthood.[24] We learned this partly from studies of women in Scandinavia and Holland who were in their first months of pregnancy during a period of severe food shortage. It was later found that their female offspring were consistently obese and diabetic.[25] In another intergenerational study, young boys who gorged after a famine were found to have had grandsons who'd died prematurely of diabetes.[26] These are the profoundly disturbing potential genetic consequences of our own similarly extreme eating practices. In fact, we're already seeing these consequences lived out in our children. Can we stop the progression?

We can prevent any new genetic damage caused by the continued overeating of nutrient-stripped food and low-calorie dieting with the help of the amino acids and traditional eating practices. It seems to me that we can also affect genetic tendencies that are generations old. We have seen this with many of our clients who are the children of alcoholics and have inherited strong familial neurotransmitter deficits that show up as cravings, addictions, and mood problems. After taking the aminos and the *support nutrients* along with healthy foods, these clients no longer experience those clearly inherited cravings or mood problems. Although these clients have needed to take the aminos and other supplements for at least one year (longer than most other clients do) this seems to have accomplished positive genetic adjustments that have held long term, even long after they have discontinued their aminos.

I have always assumed that this could only have been made possible by the presence of the targeted amino acid concentrates and other nutrients in the brain areas where the addictive genetic defects were being expressed. Dr. Kenneth Blum, the neuroscientist who pioneered the research on amino acid therapy for neurotransmitter restoration, has done extensive research establishing the genetic influence of amino acid precursors on neurotransmitter functions, particularly in the dopamine D-2 receptors.[27] It seems likely that not just aminos, but other key nutrients taken as individual concentrates, combined with a similar diet and broad multivitamin/mineral supplementation, could reverse many epigenetic faults resulting from over- or undernutrition, including those that contribute to stubborn weight retention.

What do I mean by genetic *faults*? Aren't genes fixed? Aren't we stuck with the genetic hand we've been dealt? The good news and the bad news is that we aren't. When well-supplied with particular nutrients and not subjected to too much stress or chemical toxicity, our genes express themselves well. They behave nicely. But when they are nutrient-starved, overstressed, or subjected to toxins (or all three, as they are so often now), they can't behave themselves anymore.

They become *skewed* in the way that they express themselves. This is what the term "epigenetic" refers to: the potential of genes to vary their expression from positive to negative or vice versa depending on nutritional and environmental influences. If the factors, notably malnutrition, stress, and exposure to toxins, that can alter our genes are eliminated, we can be altered, and that alteration can include how we'll burn calories properly or attain and maintain an appropriate weight.

How Long Does it Take to Change Genetic Expression?

How genes express themselves can influence whether our immune system is able to protect us from illness or not. In a study of men with prostate cancer, the genes that programmed the men's immune systems were assessed before and after the men joined the study. Hundreds of genes were found to be negatively expressed by the first test. They studied the same set of genes again, after the same men had been put on a mostly whole-foods diet, extensive nutrient supplementation, and improved lifestyle. The results? Positive expression replaced negative expression in hundreds of the formally "faulty" genes. This genetic transformation was accomplished in just three months.[28]

Unfortunately, the study authors were unable to assess progress at one year to track and document the value of this potentially life-saving experiment. Why? Because so few of the participants had continued on the diet, which was close to vegan and too low in protein, fat, and calories (participants ate 2,200 calories per day) for most men. This is another reason that combining the amino acids with traditional eating practices can be so vital: by wiping out our cravings for toxic and nutrient-void Techno-Karbz, they allow us to *stay* on a diet that can improve our genetic expression.

A group of Scandinavian researchers studying the impact of diet alone on genetic expression found that the adoption of traditional eating habits (like those advocated in *The Craving Cure*) could start reversing negative genetic expression *in a week*.[29] But the authors caution that these genetic improvements can be *lost* just as quickly. For example, if sugar returns to the diet, negative genetic expression can be reinstituted in only *six hours*.[30] The aminos can protect us from such returns.

There is one nutrient that seems to play a particularly pivotal role in reversing negative genetic expression of all kinds: folic acid, vitamin B_9. The studies that I've found on the use of this methylation-promoting nutrient supplement for weight reregulation were done on mice and fruit flies. The results were stunning. For example, the supplemented mice, though they themselves had been bred for generations to be freakishly obese (and blond), produced perfectly normal-sized, brown-haired offspring.[31] Folic acid was the key nutrient consumed in both studies, *but it was provided only in moderate amounts and only* <u>along with</u> *other B vitamins in their methyl forms and a few other key nutrients,* notably *phosphorylated choline,* a major "methyl donor."

Your anti-craving diet plus your multivitamin/mineral and the other Support Nutrients recommended in Chapter 12, page 195, provide the nutrients that transformed the mice, in safe (i.e., *low to moderate*) amounts that can be well utilized. Those with the now common MTHFR genetic defect can't utilize even food-form folic acid, let alone the generally poorly absorbed form found in most B-vitamin supplements and those added to processed foods. They *can* benefit from the now more widely available methyl-folate form (which all the supplements I recommend in Chapter 12 contain). But there are other supplemental nutrients that may be as, or even more, beneficial. This is a genetic cliffhanger. We're just at the edge of this extraordinary development in nutritional gene therapy. Stay tuned for human study results.

Genetic Testing

The entire genome is immense, but we have easy access to a test for at least twenty-three genes that are often faulty (including the gene that controls the utilization of folic acid). The "23 and Me" test and interpretive information can be ordered at 23andme.com. Other tests, including at least one that is insurance-reimbursable (the *predictive genomic test*) are available through physicians. More will come.

Although you couldn't have known it, none of the weight-loss efforts you've probably made up to now could have worked long term. Weight loss has to begin with craving elimination, and the one thing guaranteed to accomplish *that* is nutritional brain repair, which has probably *not* been on your weight-loss radar. The next two sections of this book are going to put that right. In Part II, Understanding Your Craving Type, you'll go behind the scenes in your brain to find out what is really interfering with your efforts to control your eating. Then, in Part III, The Amino Breakthrough, you'll learn how to use the simple nutritional tools that will quickly give you back that control.

Understanding Your Craving Type

5

Your Brain: Craving Control Central

BEFORE THE EXPLOSION OF THE Techno-Karbz and the new dietary trends of the 1970s, we really did live in a land without weight problems. That was mostly because our brains were in such good shape then, thanks to our diet. High-quality brain fuel, served three times a day, was all it took to keep our appetites properly aligned. Did it take every cell in the brain to accomplish this feat? No. Only a few kinds of specialized brain cells called neurotransmitters, well-fueled and maintained, were required. Fortunately, they're still there, but most of us these days do need a neurotransmitter tune-up.

The purpose of Part II, Understanding Your Craving Type, is to prepare you to perform your own personal brain tune-up. This first chapter is intended as an introduction to your brain's extraordinary pleasure- and appetite-regulators: what they are, how and why they may be malfunctioning, how amino acid brain repairs and dietary improvements can put things right, and the clinical and scientific basis of this whole enterprise. The particulars of each Craving Type and its specific nutritional tune-up needs will be the focus of the five chapters that follow.

Your brain, when fully functioning, acts as Craving Control Central. If that central control falters and the levels of any of the brain's primary appetite-regulators drops too low, cravings automatically crop up. Once they do, no diet plan will work long term.

You're going to learn a lot here about appetite dysregulation, but you're also going to get acquainted with what it will be like when that dysregulation is corrected. The first astonishing sign that you've restored your brain to its optimal craving-control capacity will be the sudden silencing of your cravings. But there will be other quick benefits, too. For example, your mood and energy are likely to improve right along with your ability to ignore a corn chip. When your appetite control capacities are refurbished, be prepared to feel like the Sleeping Beauty; suddenly awake and enjoying your life in many nice new ways. Here's the true tale of one such beauty and what happened after she was awakened by her amino acid tune-up.

Claire started every day with a Starbucks vanilla spice latte. She had half a sandwich, chips, and a Coke for lunch. In the afternoon she had a chocolate candy bar . . . or two, if it was a stressful day. At night, her go-to meal was a burger and fries or pizza with a soda, followed by an evening that typically included chips and salsa, ice cream, and cookies.

She had been a regular low-cal dieter but had become so addicted to sweets and starches that she was no longer able to stop long enough for even a brief "starve it off." By age thirty, she was borderline diabetic with high blood pressure. She had quit weighing herself when she reached 200 pounds. Desperate, she at one point created her own low-carbohydrate, Atkins-type diet and tried one more time: eggs and sausage for breakfast, a salad with a chicken breast for lunch, and a steak with vegetables for dinner. She lost weight, felt good, and her blood sugar normalized. She reported that her carbohydrate cravings had been cut in half, but that half the time her cravings still called to her.

Unfortunately, being half addicted is like being half pregnant. Over time, the nagging urge for the sweets on her officemate's desk and the fast-food drive-through on the way home eroded her resolve. She decided to just have a treat once a week. That lasted for two weeks. By week three her habit had fully taken hold again. A year later—after weeks of on-again, off-again efforts at self-control and six pounds heavier than when she started—Claire called our clinic.

Claire hasn't had sweets or starchy Techno-Karbz since the day of her first appointment with us. More important, she hasn't wanted them. How did she do it? She changed her mind! Actually, she changed her brain—specifically the two parts of her brain that were forcing her to eat toxic foods. How long did it take? It started twenty-four hours after she added the right amino acids to her life.

Claire's Craving-Type Questionnaire showed her to be a Type 1 Depressed

Craver and Type three Comfort Craver. Her Type 1 serotonin deficiency caused
her cravings to hit her hardest between three pm and midnight. (Serotonin
levels drop off after noon because they are stimulated by sunlight and sup-
pressed as the day gets darker.) Without the aminos, because of her depleted
brain reserves of serotonin, she hadn't been able to get to sleep without her
bedtime Cap'n Crunch. Winters were especially bad. Her cravings and her
moods deteriorated as the days got shorter and darker. She was anxious and
worried, and even experienced some panic attacks.

The Techno-Karbz had taken the edge off, but she had also been on and off
of serotonin-targeted antidepressants for years, despite their tendency to cause
her to gain even more weight. She was also a Type 3 Comfort Craver, with
endorphin deficiency, so chocolate, with its legendary pleasuring capacity, was
her best friend. She felt she couldn't experience joy in her life without it.
Chocolate kept her heartache at bay, including the pain of having been overweight
for so much of her life. She had always been the ultrasensitive one in her family,
even as a child. Like many Type 3s, she'd probably inherited a tendency to
produce too few naturally comforting endorphins. Even with three craving strikes
against her, by day two on her Craving Cure, Claire had lost every urge for her
former favorites and no longer regarded Techno-Karbz as her "best friend." This
made it easy for her to stick with a healthy diet for the first time and to find a
sense of peace she hadn't experienced since early childhood.

NATURAL AND UNNATURAL APPETITES

The brain's appetite-control center is supposed to automatically keep us on the right dietary track at all times. Our survival depends on it. Our bodies and brains are actually studded with dozens of separate but interacting appetite enhancers, inhibitors, and monitors. For example, when, for whatever reason, we go too long without eating, the appetite-regulating squad sends out a unified signal that we experience as *hunger*. The stomach growls and food suddenly begins to smell and look appealing. If there is no food available, we start imagining some. This is the healthy hunger signal that is sent out to remind us to eat. Then, a second signal, one of pleasure, is sent out *during* our eating experience. These signals are built into our genetic makeup and are required in order to make us eat. We'd never do it otherwise. What else could motivate us to do all that hunting, planting, harvesting, shopping, cooking, chewing, and cleanup?

If we are presented with a nice array of wholesome, largely unprocessed foods, we are programmed to instinctively choose the balance of proteins, fats, and carbohydrates that best suits our nutritional needs at that particular time.

The right balance of nutrients from all three fundamental foods—protein, fats, and carbohydrates—makes us feel satisfied. That experience of satisfaction indicates that our appetite chemistry has just transmitted a third life-preserving appetite signal: "You've had enough." At that point, we find ourselves saying things like, "That really hit the spot." No longer hungry, we easily turn away from the plate, ready to focus on other things.

When all of our appetite-regulators are functioning as they should, we don't tend to overeat or undereat, and we don't tend to gain or lose weight. It's almost impossible for us not to be moderate and normal-weight eaters if our appetites' natural checks and balances are in order.

Unfortunately, many of us live with a brain whose appetite-control system has been disabled by foods designed to do just that. Earlier, I mentioned Sleeping Beauty; Techno-Karbz have literally cast a paralyzing spell on us. They have put our vigilant food regulation guardians to sleep at the switch. They are no longer able to turn off our cravings for unhealthy food.

After a healthy meal, your brain's five primary appetite-regulators would ideally generate moderate sensations of pleasure and satisfaction that last for hours, leaving you free of any thoughts about food at all. However, a big dose of Techno-Karbz can impact all five appetite factors. The result? A collectively generated drug-like level of pleasure. This brief thrill is followed sooner or later by a crash. That's when the cravings set in. Over time, the amount of Techno-Karbz needed to appease the stepped-up cravings increases, leading to all the "cheats," bingeing, yo-yo dieting, and the inexorable, unnatural weight gain.

NEUROSCIENCE TO THE RESCUE

But what can we do if knowledge, willpower, counseling, peer support, mindfulness, and other spiritual practices have failed? That's the question I asked myself as the new director of an addiction treatment program in San Francisco when the crack epidemic hit us in the early 1980s. We'd gotten used to a 50 percent recovery rate with our alcoholic clients in the '70s. But with crack addiction, the recovery rate had suddenly plunged to zero, despite the fact that we were providing intensive and long-term counseling and education for the whole family, twelve-step meetings, spiritual and meditative practices, and both residential and outpatient care. What more could we do?

Fortunately, the new field of neuroscience gave us the answer. In the mid-1980s it gave us just the information we so desperately needed. I was astonished and chagrined to learn, first of all, that the problem was primarily biochemical. This explained why our psycho-spiritual programs weren't working better. However, not knowing anything about biochemistry, especially about brain biochemistry, I had to spend a few years learning what I'm about to share with you now.

First we discovered that all addictive substances (including, we now know, Techno-Karbz) target the same five brain functions, functions that are intended to regulate our appetite and to produce, between them, a wide variety of positive feelings, thoughts, and sensations on an almost constant basis. This includes pleasurable responses to the smells, tastes, textures, and thoughts of foods.

Mundane experiences like having an apple, getting a hug, reading a good book, seeing a rising moon, taking in a ball game, or having a dream or a shower, and *many* more daily events that we aren't even aware of become pleasurable largely by the action of this small collection of neurochemical functions. In fact, this five-part production is responsible for most of the emotional and sensual tone of our lives.

Four of the brain's five primary pleasure- and appetite-regulating functions are cellular signal centers that produce and relay amazing molecules called neurotransmitters. These specialized nerve cells (*neuro* means "nerve") transmit their four types of messages in bursts of signaling that reach outward from neuron to neuron through your brain and nervous system, almost instantaneously. Each neurotransmitter sings a difference song. Serotonin sings a hopeful, happy tune, for example.

When it comes to pleasure, specifically the pleasure of eating, we can hear these four neurotransmitter songs loud and clear. Together, they're intended to convey very positive messages, like "relax" and "enjoy your meal."

These four neurotransmitter wonder-workers are themselves strongly supported by a fifth function: your brain's critical blood sugar fueling system, or glucose supply line, which is responsible for fueling your brain cells with a constant stream of exactly the right amount of glucose—not too much, and not too little.

There are several things that can sabotage this five-part miracle. The most critical one has to do with the effects of drug-like substances (including Techno-Karbz and some other foods), which can hijack the brain's natural pleasure-producing powers. They can briefly overamplify the neurotransmitters' output of pleasure sensations, but in the long run, by interfering with the natural function and production of our neurotransmitters, they end up reducing their ability to transmit these positive sensations. That leaves us with increasingly negative thoughts and feelings, and more powerful cravings.

Addictive substances tend to have molecular structures so similar to those of our neurotransmitters that they can masquerade as, and directly substitute for, them. This is the case, for example, with the unusual proteins gliadin and casein found in wheat and milk products, respectively, which plug right into the cellular receptors for the neurotransmitter endorphin, our natural opioid. Sweetened foods can quickly activate all of the neurotransmitters at once as they briefly raise our blood sugar levels too high.

By whatever means, when such substances set off exaggerated pleasure-charged sensations by overstimulating our key neurotransmitters, this, in turn, can lead to the automatic formation of additional receptors to accommodate the increase in active neurotransmitters. Since this excess, drug-stimulated neuro-transmitter activity cannot be maintained, these new receptors go empty and a depletion reaction results. This contributes to the quick loss of the exaggerated sense of well-being that the drug had caused and a strong need to have more of the drug and the lost pleasure. Often the neurotransmitter function that the brain had been maintaining naturally, before the substances interfered, cannot recover, so more and more, only drug-substances can provide any pleasure. For example, the excess fructose in a cola, though it briefly inflates many pleasurable sensations, specifically reduces our access to both serotonin, our natural anti-depressant, and tryptophan, the amino acid from which serotonin is made. Several substances, notably alcohol, cannabis, sugar, and flour, can interfere with *all* of the neurotransmitters simultaneously!

This forced overactivity eventually exhausts our neurotransmitter functions. It doesn't help that the supply of nutrients needed to assemble neurotransmitters is typically low in the first place in the current American diet. This alone can make it easier for neurotransmitters to become depleted and their signals weakened. We can easily start to feel unsatisfied because of the reduced sensation of pleasure they're able to transmit and begin to experience more negative moods and cravings for the unnatural, drug-induced thrills. If you were raised before 1970 on a better diet, you may have forgotten how satisfied your drug-free brain used to naturally make you feel. And even if you do remember, like most of us, you've probably lost your way and can't find your way back to the good feelings that we used to take for granted.

Fortunately, in the 1970s—the decade wasn't *all* bad!—a group of neuroscientists devoted themselves to the problem of addiction and the brain. Through hundreds of studies, they discovered how addictive substances, initially alcohol, cocaine, and opiates like heroin and morphine, were impacting the brain. Their study of addictive *foods* didn't come until later; until the announcement of the obesity epidemic in the twenty-first century. Before that, the prevailing opinion, even among neuroscientists, had been that food cravings were entirely psycho-logical (though they'd said the same thing initially about cocaine cravings!). But when the *majority* of American adults became overweight, it became obvious that something beyond weak willpower or emotional upset was at the root of the problem. The sudden virulent spread of the overeating epidemic ruled out an in-herited cause, too. As a result, neuroscientific interest in the role of the brain in eating behaviors began to quickly heat up.

Leading figures in the field, like MIT researchers Richard and Judith Wurtman, found early on that inadequate brain levels of the antidepressant neurotransmitter serotonin could trigger cravings for sweetened foods.[1, 2] Other early research showed that sugar, chocolate, and fat could raise levels of endorphin, our natural opioid.[3] In the past fifteen years, it has become clear that sugars and other ingredients in Techno-Karbz, like the more obvious ad-dictors, alcohol, cocaine, and heroin, could deplete not only serotonin and endorphin, but other major neurotransmitters, like dopamine, as well. Nora Volkow, Ph.D., head of the National Institute on Drug Abuse (NIDA) and a neuroscientist herself, acknowledges the role of all these neurotransmitters in generating addiction, including food addiction.[4]

MEET YOUR BRAIN'S FABULOUS FIVE
APPETITE AND PLEASURE-REGULATORS

In your Craving-Type Questionnaire, you learned that depleted levels of any of the brain's five appetite factors—serotonin, blood glucose, endorphin, GABA, and catecholamines—can prompt specific distress signals that we experience as distinct kinds of negative sensation, including a particular kind of craving. When even one of the five parts of this interconnecting food response system isn't functioning properly, aberrant appetite signals, notably cravings, almost inevi-tably result. But when they're all tuned up and transmitting in top form, we feel great and craving free.

I see this dynamic as a concert by a five-member ensemble, a quintet. Each of the five brain functions is like a musical instrument with a tone of its own. When all instruments are in tune, the ensemble sounds lovely. When any one of the instruments has become defective, jarring notes of craving and negative mood distort the sound.

Allow me to introduce you to your brain's "ensemble" members in the order of their appearance on the Craving-Type Questionnaire.

Serotonin is your brain's natural antidepressant, potentially so sunny and strong that it can light up your entire life. This most well-known of the neuro-transmitters broadcasts messages that are designed to *make* you feel optimistic, confident, humorous, ready for sleep by ten o'clock at night, and satisfied by foods other than Techno-Karbz. Serotonin is your inner sunshine, capable of making you feel perfectly happy without a cookie. Think of the golden sound of a harp. Generous amounts of dense protein, natural light, and low-stress living are the basic means of keeping your serotonin production optimal. But if your serotonin-producing brain sites are undersupplied with high-quality food and oversupplied with dim light and stress, those happy messages can be stifled, and negative directives will start to filling the void—directives like "eat sugar" or "get depressed" that sound more like a broken record than a harp trill.

Glucose, when available in a steady supply from regular meals that include whole carbohydrates, provides essential fuel to all of your body's and brain's functions. Think marimbas, gently keeping it all in flowing motion. Skipped or delayed meals and a diet high in Techno-Karbz guarantee the blood sugar dissonance that results in cravings.

Endorphin is your comforting neurotransmitter. It's thousands of times better at generating pleasure and killing pain than morphine—or chocolate. Fully functioning endorphins can provide the beautiful sounds of soaring violins. But if levels drop, there goes the quality of your life and here come the sour notes, the lonely, sad, hurt feelings and the cravings for comfort foods.

Gamma-amino-butyric-acid (GABA) is your natural tranquilizer. It keeps you from eating doughnuts or biting your children when you're stressed. Relaxing and calming GABA softens your neck and shoulders and clears away the tense thoughts. Think of a gentle acoustic guitar strum. Caffeine and stress put big demands on the GABA supply, but regular wholesome protein-rich meals can allow GABA to perform its gentle magic for you.

Catecholamines (I call them the Cats) are four closely related neurotransmitters, a family of tigers that give you energy and excitement plus the ability to concentrate and focus, without coffee or energy drinks. One of them, dopamine, is addiction neuroscience's very favorite neurotransmitter because it can produce the ultimate sensation of "reward." These Cats are definitely the percussion section of the brain's neurotransmitter consort. Without their beat, you drag and lose focus.

These four neurotransmitters and your brain's glucose supply have all sorts of interrelationships. Your brain is conducting a concert at all times, complete with harmonies, counterpoints, and the occasional solo or duet. Dr. Kenneth Blum, a leading neuroscientist in the study of the brain's response to addictive substances, describes this concert as "The Reward Cascade."[5] He, and most of his colleagues who specialize in addiction, regard the process of appetite satisfaction as reaching a crescendo when an adequate supply of amino acids and blood glucose allows the brain's neurotransmitters to play in perfect harmony, culminating in an elevation of dopamine which provides the ultimate sense of reward—the sound of the cymbals.

Your brain may need to refurbish one or all of its instruments to keep its music flowing. Fortunately, it can accomplish any necessary repairs using key amino acids to quickly restore the natural, craving-free cascade of music that your brain was designed to play.

AMINO POWER: MEET YOUR BRAIN'S APPETITE-REPAIR TOOLS

There are a total of twenty amino acids in protein-containing foods, all with long and awkward-sounding names. These aminos have innumerable tasks in the body. Everything in the body is built out of them, which is why they're always referred to as the building blocks of protein. Various aminos combine with each other in extraordinary complexes to create all our tissues, from bones to hormones. The name says it all: *pro* means "first, primary." Protein is certainly primary when it comes to the brain. Although brain cells need special fatty coats, the neurotransmitters within, which produce things like pleasure, thought, and sleep, can only be made from very particular amino acids.

All twenty amino acids can be provided most readily and generously by a food that we're not eating much of now, though prior to the 1970s, when we had neither weight problems nor food cravings, it was our primary food source. That food is the complete protein found in meat, poultry, seafood, and milk products. Nuts, seeds, beans, and grains also contain protein, but less of it, and with a low, uneven, or incomplete amino array. Combining animal and plant sources of protein has been our habit for about two million years, since we first began to eat meat (more on this in Chapter 14).

There is a commercial source of amino acids, too. In Japan, in particular, companies like Ajinomoto, now a huge international enterprise, have mastered the art of breeding yeasts that produce individual amino acids in the lab. (These yeasts are not the often invasive yeasts like *Candida albicans*.) Individual aminos and blends of aminos in supplement form have gradually attracted a massive public market as people have discovered their remarkable benefits for themselves. Aminos are also flourishing as ingredients in a broad range of consumer products, from toothpaste (arginine) to cosmetics (tyrosine).[6, 7, 8]

Are aminos in supplement form different from the aminos in food? No and yes. They are composed of easily digested nutrients, but yeast-derived aminos have a therapeutic advantage over whole food sources of aminos (like steak or whey protein powder). They've been bred to produce *individual* aminos in the "free" form. That means that they are not bound to many other aminos as they are in protein-containing foods or powders. That means that we don't have to go to the digestive effort to break apart all the bonds in order to access a particular amino. As freed individual amino acid concentrates, they act quickly, allowing us to clearly observe their unique effects. They have been an invaluable technological gift to our protein-malnourished, craving-ridden clients. We've seen thousands of our clients rapidly restored to complete appetite-sanity by the temporary use of these amino acid supplements. After an initial period of taking the amino supplements therapeutically, the protein from regular, healthful meals becomes their permanent source of aminos. The protein-rich Craving-Free foods (fully laid out in Part IV) eventually provide all the aminos that the brain and body need, just as they were designed to do.

How many of which amino acids will you need in order to turn off your own cravings? Some clients accomplish this miracle simply by eating more complete (animal) protein which they need to eat along with good fats, whole carbohydrates, and adequate calories (low-calorie dieting starves the brain!). Most clients, though, also need to take amino acids as supplements for a while, to get jump-started.

DISCOVERING THE AMINO-ADDICTION CONNECTION

As I mentioned earlier, one of the pioneers in the international group of addiction-focused neuroscientists was Kenneth Blum, Ph.D., author of hundreds of scientific papers and several books.[9] Early on, Dr. Blum made many important discoveries about how cocaine, alcohol, and opiates interacted with the brain's neurotransmitters. Then he turned his attention to the possibility of using supplementary amino acids to improve the brain neurotransmitter dysfunction that resulted from that interaction (and the genetic dysfunction that often contributed to it). Aminos had already been used experimentally in studies on blood pressure, mood, and other conditions, and Dr. Blum wanted to find out if they might be used to correct the neurotransmitter deficits caused by drugs, alcohol, and addictive foods.

In fact, using amino acids to stop addictive brain activity turned out to be a simpler and more successful project than anyone could have imagined. As magical as neurotransmitters are, their construction is surprisingly simple. Each neurotransmitter is made out of one special amino acid called a precursor. (A few vitamins and minerals must also be present to accomplish the transformation.) Basic brain biochemistry indicated that the neurotransmitter dysfunctions at the core of the addiction problem could be corrected by the use of just a few "precursor" amino acids. Of the twenty total available amino acid building blocks, only five turned out to be needed. Once Dr. Blum had identified the specific aminos needed, it was time to find out exactly what their effects on the depleted neurotransmitter supply would be and how that would change the behavior of the addicted study subjects.

The results were clear: more normal neurotransmitter function quickly resumed. "Normal functioning" meant that the subjects experienced more positive mood and that their sensations of deprivation, craving, agitation fatigue, and other discomfort were much reduced or eliminated. In an early study of addicts on a cocaine-addiction-only inpatient treatment unit, Dr. Blum's simple cocaine-targeted amino acid formula reduced the number of patients who left treatment prematurely from 40 percent to 4 percent.[10] This approach was elegant. It simply provided emergency supplies of a few select nutrients to specific nutrient-starved brain sites.

Dr. Blum's studies used aminos chosen to target particular addictions. In the case of addiction to food, he used four of them. My favorite of his food addiction studies followed 250 Optifast dieters for two years after they had completed the required extremely low (500-calorie) medically monitored fast. The results were astonishing, especially in light of the Biggest Loser study and the other studies I mentioned in Chapter 4 that have now documented how such extremely low-calorie diets can dramatically increase cravings and weight regain. In spite of the fact that the amino doses were quite low compared to the doses we typically use at our clinic today, and that no dietary guidance was provided, the post-Optifasters lost 70 percent of their cravings. Those in the no-amino control group, who had started out with the same high level of cravings, showed no improvement *at all* and had steadily regained over 40 percent of their weight in two years, with no sign of letup. The amino-takers regained only 15 percent in the same two-year period.[11]

HOW MY CLINIC APPLIED THE NEURONUTRIENT RESEARCH

In 1986, I asked the Ph.D. nutritionist at my nonprofit outpatient addiction treatment program to research and begin integrating the amino acid recovery process into our program. We found that it immediately improved the moods and the cravings of our clients regardless of their type of addiction! Whether in trouble with crack or cola, this was the missing key that our addicted clients had been searching for. A group of addiction professionals who are experts in the nutrient therapy approach have now formed an association (the Alliance for Addiction Solutions) to help spread the word. Several of them have written fine books on the use of aminos with drug and alcohol addicts. See the Notes section for this page for details on their work.[12]

In 1988, I founded my own private clinic. It was the first program in the country, perhaps the world, to use these amino acid protocols to specifically stop cravings for *food*. Instead of recommending the fixed combination of low-dose amino acids that Dr. Blum's formulations contained, my nutritionists were able to tailor types and doses of amino acids to each client's needs. We were guided by our use of a neurotransmitter- and blood glucose–deficiency symptom that I gradually compiled, the prototype of the Craving-Type Questionnaire in this book. We gave the clients only the aminos that were indicated by their symptoms. We started at low doses and went up as needed until cravings and other symptoms (mood, energy, and sleep problems) were much improved or gone. Later we added the amino trialing process that allowed us and our clients to see exactly how the aminos affected them and how quickly. We also learned that several additional amino acids, beyond those that Dr. Blum's work had introduced us to, could also be helpful.

For several years, our success was too phenomenal. When I described it to my addiction and eating disorders colleagues, no one believed me! It wasn't until 2000, with my first book, *The Diet Cure*, that interest in our use of the aminos began to swell and I began training health professionals. The way had been paved a few years before by the amino advocacy of nuclear psychiatrist Daniel Amen, M.D., who had also been influenced by Dr. Blum's work. His books, starting with *Change Your Brain, Change Your Life*, and subsequent PBS presentations have been inspirational on a national and international level. My second book, *The Mood Cure*, described how our clinic was using the aminos to relieve neurotransmitter problems like depression, anxiety, and insomnia. This created another wave of interest because we are experiencing so much more emotional trouble now than ever before.

THE TRUTH ABOUT EMOTIONS, EATING, AND THE BRAIN

One of the most miraculous things about the amino acids is that, by superfueling the four neurotransmitters and balancing glucose and insulin levels, they can not only keep our appetites in order, they can also keep our moods in order! A well-nourished brain typically generates consistently positive moods: from optimism and tranquility to alertness, courage, and joy. Just as we're designed to live without sugar cravings, we are intended to go through life with built-in emotional ballast. We will inevitably experience suffering in reaction to life's blows, but our increasingly negative moods are being generated in the brain by the same depleted neurotransmitters and unbalanced blood sugar levels that are also responsible for generating most of our cravings. As you can see when you revisit the lists of the deficiency symptoms in the Craving-Type Questionnaire, there is a distinctive collection of negative moods associated with each Craving Type, moods that your Amino Breakthrough will rid you of as quickly as it will rid you of your cravings. How do I know this? I've seen it happen thousands of times, right in my office. During their amino trials, our clients typically start smiling, stop worrying, become more alert, sit back, relax, and notice colors are brighter and that their cravings are gone. All at the same time.

This may be difficult for you to accept. You can probably accept that the orgasmic taste sensations elicited by your favorite treats and your cravings for them are biochemical reactions generated by your brain. But you may be having some trouble with the idea that your *feelings* have little or no real influence on why you crave those treats and you may be understandably confused by all the "emotional" symptoms that are associated with your cravings.

Aren't these feelings of hurt, fear, anger, or low self-esteem, the ones that make you want comfort food, real? Aren't they genuine reactions to something real that is upsetting you, whether it's in your current life or left over from your past? As a full-time psychotherapist for many years, I was convinced of this myself. Now I know that there are both true feelings and false ones. True feelings are generated by life's painful realities, but they can become more intense and harder to bear or work through if we are *also* suffering neurotransmitter deficits. (Remember, neurotransmitters like serotonin govern our emotional experiences as well as our appetite.) Some upset feelings, though, can arise for no legitimate reason *at all* if your brain's mood-regulating chemistry is too depleted. Biochemically caused emotional suffering is rapidly increasing now because our brains are being so poorly fed and so overstressed. Depression, insomnia, and anxiety have been increasing right along with our cravings and overeating, (especially since the 1970s, of course).[13]

My book *The Mood Cure* is all about the clients who have come to my clinic specifically for help in becoming less anxious or depressed, in sleeping better, and in being more focused and energized. Many have come to us for help in carefully (and with their doctor's support) switching from problematic or ineffective antidepressants to the harmless and often more beneficial amino acids you'll read about in the next chapter. Most of them, though, have had *both* mood *and* craving problems, as so many Americans do today.

After 1970, likely because our incoming clients' diets were generally getting worse and worse, our psychotherapy techniques (along with those of most other therapists) were working less and less well for them. "False" feelings, those negative

emotional states generated by neurotransmitter deficiencies or blood sugar fluctuations, simply do not respond to psychotherapy. Some of our clients began to
turn to antidepressants, which often *did* help in ways that I couldn't understand
then. Now I know that these medications were reaching the *biochemical* pain
that my clients were experiencing and reducing their anxiety, their depression,
and their stress in ways that psychotherapy alone could not.

Psychotherapy for emotional distress was and still is badly needed by many
people, and it always will be. But its benefits are often limited by the lack of brain
chemistry repair. Most of the clients we work with have actually already had good
counseling before they come to see us, yet they have continued to experience negative moods and cravings for comfort foods. Their symptoms no longer make
psychological sense. But we've learned that they make good neurochemical and
nutritional sense!

---

*Jenny, a bulimic, had been in and out of counseling for years, so she was
happily disoriented after she started using her amino acids: Not only did her
frequent bingeing suddenly stop, but, as she put it, "My personality is changing,
too. I'm a lot nicer now, I get to sleep at a normal hour, and I feel hopeful a lot.
What's going on?"*

Our negative feelings these days are so often a mix of brain error and genuine psychological distress. This can make for an emotional double whammy, an
often intolerable inner state, one from which you may have naturally looked for
relief wherever you could find it. Most people discover as children—long before
they ever try a beer, a joint, or an SSRI—that Techno-Karbz can very effectively
drown out their negative feelings for a little while. Most of us have been Techno-
Karbz addicted to some extent ever since. Whether you're struggling with bad
moods, bad cravings, or both, the amino acids in your Craving Cure can help you
handle it all.

Each of the next five chapters is devoted to one of the five Craving Types, the
brain deficits behind it, the symptoms including the specific kind of cravings—
and the amino solution to it. Choose which chapters to read depending on which
Types of Craving you have (as identified on your completed Craving-Type Questionnaire and Profile on page 12). As you read through the relevant Craving Type
chapters, think about which type of craving you'd like to get rid of first. Then
you'll be ready to launch into your amino breakthrough.

6

Are You a Type 1 Depressed Craver?

If so, your cravings are caused by a dearth of serotonin, your brain's inner sunshine, and can only be dispelled by an amino acid called tryptophan.

PERHAPS THE MOST PRECIOUS OF our brain's neurotransmitters is sunny serotonin. It prevents the particular kinds of food cravings that hit hardest as the light fades in the afternoons, at night, and in winter. Serotonin is most famous as our natural antidepressant, but provides us with many other benefits too, more benefits than do any of the other neurotransmitters. It provides the positive opposites of all the deficiency symptoms listed below. For example:

- If you are feeling worried, negative, or irritable, having adequate serotonin can give you feelings of optimism, self-confidence, courage, flexibility, patience, and humor.
- If you sleep poorly, serotonin can convert into the natural sleep potion, melatonin (which also seems to be a weight-loss aid!) and optimize your sleep time.

Increased food cravings are a proven consequence of serotonin depletion.[1] My clinics have conducted thousands of symptom assessments on people with every type and degree of food craving. We have consistently found that more of our clients identify with the symptoms of Type 1, serotonin deficiency, than with

Type 1 Depressed Cravers: A Short List of Symptoms

Here are the key serotonin deficiency symptoms.
Type 1s have:

- afternoon and/or evening cravings for foods or other substances
- negativity, depression
- winter blues
- worry, anxiety
- hyperactivity
- obsessive thoughts or behaviors
- perfectionist, controlling tendencies
- phobias (fear of heights, snakes, small spaces, etc.), panic attacks, irritability, anger
- "nervous" stomach (knots, butterflies)
- fibromyalgia, TMJ, migraines
- night owl tendencies, trouble falling asleep, difficulty staying asleep

those of any of the other four Craving Types. The number of symptoms checked off tends to be higher and so do the severity scores.

WHY ARE SO MANY OF US SEROTONIN DEPRIVED?

We actually seem to be in a national serotonin-deficiency crisis, with epidemics of craving and other serotonin-deficiency conditions, like depression, anxiety, and insomnia, ever on the rise. Sufficient serotonin is essential—not optional—for allowing the brain and the body to regulate appetite, mood, sleep, digestion, and more. This neurotransmitter has a huge job, so we have to be able to produce lots of it on a daily basis (no days *or* nights off!).

Unfortunately, serotonin is also the neurotransmitter hardest for us to produce.

The main obstacle to our enjoyment of the benefits that adequate serotonin can bestow has undoubtedly been our *anti-serotonin* diet. We have to eat lots of a very specific type of protein to extract enough of the one and only amino acid that can be used to make serotonin. That amino acid is called tryptophan. Tryptophan is the hardest of all the amino acids to find in quantity, even in the highest-protein foods. And even once it is ingested, it's the hardest to maneuver into the brain.

Tryptophan is relatively scarce even in the densest animal protein sources (I'll explain why in a minute), and we're not eating much animal protein these days. Of the top ten foods eaten in America, eight are Techno-Karbz.

And then there are the high-fructose syrups present in sodas and in so many other corn-, agave-, or fruit-sweetened drinks and foods. Our massive exposure to high amounts of fructose has created a now common condition called "fructose malabsorption." Glucose actually enhances our absorption of tryptophan. But when fructose dominates, it is well known that decreased tryptophan levels in the blood result.[2]

And there's another corn factor: most poultry and cattle can't make adequate amounts of tryptophan themselves unless they are range fed.[3] Since feedlots have largely replaced range feeding (another "innovation" of the '70s), the animals we do eat have mostly been fed on tryptophan-*poor* corn. Corn became notorious for its low tryptophan content in the early 1900s when a high-corn diet caused an outbreak of pellagra among poor Southerners who could afford nothing more nutritious to eat. Pellagra, like scurvy, is caused by a radical nutrient deficiency. In the case of pellagra, the deficient nutrient is tryptophan.

We're all eating lots of corn now. Even though we rarely develop the symptoms of *full-blown* pellagra (dementia, diarrhea, and dermatitis) many of us do show the early-stage symptoms: depression, anxiety, irritability, insomnia, *and cravings*. Eating corn chips or popcorn (and who doesn't?) can quickly reduce tryptophan levels by as much as 50 percent. (This study also found gluten to reduce tryptophan levels by 25 percent.[4]) Tortillas and hominy, on the other hand, are made from masa, cornmeal processed using the ancient lime-soaking method that allows us more access to this grain's tryptophan and other nutrient contents. (This is not an endorsement of fried tortilla chips, of course!)

As if all this didn't make it hard enough to access tryptophan, there's another problem. This elusive amino is one of the nine (out of twenty) aminos that are considered "essential." This means that your body can't manufacture any of them out of other aminos. Tryptophan and the eight other "essential" amino acids must be delivered directly into us in daily servings of *complete* protein, meaning protein that includes at least all of the nine essential aminos. Most plant-derived proteins contain *in*complete protein and many, like corn, contain particularly little tryptophan. Our current trend toward plant-based, low-protein diets can't help but slow down the "essential" amino deliveries to the brain.

Vegans, vegetarians, and low-calorie dieters are particularly handicapped when it comes to tryptophan. The latter practice robs us of the very thing that, as Type 1 Depressed Cravers, we need most for eradicating our cravings for weight-producing sweets and starches. Much of the protein allowed on low-calorie diets is burned up as emergency fuel (to replace the carbohydrate calories which are often even lower). That doesn't leave enough to build more serotonin into the brain (or muscle mass onto the body). This is a big reason for the cravings (and muscle loss) that increase during or after periods of calorie slashing.

Eating Disorders Are Low-Tryptophan Conditions

A joint U.S./UK research project on bulimia found that when no tryptophan was consumed for up to twenty-four hours, bingeing became much more violent and that even bulimics who had been in recovery began craving, bingeing, and purging again. According to experts like Oxford University's Katherine Smith, chronic depletion of tryptophan by "persistent" low-calorie dieting can not only lead to bulimia, but to other eating disorders of all kinds.[5]

Our clients have often developed their Type 1 symptoms as a result of one or more of the following serotonin-blocking lifestyle factors:

Too many antiserotonin drugs. Caffeine—whether in coffee, colas, or energy drinks—other stimulants like diet pills, Ritalin, or Adderall (for ADD); and aspartame-sweetened diet drinks (even without caffeine) suppress serotonin.[6]

Overstress. The primary stress-response chemicals, adrenaline and cortisol, suppress serotonin, which is how your brain decides that tax time is no time for cracking jokes or taking a nap, but a good time to eat sugar.

Not getting enough serotonin-stimulating light. Sunlight or any bright light (over 300 watts) signals your brain to make more serotonin. But most people are indoors most of every day, where the light is always too dim to give the serotonin-boosting signal. There's much more light outside, even in winter. If increased protein, tryptophan supplements, and the great outdoors still leave you glum and craving in the winter, adding a therapeutic lamp (3,000 to 10,000 lumens) should do the trick.

SEROTONIN AND CARBOHYDRATES

How can a protein deficiency condition—specifically a lack of tryptophan—lead to cravings for carbohydrates? After all, sweets and starches can't be made into serotonin, only proteins that contain tryptophan can. Why don't we crave steak, instead of cake, if it's an amino acid our bodies are after?

Two of the world's most prominent serotonin researchers discovered the answer to this question. MIT professors Richard and Judith Wurtman became intrigued in the 1970s with serotonin's powerful ability to turn off food cravings (as well as depression and insomnia). They eventually discovered how the brain could be easily tricked into activating more serotonin.[7] Judith wrote several books and toured the country touting her breakthrough method: a teaspoonful of jam every afternoon![8] The body has an automatic response when we eat at least this much sugar: an instant insulin release. The insulin sweeps most of the amino acids out of the bloodstream along with most of the available blood sugar. But this insulin surge bypasses tryptophan. Instead, it gathers up the other aminos, the ones that typically compete with tryptophan for the limited entry slots into the brain. This allows more tryptophan to suddenly glide through. When this illicit tryptophan arrives, extra serotonin is instantly converted from it. Cravings are temporarily dampened, and more positive feelings are generated.[9]

Unfortunately, this seemingly cheery process is a big part of the mechanism by which an international public health crisis called *diabetes* is being perpetuated. Most of us now can't stop with just one teaspoon of jam. We're raising our levels of serotonin, blood sugar, and insulin by downing sugary and starchy Techno-Karbz all day long. The excess glucose, fructose, and insulin eventually erode our body's ability to cope and diabetes results. Diabetics have doubled rates of depression and overwhelming Techno-Karbz cravings, at least partly due to the fact that they are known to be deficient in tryptophan *and* low in serotonin.[10] Type 1 Depressed Cravers, like all Cravers, are at high risk for diabetes, but tryptophan supplements will pluck them from the fast track to this modern plague, or, if they have arrived already, it will help halt or reverse their course. (Much more on diabetes in Chapters 7, 12, and 14.)

Type 1 Aminos and Phen-Fen

By raising serotonin levels so effectively, tryptophan can provide many of the benefits of the most stunning food craving eradicators ever known: the drugs phentermine and fenfluramine. This beloved duo was called Phen-Fen. Fenfluramine (an antidepressant) raised serotonin levels very nicely. Phentermine raised serotonin too, but it also acted as a stimulant and an appetite suppressant by raising Cat levels. So all Phen-Fen takers became happy and energized, as well as thinner. When the purely serotonin-targeted

drug, fenfluramine, turned out to have deadly side effects, it was permanently withdrawn from the market. Phentermine alone did not work
nearly as well and millions went into mourning. For those who have Type 5
Cravings as well as Type 1 Cravings, a combination of Type 1 tryptophan with
Type 5 tyrosine can work well to duplicate the Phen-Fen effect.

TRYPTOPHAN'S HISTORY AS AN AMINO ACID SUPPLEMENT

Serotonin has long been our most-studied neurotransmitter. Hundreds of researchers worldwide launched into a fervid study of serotonin and tryptophan in
the 1970s, many of them supported by the pharmaceutical industry, which was
eager to develop new drugs for the increasingly depressed American public.

The demand for the new serotonin-boosting drugs increased after 1970 as our
traditional brain-fueling, protein-rich diet was being traded in for brain-starving
Techno-Karbz on the one hand and low-calorie diets on the other. These two
tryptophan-depleting activities also deprived us of the brain-supportive vitamins
and minerals that aid in the conversion of tryptophan to serotonin. (That's why
you'll be taking a vitamin and mineral supplement and eating lots of fresh produce
along with your amino acids and high-quality food protein.)

All neuroscientists, worldwide, are familiar with the same basic facts of brain
biochemistry: serotonin can be made out of one thing, and one thing only: the
amino acid tryptophan. Tryptophan was the most studied of all brain nutrients up
through the 1980s. Several studies found that raising tryptophan supplies, through
diet or through supplements, raised levels of serotonin as much as 100 percent.[11]
These studies also found that the tryptophan supplements specifically helped
reduce overeating by raising levels of serotonin.

The public's response to tryptophan supplements as mood and sleep promoters
was enthusiastic. Psychiatrists too discovered the mood and sleep benefits of
tryptophan early on and began recommending it, very successfully, for their
patients. As a result, when the first SSRI, Prozac, came out in 1987, many psychiatrists were indifferent. One told me that she would tell the drug reps that she
didn't need Prozac because tryptophan was working so well. They eventually came
back to try to sell her a very low-dose (5 mg) version of Prozac "to make the tryptophan work better." That she *was* interested in.

After 1989, though, neither she nor anyone else in the United States had
much choice. In that year, a bad batch of tryptophan, made in Japan, was sent to
the United States. Over a thousand people were poisoned by it and at least ten
died. This understandably prompted the FDA to ask for a voluntary ban on all

tryptophan sales. But even after the source of the bad batch was identified and the guilty company had admitted its responsibility in court (and stopped making it altogether), the ban remained mysteriously in effect. Prozac sales leapt forward, and, as depression rates continued to rise into the '90s and beyond, it was joined by many other serotonin-targeted antidepressant drugs called selective serotonin reuptake inhibitors (SSRIs).

Type One Aminos and SSRIs

Are you taking a serotonin-targeted antidepressant? If you are taking an SSRI, please do not try a Type 1 amino until you have read the section on this subject in Chapter 12, page 172. I don't want you to run the risk of raising your serotonin levels too high. On the other hand, these aminos are often very helpful for those wanting to go off SSRIs.

The voluntary ban was gradually relaxed after years of protest and became available by prescription and under the guise of a supplement for pets. The ban was not formally lifted, though, until 2005. Since then, many companies have started offering tryptophan supplements again, *with no adverse reports*.

Unfortunately, the ban had meant not only that the public lost access to tryptophan, but that all scientific studies on tryptophan in the United States were halted as well. Scientists in other countries had continued to study tryptophan and published their findings in the *International Journal of Tryptophan Research*. Tryptophan research is again picking up in the United States, too.

THE ARRIVAL OF A SECOND FORM OF TRYPTOPHAN: 5-HYDROXY-TRYPTOPHAN (5HTP)

In 1997, after eight years without tryptophan supplements, the serotonin-starved were blessed. Although tryptophan was still only available by prescription, a different form of tryptophan, which had almost identical effects, was approved for use in the United States. It was called 5-HTP (five-hydroxy-tryptophan).

When tryptophan, whether from high-protein foods or from capsules, or both, arrives in the body, it is quickly converted into its sister form, 5-HTP, which is then converted directly into serotonin with the help of a few vitamins and minerals. 5-HTP itself can be extracted, not from a yeast, as tryptophan is, but from an African bean. It was available for many years in Europe before it was sold in the United States. Italian researcher Carlo Cangiano, and others, conducted several 5-HTP studies, all showing how well 5-HTP works for food-craving elimination and weight loss in overweight overeaters and diabetics. 5-HTP quickly became a big seller stateside, after its introduction in 1997.[12, 13]

Now that 5-HTP and tryptophan are both widely available, millions of people are using them. Our clinic has been using them both since the mid-'90s. These two forms of tryptophan have an almost identical impact on serotonin levels and, therefore, on appetite: they're both marvelously effective at turning off Type 1 cravings. (Chapter 12 will help you choose between them based on some secondary differences.) Here is the story of someone who hit the jackpot with 5-HTP.

Kenny, at forty-nine, was a tech professional who was serious about working out. But he could not stop eating M&M's, cookies, popcorn, and chips. This was a lifelong habit, but he had stopped being able to burn off these extra calories like he could when he was younger. His cravings hit him at night only, and went along with having some trouble getting to sleep and a tendency to be obsessive.

When his nutritionist gave him trials of both aminos, it was ten am so his cravings hadn't hit yet and he had no particular response to either tryptophan or 5-HTP. After one week on a regimen of 5-HTP, though, Kenny declared it "a miracle." No more nightly debates or guilty indulgence. After a month, it was clear that Kenny had no further need of our help at all! His Type 1 scores were all zeros, which meant that his mood and sleep problems were just as "miraculously" eliminated as his cravings were.

INSOMNIA, WEIGHT GAIN, AND TYPE 1 CRAVERS

In addition to the kind of food cravings that Type 1 Cravers experience, many Type 1s also share a characteristic kind of insomnia. Many of the Type 1 clients who come in seeking release from their cravings are happily surprised to find that they get an insomnia cure as a free bonus! For all those struggling with weight gain, an insomnia cure is a particularly good thing to acquire. Why? Because the research is clear: sleep disturbance is associated with weight gain. Among our clients, insomnia has become such a common client complaint, right along with craving, weight gain, and depression, that my staff is actually shocked when we interview a client who does *not* have some sort of chronic sleep disturbance. In our experience, there are three primary causes of insomnia. Two of the three are low GABA and high cortisol, both Type 4 Craving factors that I'll cover in Chapter 9. By far the most common cause, though, relates to Type 1 Cravers.

Serotonin is our inner sunshine, but it is also our inner moonlight. That's because it has sleep-promoting as well as mood-enhancing properties. As the sun drops and its light fades at the end of the day, some serotonin is gradually converted into melatonin, the hormone that gets us to sleep. Sleep is vital for all of us, but we have epidemic rates of insomnia now. Late-night exposure to light sources (including phones, computers, and e-books) interferes with the adequate conversion of tryptophan and serotonin to sleep-regulating melatonin, which, it turns out, is also a weight regulator. We've seen thousands of under-sleepers and most of them have clearly had low-melatonin insomnia. How do we know? We've been able to turn them back into normal sleepers by giving them bedtime doses of tryptophan, melatonin, or both.

Weight gain can be triggered if, for *any* reason, we sleep less than eight hours per night on a regular basis. Most of our weight-gaining clients are among the 40 percent of Americans who are trapped in a sleep pattern that gives them less than *seven* hours a night![14] What causes the weight problem is that the function of hormones like ghrelin, leptin, and insulin, which regulate appetite and fat storage, are *dysregulated by inadequate melatonin release*. This means that the less we sleep, the more biochemical commands like "eat more" and "store more fat" are sent out.[15] *Those commands shut off when melatonin output, and sleep, increase.* Keep in mind that fructose also flips the same switch on these three hormones, so we're in double trouble after years of high-fructose corn, agave, and fruit syrup consumption, on top of insufficient sleep.

But for you, insomnia and high-fructose syrups are both about to become things of the past.

7

Are You a Type 2 Crashed Craver?

Type 2 Cravings can erupt whenever blood sugar levels drop too low. Fortunately, this crash-and-crave syndrome can be smoothed out in minutes by the amino acid glutamine and a few co-nutrients.

AMERICA'S BLOOD SUGAR BEFORE AND AFTER 1970

Most people used to wake up, have a "decent breakfast," and not think about eating again until lunchtime. Even then they were not famished. In the afternoon, maybe they would feel like having a piece of fruit around three o'clock or some nuts on the way home from work. If they hadn't had a good lunch, they might be grouchy when they got home and prowl for snacks, but usually, the "square meal" people of the pre-1970s could wait comfortably until dinner was served—and that usually happened around six PM. Square meal eaters are rare now, but in the decades before 1970, they were the norm. Since then, most of us have become Type 2 Crashed Cravers instead. Blood sugar control is literally now a thing of the past. In the '70s, as our diets deteriorated, many of us started complaining about being hypoglycemic (having frequent low-blood-sugar symptoms). That meant feeling stressed, headachy, edgy, and weak and craving a quick sugar fix. Whatever the nature of your own blood sugar–related cravings, they'll respond beautifully to the nutritional remedies I describe in this chapter.

Type 2 Cravers' blood sugar supply problems start in the brain. This is the most crucial, yet the most difficult, part of the body to keep supplied with

> ## Type 2 Crashed Cravers: A Short List of Symptoms
>
> Here's a list of common symptoms of Type 2 Cravers, which you'll recognize from the questionnaire you completed at the start of the book. 2s:
>
> - Are irritable, shaky, stressed, tired, fuzzy-headed, dizzy, flushed, nervous, or headachy, especially after you eat high-carbohydrate foods or go too long between meals.
> - Crave sugar or starch (or alcohol) frequently, especially if you skip or delay eating.
> - Are aware that you have hypoglycemia, prediabetes, or diabetes.

glucose. The brain requires far more glucose than any other organ of the body. Every one of its 200 billion neurons is dependent on a constant, uninterrupted supply. That's because our brain contains none of the *stored* glucose that the rest of the body can quickly access. Without regular, substantial, healthy meals, our brain's critical blood sugar supply can be interrupted several times a day, every day. Each time this happens, as the brain becomes desperate for fuel, cravings can erupt.

It often starts in the morning when you, like most Americans now, skip breakfast. Your brain sends out overwhelming craving signals by ten AM and again in the afternoon. Whether you eat lunch or not, the glucose supply process has often been thrown off for the whole day. This means that Techno-Karbz will start calling to you. You'll walk into the store for some healthy food to prepare after work, and you'll walk out eating the candy from the checkout counter. You may not get around to preparing the healthy dinner you planned because you've had so many Techno-Karbz by dinnertime that you're no longer hungry. You're also probably too panicked by the calories you've just overconsumed to add any, even real-food, calories. Your "solution"? You flip into starvation mode. You decide to fast the next day—which triggers a really shocking drop in blood sugar. The intense Type 2 cravings that result force you to helplessly consume big batches of Techno-Karbz.

What about a day that starts with a tall, sweet Starbucks drink and a scone? That creates a different blood sugar crisis: Your system is so traumatized by the glucose plus caffeine jolt you've just administered that it sends in the emergency cleanup squad to spray insulin on the blood sugar conflagration. Presto, the insulin clears the blood sugar. But then there's no more glucose available *at all*. Again, your brain sends out a desperate cry for glucose. You obey by eating something sweet or starchy, insulin again responds to the alarm, and the cycle starts all over again. Most of us are skipping or skimping on real-food meals and living on Techno-Karbz. That's why the second most common cause of cravings is this crash-and-crave syndrome I call Type 2.

Even if you avoid sugars and instead go for artificial sweeteners, that won't help much because fake sugars, too, can set this blood sugar debacle in motion, as we saw in Chapter 2.

Skipped meals, Techno-Karbz consumption, caffeine, and artificial sweeteners are the top four contributors to the problems of Type 2 Crashed Cravers, but there are a few other contributing factors. One kicks in after you eat particular foods to which you may be intolerant. One of our new clients told us that she had Type 2 craving symptoms even though she ate regularly and well. She'd brought in her baseline Food Logs and they came in very handy. They showed that she got headaches, had cravings, and felt drowsy after every meal that included sandwiches, toast, or pasta—in other words, wheat flour. When she removed the wheat from her life, all of those symptoms went away. (More on wheat and gluten sensitivity in Chapter 14.) This is an example of what's called *reactive hypoglycemia*. Stomach surgery and low thyroid states can also trigger blood sugar crashes. Hypoglycemia among diabetics on insulin is often dramatic. This glucose nosedive has been immortalized in many movies. All show a glass of orange juice saving the day. What they don't show is the increase in the risk of death within three years after a single such incident.[1]

Some Type 2 Crashed Cravers have a genetic tendency to chronic hypoglycemia; they have inherited some difficulty in keeping their brains' blood sugar levels in balance. If you were born with this tendency, you are probably subject to extreme, unpredictable, and frequent crash-and-crave episodes. You also probably come from a family in which hypoglycemia, diabetes, alcoholism, or all three have been common for generations. You may have cravings for alcohol as well as for Techno-Karbz. Low blood sugar is a tragically underappreciated cause of alcoholism.[2] In fact, in hundreds of cases at our clinic, the most common cause of relapse into either Techno-Karbz or alcohol use has been a skipped meal. Neurotransmitter deficiency problems underlie most addictions to alcohol, but hypoglycemia is always present as well. Many people with bulimia are Type 2 Crashed Cravers, who ricochet between sugar bingeing and alcoholic drinking for precisely this reason.

One of our clients, a college administrator, had been a binge drinker (like others in her family) and bulimic from age fourteen, and had a long history of alcoholism in her family. She was in her late thirties when she came to us. She had been quite an athlete, but now she felt so tired she could barely walk her dogs. After beginning her aminos, the cravings for both the alcohol and the

binge foods were totally gone within two weeks—although it took three months
for us to fine-tune her mood, her energy, and her ability to tolerate stress.
Stabilizing her blood sugar to eliminate Type 2 cravings was our first and most
fundamental job, but she had all of the other craving types as well, so she took
five aminos plus her support nutrients, at slowly reducing doses, for two years.

TOO MANY CRASHES LEAVE US STRANDED IN HIGH BLOOD SUGAR

The human body was not built to withstand the twenty-first-century blood sugar roller coaster. Our current intake of Techno-Karbz raises our blood glucose and insulin levels, often too rapidly, and too high. Insulin is always present in our bodies. Ideally, levels rise gently when we even think about or smell food. It rises higher, but still moderately, after real meals, but sweet or starchy Techno-Karbz consumption leads to an immediate and exaggerated insulin release that pulls the excess glucose out of the bloodstream to reduce the damage from the overdose.

INSULIN, GLUCOSE, AND FRUCTOSE IN COLLISION

Insulin can regulate glucose levels, quickly escorting criminal amounts of glucose to the cells in your muscles and depositing it as a fat that will be burned to fuel those muscles. So far so good. But when this happens too often, the process gluts your arteries with the triglycerides that the excess glucose is converted into for its trip through the bloodstream to cellular storage sites. This almost constant stream of triglycerides contributes to our heart disease rates, which are at an all-time high, especially among diabetics.[3, 4] Even more serious is the fact that, at some point, for reasons that researchers cannot yet explain, muscle cells eventually refuse entry and the glucose-turned-to-triglycerides must be dumped into fat cells, especially the ones around the waist, from which it cannot be easily accessed and burned off. This shunting is called *insulin resistance*, a central feature of our epidemic of weight gain.

The demand for emergency insulin that is created by our frequent consumption of Techno-Karbz inevitably leads us toward diabetes as well as weight gain. Insulin levels eventually begin to stay high all the time, though they no longer direct glucose traffic effectively. In late stages, the pancreas can no longer even make insulin.

Fructose slowly converts into glucose over time, so it does not directly stimulate insulin, as glucose does. Instead, it rampages, *unregulated* by insulin (or other appetite-regulating hormones), increasing the production of AGEs (glycation-damaged cells) and raising triglyceride levels. It actually impairs insulin signaling.[5] All this increases our cravings for fructose-sweetened Techno-Karbz, specifically (and remember that fructose is twice as sweet as glucose to begin with.) Much more on fructose in Chapter 2, page 43.[6]

FOODS, AMINOS, AND OTHER NUTRIENTS THAT STOP TYPE 2 CRAVINGS

The traditional foods that are the quickest glucose suppliers are the higher-carbohydrate foods like fruits, beans, and yams. Proteins and fats provide the slowest and steadiest cellular fuel-supplies because they convert, not quickly into glucose, but gradually into alternative fuels like ketones and lactate that the body often actually prefers to glucose. Eating a balance of protein, fat, and emphasizing lower carbohydrate vegetables stabilizes blood sugar levels nicely, as you'll discover in Part IV, Craving-Free Eating.

If you, like many Type 2 Cravers, need to add snacks to keep your blood sugar from crashing between meals, don't worry. Snacking is associated with weight loss! You read that right. Of course, you're not going to be snacking on potato chips or cookies. Instead, you'll be satisfied with healthier snacks and you'll get plenty of ideas for them in the Recipes and Menus section.

"All very interesting," you say, "but I can't just decide to change my diet permanently, no matter how good a whole-food diet would be for me. My cravings won't let me." No problem. There is a miraculous amino acid and a magnificent mineral and vitamin combination that we've seen transport thousands of our clients right back to the stable blood sugar state that is their birthright.

Glutamine—The Type 2 Craver's Glorious Amino

What your brain needs first to stop the cravings caused by hypoglycemic fuel outages is an amino acid called *glutamine*. When glucose levels crash, your brain can use glutamine to pinch-hit. And your brain won't skip a beat because brain cells are used to burning glutamine as an alternative fuel to glucose. Too often, though, the brain runs out of both fuels. With glutamine supplements, that never has to happen again.

Glutamine has an amazing capacity to restore the insulin response.[7, 8] Diabetics, who are known to be profoundly depleted in glutamine, have lost their ability to respond to insulin. It's been found that the greater their glutamine deficiency, the more progressed their disease.[9]

Glutamine can be made in the body from several different amino acids. However, the amino-rich, high-protein foods that should be supplying these aminos aren't being consumed in the necessary quantities by most people now. In addition, aging, illness, and injury greatly increase our need for glutamine. The result is widespread glutamine deficiency.

Our clients empty a 500-mg capsule of glutamine into their mouths (it is pleasant-tasting) during their amino trials. Minutes later, they squeal with delight: they suddenly have no more hypoglycemic headache, edginess, or desire for a stick of gum or a candy bar. They're delighted all the time once they start taking glutamine capsules daily, because glutamine wipes out *all* Type 2 Crashed Craving and the other symptoms of uneven blood sugar.

Try not to trial glutamine when you've just eaten. It makes it hard to know what its effects are. I did an evening workshop once at a seminar center that had just served dinner. No one had cravings at the moment, because they'd just had a nice meal, but they all commented on how "even" and "balanced" they felt. Our clients adore glutamine and take at least a couple of capsules with them wherever they go so that they can open one if a sudden need arises and instantly dispel any cravings or other threatening hypoglycemic symptoms.

Research has found that glutamine is effective for people on the whole spectrum, from hypoglycemia to diabetes.[10] In a spectacular study of overweight, prediabetic overeaters who were told *not* to try to restrict their food intake, glutamine supplementation reduced their calorie intake by 500 calories a day, resulting in a quick loss of both weight and inches (especially around the waist). It also reduced insulin levels by 20 percent.[11]

For hypoglycemia elimination, we don't need much glutamine. Just a few (one to three 500-mg capsules) between meals typically keeps the brain in balance and Crashed Cravings at bay. The glutamine secret is common knowledge in many alternative health circles. Just from customers who are sugar cravers and muscle builders, the supplement industry is guaranteed millions of dollars' worth of glutamine sales annually.

A forty-year-old mother of two with all of the Type 2 Crashed Craver symptoms came to our clinic to try to stop her afternoon and evening "splurges" and resultant weight gain. We started her on two capsules of glutamine in the afternoon, right when her cravings typically started. She was amazed to report that from the very first day, she never even thought about her large, sweet, Starbucks lattes or, during dinner, about the ice cream in the freezer, let alone ate any of it, except when she forgot her glutamine! Like so many of our clients, she already knew how to get healthy foods into her diet. Finding a way to drop the sugar was all she needed.

Glutamine supplements have been used and studied extensively in the medical field for many years. There it is routinely used in large doses (up to 50 grams, or 100 capsules a day!) for muscle-building in the acutely ill. Glutamine at 30–50 grams a day has also been found to be life-saving in *relieving the diarrhea associated with HIV* through its undisputed capacity to heal the lining of the digestive tract.[12] Cancer treatment relies on the use of glutamine to *support the immune system,* to *heal the tissue damage caused by radiation and chemotherapy,* and to limit post-operative muscle wasting.[13] It's used with critically ill patients to "prevent infections, decrease oxidative stress, and *improve survival.*"[14] Roger Williams, Ph.D., discoverer of glutamine, wrote two books on its use in alcoholism recovery, something I have witnessed countless times.[15]

Chromium and Biotin—The Type 2 Craver's Mineral and Vitamin

Alone and in combination, these two nutrients have proved very helpful in studies of diabetes and insulin resistance. Our clinical experience with them confirms these positive research findings. They've been tremendously helpful with both our hypoglycemic and our diabetic clients. For one thing, the mineral chromium and the vitamin biotin are both often depleted, especially in obese and diabetic Americans.[16] Together with glutamine, they reliably support the rescue of our clients from the blood sugar fluctuations that lead to so much suffering, including cravings. (Ironically, Techno-Karbz consumption is the most common cause of both chromium and biotin deficiency.) Chromium is required for insulin function in our cells, but its levels are 40 percent lower in diabetics than in those with normal blood sugar function. Biotin activates optimal genetic programming of glucose metabolism. Our clients have been using a multivitamin/mineral for twenty years that contains high doses of both. (You will be using it too, as it's the central feature of the Support Nutrients for all cravers that are detailed in the last section of Chapter 12, page 197.) When we have occasionally run out of it and have had to suggest that our clients use different multis that contain less chromium or biotin, yet similar amounts of the other nutrients included, they have noticed the difference right away.[17, 18, 19]

DEALING WITH DIABETES: THE ADVANCED STAGE ON THE TYPE 2 CRASHED CRAVER CONTINUUM

After years of riding the blood sugar roller coaster, you may have contracted prediabetes or type 2 diabetes, along with over 50 percent of Americans today. Those on this diabetic spectrum, trying to improve their life-threatening diets, almost always hit the same wall that all Techno-Karbz cravers hit—the wall of addiction. Though they know that they're fighting for their lives, they cannot eat moderately. Why not? Because they're trying to follow the conventional diabetic diet, a diet that consists mostly of "moderate" servings of highly addictive sugars, starches, and artificial sweeteners, all known to raise glucose and insulin levels. This diet is also low in the proteins, saturated fat, vitamins, minerals, and fiber that are required to prevent Techno-Karbz cravings and stabilize blood sugar and insulin levels. It is typically too low in calories, as well.

Actually, scores of diabetes studies have now confirmed the superiority of the low-carbohydrate,[20] higher-protein and -fat diet advocated by the much embattled but now vindicated cardiologist Robert Atkins. They've been found to lower weight and levels of cholesterol, triglycerides, glucose, insulin, and hemoglobin A1C, as well as blood pressure. Unfortunately, diabetics can have trouble following these proven diets long term because of their untreated food cravings and because these diets tend to be too low in calories and allow some trigger food.

Years ago I read an article in the *New York Times* about a leading American diabetes researcher who was asked why he had closed his university clinic where diabetics had come for years to meet with dietitians. His answer was that their patients *never* followed the clinic's dietary advice, so there was no point in continuing to give it. This kind of bitter complaining about the "unwillingness" of diabetics to "cooperate" is rife throughout the diabetes treatment world.[21] But how can diabetics possibly follow advice to limit their sugar and calorie intake when their *addiction* to glucose bombs is never addressed? They have had no chance without supplementary nutrients, especially the amino acid glutamine. With the help of the aminos and certain other blood sugar–regulating support nutrients, diabetics now have a real chance. Here is the story of someone who took that chance.

A few years ago, I held a community workshop. One of the attendees was Carolyn, a fifty-seven-year-old nurse with diabetes. Since she could rarely limit her Techno-Karbz intake, Carolyn's glucose levels always ran at least 100 mg/dL above the top of the normal range. The 200 mg/dL level was average for her. Like most nurses, Carolyn almost never had time to stop and have a meal, but she didn't mind. Techno-Karbz snacks were all she wanted, despite her certain knowledge of the consequences. She had made her peace with eventual heart disease, kidney dialysis, and worse. She'd had to accept that future for herself because she had no choice. Worse for her, she'd had to accept that future for her son, already diabetic at age twenty-seven.

Three things happened to her that Thursday evening:

She discovered that she was as a Type 2 Crashed Craver and a Type 5 Fatigued Craver. She immediately (that night) started taking the two indicated amino acids: tyrosine (for her Type 5 cravings) instead of the chocolate and coffee (with lots of sugar) she typically used to stay awake on her night shift, and, even more important, glutamine, which completely stopped her urge to graze on candy, cookies, chips, and soda. She also started to take the high-chromium multivitamin/mineral supplement with the healthy meals that she was suddenly hungry for. When she saw that her glucose level was dropping, she rushed some glutamine to her son. Both dropped from their usual glucose levels of over 200 to safe levels under 100 in forty-eight hours.

In our second followup workshop a few months later, she reported that they'd both easily maintained those lovely blood sugar levels.

DIABETES: NUTRIENT SUPPLEMENTS THAT FIGHT BACK

An immediate and permanent improvement in diet, compliments of glutamine (and perhaps other aminos) delivers the most powerful counter-punch. See the end of Chapter 14 for my proposed anti-diabetes cuisine. If you have already developed serious "complications," I want you to know that many studies show that you can multiply your benefits by adding supplements of other nutrients that diabetics are now known to be specifically and deeply deficient in. Diabetes seems to be a disease of sugar toxicity combined with pathologically low levels of *many* nutrients. What are they? A deficiency of glutamine is one. No surprise here, but higher doses than we typically use may be helpful. Some studies provided 30 grams a day of glutamine, in three 10-gram doses during or after meals.[22] This resulted in lowered blood glucose levels, blood pressure, and HbA1C percentage and a loss of fat at the waist (in six weeks).[23] (*Note:* Up to 30 grams a day of glutamine has been repeatedly proven safe.)[24] The aminos carnosine[25] and taurine[26] are also deficient, as are the minerals chromium, magnesium, and zinc,[27] the phospholipid choline, and vitamins C, D, B_1 (thiamin), and biotin.[28, 29, 30] The studies on these individual nutrients that I cite in the Notes section for this chapter and Chapter 12 are stunning in their potential. For example, a low dose of zinc (30 mg/day) lowered HA1C percentage significantly.[31] Taurine and carnosine can help with AGE damage, and chromium lowers HA1C and both fasting and post-prandial glucose levels. Studies on the omega-3 fats DHA and EPA[32] also show good reduction in HA1C and there are promising findings for the use of several other individual or combined nutrient supplements, as well. Most of the above nutrients are provided among the *Support Nutrients* that I recommend to all cravers at the end of Chapter 12, page 197. Additional nutrient support for diabetics is laid out in the Type 2 Craving section of that chapter, on page 179. Keep looking at the human research (animal and human results may not correlate) that is increasing fast and is increasingly nutrient-focused and so exciting.

For Cravings and Fatigue During or After Meals

This is an unusual type of craving that is common among those on the diabetic spectrum. Taking some extra glutamine right before meals (as well as the usual between-meal doses) can help. Taking Metformin (or the similar-acting herb berberine) with meals typically helps with this, but I'm hoping that the supplements and diet changes will make them less needed.

8

Are You a Type 3 Comfort Craver?

If you are a Type 3 Comfort Craver, you are missing out on the pleasure in life that should be naturally provided by your internal joy-promoters, the endorphins. Fortunately, that lack can be quickly supplied with the help of an unusual amino acid called DPA (d-phenylalanine).

The Type 3 Comfort Craver: A Short List of Symptoms

Here's an abbreviated list of the key endorphin deficiency symptoms. You'll recognize it from the Craving-Type Questionnaire you completed at the start of the book. If you have Type 3 cravings, you:

- Are very sensitive to emotional or physical pain.
- Cry or tear up easily.
- Have a history of chronic pain or sadness.
- Crave substances or behaviors that give pleasure, comfort, reward, or numbing.
- Particularly "love" chocolate, doughy, or creamy foods, alcohol, or painkilling drugs, or can't stop certain behaviors that give pleasure or relieve pain, like overexercising, pornography, or gambling.

THE NEUROTRANSMITTERS CALLED ENDORPHINS ARE from heaven. They can *erase* discomfort and pain, whether physical or emotional. They are defined as "endogenous opiates," meaning that they are powerful painkilling substances made by the body, not by a lab. These inner narcotics come in several forms. One of the most potent endorphin subtypes is called enkephalin. Did you ever think you'd hear about a heavily funded scientific study on the effects of M&M's? Since M&M's are the number one candy consumed in America, the subject was actually well chosen. The finding? M&M's caused enkephalin activity to increase 150 percent! The study found this sugar- and chocolate-fueled surge to be comparable, in brain effect, to that elicited by the drug opium.[1] But if we can make our own potent enkephalin and other endorphins, why do we need chocolate for a pleasure surge? We don't, unless our natural endorphin output is inadequate. In that case, we need an external supply in order to make life seem worth living.

If your consumption of M&M's or other chocolate treats is out of control, the above study should help you to understand why and to forgive yourself for succumbing to the overwhelming force of your cravings. It certainly explains why we're consuming at least 3 *billion* pounds of chocolate and spending 31 billion dollars on it every year in the United States alone![2] In fact, there is some concern that the chocolate supply is running out because of our ever-increasing addiction to it. Of course, chocolate is not the only food that can be irresistible to Type 3 Cravers, as you'll see.

THE CHEMISTRY OF COMFORT

The enjoyment and the numbness we can derive from chocolate and other narcotic foods can only be elicited by a member of a single family of potent endorphin-activating drugs called opiates or opioids.

Technically, "opiate" refers only to substances like heroin and morphine that are derived from opium poppies, while "opioid" is a more general term for synthetic painkillers like oxycodone and food-derived painkillers.

Opioid foods, like opioid drugs, work by magnifying the effects of our natural endorphins, which are produced by the brain. The cocoa bean concentrate called chocolate contains its own unique pleasuring opioid chemicals, but it's usually combined with sugar, fat, and milk, each of which has additional, somewhat different endorphin-boosting powers. By adding the endorphin lookalike gliadin (from wheat flour) to the mix, we get chocolate chip cookie dough ice cream, an opioid avalanche. In fact, chocolate and its fellow comfort foods are the top-selling painkillers in America.

If you're a Type 3 Comfort Craver, you long for more of the natural solace provided by the endorphins. We're all designed with an endorphin buffer zone to help us survive the sharp edges of life—a cocoon when the going gets tough. But it's quite possible for your legitimate need for that comfort not to be fully satisfied by your own production of natural pleasure-enhancers. Endorphins should automatically be released, both to help you have a good time, and whenever you are feeling sad, hurt, or stressed. They should release massively when you are seriously injured. The father of a friend of mine was badly injured in a car accident in his home town. Raised long before 1970, eating meat and other high-protein foods daily, the man's endorphin resources were naturally strong. He walked home, lay down, assured his wife he was not seriously injured, and died. An ER doctor later explained that this extraordinary level of naturally induced numbness was a part of the automatic shock reaction made possible by the power of our endorphins.

Endorphins are the largest and most complex of all the appetite-regulating neurotransmitters. Molecule for molecule, they are thousands of times stronger than heroin. It takes lots of protein, consumed at least three times a day, to provide adequate supplies of all the amino acids required for assembling this complex molecule. Our need for it is always high, because, as the great comforter, it is part of the stress response reflex that is automatically activated by *any* disturbance. Even in response to a loud noise, endorphin must go to work.

ENDORPHINS AND APPETITE

In the 1990s, news reports about fashion models who were using heroin to turn off their appetites started coming out. I understood this because years earlier I had visited the home of a famous musician who'd been addicted to heroin for years. His floor was littered with small dishes containing half-eaten hard-boiled eggs and half-empty Coke cans. He knew he was too thin and was trying to eat, but he couldn't. Your own naturally produced heroin-like neurotransmitters, the endorphins, don't eliminate your appetite *altogether* this way; instead they allow you to enjoy healthy foods but become satisfied by moderate amounts of them. Enjoyment and satisfaction are endorphin's signature endowments. The trouble is that many of us are now much too low in endorphin to enjoy any food but narcotic Techno-Karbz.

We need as many as nineteen different amino acids to make one molecule of an endorphin, while to make a molecule of any of the other neurotransmitters requires only one or two. Your current diet probably does not supply enough aminos from protein-rich foods to fill your body's needs, for all of the reasons that I gave in Chapter 3. So you reach for the comfort foods that can temporarily force a surge when you're feeling upset, lonely, or that there's nothing to look forward to. Any *chronic* pain of a physical *or* emotional nature can make you especially vulnerable; for example, an unresolved back injury, a custody battle, prolonged unemployment, or early childhood sexual abuse. You might also have a *genetic tendency* to produce too little endorphin, Does addiction to painkillers (like alcohol or chocolate) run in your family? Did your mother eat a lot of junk food while pregnant and/or nursing? If so, you could have inherited her addicted, "desensitized" opioid system, which would program you also to crave and overconsume comfort foods.[3] Whatever the causes, your levels can eventually bottom out, leaving you with no rewards but the edible ones.

How do we know that comfort foods can turn us into junkies? Shall I tell you about the heroin users who've told me that they could turn off their withdrawal symptoms with a piece of pie? Or would you prefer to hear it from PubMed? Research does confirm the addictive effect of sugar and other foods on our endorphins. Early in the 1980s, I started reading studies showing that the enjoyment brought on by eating sweets, like a heroin rush, could be turned off by drugs like naloxone or Naltrexone. These drugs block endorphin receptors in the brain, making it so that opioid drugs and drug-foods cannot activate the endorphins. A study on chocolate-chip cookies showed that blocking the endorphin receptors this way made even this iconic treat a big flop.[4] Other studies on sweet (and fatty) foods have also shown that the charm is lost when the brain's endorphin reception is sealed off.[5]

Ever-more precise methods, such as brain scanning, are being developed that can confirm the effects that well-designed Techno-Karbz can have on our neurotransmitters. A much-coveted prize in the advertising industry was awarded to a company whose ad had increased Cheetos sales by 20 percent. It had done so by giving audience members a brain device that identified their responses to the images in a potential ad for Cheetos. The images that elicited the most endorphin activity had been included in the ad.[6]

HOW ARE YOU GETTING *YOUR* OPIOID HIGH?

There are many foods that can trigger moderate, naturally pleasurable endorphin boosts: *Any* food can have that effect when you're really famished. Hot food does it when it's cold and cold food does it when it's hot. But then there are the endorphin slammers that can *always* induce swoony pleasure, especially in Type 3 Cravers:

1. Anything chocolate
2. Sugary products of all kinds
3. Doughy treats made from refined wheat flour
4. Creamy treats made with butter, cream, cheese, and other full-fat milk products

As we've just seen with the Cheetos experiment, the effects of any opioid-like substance or activity on the brain can be measured. For example, fat has been found to have a mildly opioid effect, while sugar's effect is so powerful that many studies are comparing it to the impact of "hard" opiates like morphine.[7] Mindfulness can raise endorphin levels and temporarily reduce "reward-driven eating."[8] Eating disorders (bingeing, purging, or starving) are known to trigger endorphin elevations.[9] Some other behaviors, too, can force endorphin releases so powerful that they can lead to addiction. For example, pornography, self-harm, and prolonged aerobic exercise.

One of our clients was a former Olympic contender who could not imagine life without a long, heavy-duty daily workout, or the "carb-loading" that came before and after it. She eventually got a pelvic fracture from repetitive exercise and the nutrient-poor quality of her diet. This forced her to stop exercising altogether and put her through a prolonged depressive withdrawal period in which she found herself even less able to stay away from the pasta and cookies. In fact, she was Techno-Karbz-loading ever more heavily, trying to re-create the sense of well-being she had lost along with her daily workouts.

As a result, the numbers on her scale kept increasing, on top of the endorphin-less emotional void that was not letting up. Eventually she landed in our clinic.

Sure enough, she was a Type 3 Comfort Craver. She responded nicely to adding more animal protein to her diet and was able to cut out the bagels and the pasta entirely. When she added the right amount of the amino acid supplements that built up her brain's depleted endorphin stockpile, she felt comforted and happy even without the exercise or the doughy foods. (It helped that her weight gain stopped right away, too.) With her endorphin levels rising, she began to really enjoy reading and writing. Quiet walks became fulfilling. When she'd healed from her injury and added some biking into her program, she found that her new, higher-protein diet had improved her natural athletic ability and she was easily out-pacing her experienced cyclist friends. However, while she enjoyed cycling, she no longer exercised for the high. Instead of serving as a drug, exercise had become a pleasant, but not addictive, expression of her natural athletic gift. She was just as happy on her quiet days.

Which of the four top opioid foods—chocolate treats, sugary treats, doughy treats, or creamy treats—do you find it hard or *impossible* to do without? You already know that sugar and white flour will have to go. But will you also need to jettison potentially healthful foods like whole wheat bread or cheddar cheese? It depends on your unique endorphin chemistry. As I explained in Chapter 3, flour-based foods are now loaded with extra concentrates of an endorphin lookalike called gluteomorphin l, while milk products, especially cheese, contain lots of an endorphin mimic called casomorphin. Listen to your body's reaction.

Note: When it comes to dough and milk products, there are other factors, beyond the craving they can elicit, that I'd like you to watch for, health factors that may be additional reasons for you to avoid them completely. Ironically, these two endorphin-boosting foods are more likely than any others to cause unpleasant intolerance reactions, notably digestive or respiratory problems, such as chronic constipation, diarrhea, postnasal drip, or asthma. (Chapters 14 and 15 will help you to determine your tolerance of these foods.)

Scan for any foods that give you that insatiable Type 3 craving. Once you begin your targeted aminos, you won't miss them. You may experiment later to discover whether you can tolerate any opioid-food without re-addicting yourself. Like so many of us, though, you'll probably just be reminded that you still can't have *any* without losing control. (The aminos will always be there to make withdrawal easy if you should get re-addicted.)

RAISING YOUR ENDORPHIN LEVELS NATURALLY: THE AMINO SOLUTIONS

The amino acid solutions for Type 3 Comfort Cravers are particularly well-researched, thanks largely to a compassionate and indefatigable pharmacology professor at the Chicago Medical School, Dr. Seymour Ehrenpries. Ehrenpries found that the unusual amino acid D-phenylalanine had strong endorphin-enhancing power.[10] All amino acids made in the lab have two forms, an L- and a D-form. Dr. Ehrenpries (and later other researchers) found that the D-form of phenylalanine dramatically reduced the need for morphine among his postsurgery patients.

How does D-phenylalanine (DPA) work? Unlike the aminos that are used for the other craving types, which *directly* increase the number of targeted neurotransmitters, D-phenylalanine works *indirectly,* by slowing down the body's automatic destruction of endorphin. Certain enzymes are specifically designed to destroy each of the neurotransmitters to preserve just the right neurotransmitter balance, neither too few nor too many. In an endorphin-deficient person, that balance can be adjusted to retain more of the neurotransmitter by slowing down the endorphin-destruction process. D-phenylalanine slows the action of the enzymes that destroy endorphins very quickly and effectively. In fact, most of our Type 3 Crashed Cravers have sighed with pleasure just a few minutes after trialing a single capsule.

D-phenylalanine actually comes in two forms: DPA—as D-phenylalanine alone—and also DLPA, which contains both the D- and the L-forms of the amino acid phenylalanine. L-phenylalanine has a mild painkilling effect, as it makes up one-fifth of enkephalin, the most potent subtype of endorphin. It is also energizing (as I explain in Chapter 10). This two-amino blend often works best for Type 3 Comfort Cravers who also have Type 5 Fatigued Cravings. The simple D-phenylalanine supplement works best for those who need pain relief but don't want more energy, for example, those who crave sweets in the evening, have physical pain when they lie down to try to sleep at night, or are generally anxious.

Adding a *complete amino blend* in capsule form can also be helpful. A mix of twenty predigested aminos can supply your endorphin-depleted system with *all* the readily usable amino supplies needed for this extensive multi-amino restoration project. Addiction and nutrition pioneer Charles Gant, M.D., in his excellent book *End Your Addiction Now*[11] discusses his impressive experience treating patients based on the results of extensive plasma amino acid testing. He finds that Type 3, endorphin-deficient addicts are often low in methionine, leucine, and glycine, as well as phenylalanine, all of which are required for making enkephalin and all of which a multi-amino can provide. Total Amino Solution by Genesa is my favorite, and I helped to design it (though I do not profit from its sales). Such supplements can be important if you are not a big protein eater, or if you're pregnant or nursing and can't take the more concentrated individual doses of DLPA or DPA aminos.

Phil was a Type 3 Comfort Craver who had switched from alcoholic drinking to Techno-Karbz addiction years before, with resulting weight problems. He'd also been a martial arts fanatic who'd had many injuries and lots of pain over the years. He was on the hyper side, so he found the slightly energizing DLPA a bit too "buzzy." When we switched him to the DPA, he took a deep breath and said, "For the first time in months, the pain isn't there." The next day, when he called in with his progress report, we asked if his cravings had diminished as well. At that point he said, "I'd actually forgotten about them. I didn't even think about my nighttime ice cream last night!" And it lasted. After he'd made his diet an endorphin buttress for a solid nine months, he found that he no longer needed his DPA.

Just remember this: You may feel dependent on your opioid Techno-Karbz now, but as soon as you've raised your endorphin levels with the Type 3 aminos, you won't miss them. Try to hold on to this unlikely concept just long enough to give these nutrients a try!

9

Are You a Type 4 Stressed Craver?

Type 4s turn to soothing foods when they are under stress and their brains' supply of naturally tranquilizing GABA has run low. Fortunately, GABA supplements can quickly relieve the tension and the cravings.

STRESS IS A UNIVERSAL HUMAN experience, but we are designed with an innate capacity to survive and rebound from it. *Chronic overstress* has not been the human experience, but it is now one of the most serious health concerns of our time. The World Health Organization calls it the "health epidemic of the twenty-first century," with more than half of workers worldwide experiencing temporary or longer-term disability because of it.[1]

Too much accumulated stress from work, finances, illness, relationships, no time to slow down and rest, and other pressures of all kinds are overwhelming our brain's ability to produce enough of its chief stress-reducing neurotransmitter, GABA (gamma-amino-butyric-acid). We're also eating the most stressful *diet* ever known. Yet, ironically, 70 percent of those feeling overstressed compulsively consume harmful Techno-Karbz for temporary stress-*relief*.[2] If you are a stress-motivated eater, this chapter will help you to better understand your own stress chemistry—and how to neutralize it before it neutralizes you.

When you are in trouble of any kind, your brain and adrenal glands must instantly prepare you to fight or flee by reorganizing your stress-response forces. The feisty neurotransmitter, adrenaline, is sent to the front to mount an emergency defense, while the relaxing neurotransmitter GABA is sidelined. After the crisis is over, it is time for GABA to be called up to do its stress-recovery work by neutralizing adrenaline's agitating effects. GABA is the biochemical antidote to

Type 4 Stressed Cravers: A Short List of Symptoms

Here's an abbreviated list of the key symptoms of the Type 4 Stressed Craver, which you'll recognize from the Craving-Type Questionnaire you completed at the start of the book. **Type 4s:**

- Have stiff, tense, or painful muscles.
- Feel stressed/burned out/overworked.
- Are unable to relax/loosen up.
- Often feel overwhelmed.
- Overreact and are easily upset.
- Are too wound up to get to sleep.
- Eat (and/or use alcohol or drugs) to escape from all of the above.

adrenaline. Under its soothing influence, your blood pressure lowers, your pulse slows, the muscle tension in your neck and shoulders softens, and feelings of ease emerge. If your GABA levels are strong, you can breathe deeply, pray or meditate, and open yourself up to the peace of nature. You should be able to call on GABA anytime you're trying to minimize or recover from feelings of stress.

GABA is not only a soother of stress, it is also an excellent blocker of mental spam; it can create inner stillness by clearing our minds of clutter and chatter. GABA actually creates the silence between spoken words! It can help when attention and concentration are difficult, because adrenaline without counterbalancing GABA makes us mentally scattered, even when we're not otherwise stressed. A study that measured EEG responses to a low dose GABA supplement found that it significantly increased relaxing alpha waves.[3]

Like so many of us, you may be living under what feels like a constant emotional siege. To tolerate the forced-march pace and other stressors of contemporary life, we should always be ready with plenty of GABA. Only we aren't. On top of too many stressful circumstances most of us now are not eating enough of the high-protein foods from which our brains construct this inner peacemaker. But you'll be able to increase your protein intake with the help of aminos like GABA and the guidance in Part IV—Craving-Free Eating.

If your life stressors relent, or you begin to eat fewer Techno-Karbz and more protein, you can make lots of GABA from your diet and gain more access to its relaxing influence. You have to work at it, though, because GABA, though it is an amino acid, cannot be found directly in foods. It has to be made *inside your body from some of the other amino acids* found in high-protein foods.

THE CHEMISTRY OF STRESS-EATING

Hundreds of studies have linked stress with the onset of food cravings, and have shown that stress relief can eliminate these cravings. Neuroscience research in the 1980s showed that GABA depletion could ignite food cravings and that GABA supplementation decreased this drive for food.[4]

More recently, many studies have found that some people are more prone to stress-eating than others. Among the overeaters most triggered by stress are, ironically, food *restrictors*.[5] As we saw in Chapter 4, calorie cutting has been a popular trend for fifty years, but undereating saps our ability to cope with stress by depleting us of the aminos and other nutrients we need to create calming GABA. It also raises levels of both of the anti-GABA stress hormones, adrenaline and cortisol. Sweet comfort foods shunt GABA out of action too, partly by destabilizing our glucose supply and creating stressful low-blood sugar crashes (which, again, increase adrenaline levels).[6]

If our stressful life circumstances become protracted, adrenaline subsides but the ultimate stress-response hormone, cortisol, rises—for the long haul. Cortisol, though less jangling than adrenaline, also suppresses GABA in order to keep us ever-vigilant, which can translate into ever-sleepless and ever-craving.

USING GABA SUPPLEMENTS TO NEUTRALIZE STRESS-EATING

Fortunately, you have access to a great resource, hitherto probably unknown to you: GABA in supplement form. GABA is an amino acid that provides almost-instant relief from stress and stress-eating.

A tense, quiet fifteen-year-old craver came in with his mother one day. He was so embarrassed to be telling a stranger about how he coped with school and social stress by grazing on chips, soda, and sweets, and about his acne and weight problems. Three minutes after trialing a low-potency GABA chewable, he started twirling in his swivel chair, smiling, and chatting. When I pointed this out, he tried to stop smiling, and couldn't! He'd also lost interest in getting the candy he'd been pestering his mother for before the session, and asked to go to a real restaurant for dinner instead of the usual fast food! His mother was dazzled, but not too surprised. She'd come in herself a few months earlier and found GABA to be a revelation.

GABA is actually *both* an amino acid and a neurotransmitter. This may be why it works so well as a supplement. It is one of the top-selling antistress remedies in the supplement shops, and has been for years, because it is so effective so quickly, even in very low, 100-mg doses. We love giving stress-eaters a little GABA lozenge and watching their speech slow down and their posture soften as their necks and shoulders relax. Once we see how much calmer our clients have become, we ask if they'd still like to reach for some candy, a Xanax, a drink, or a joint to all of which they almost always say "No."

Note: There is a persistent rumor on the Internet that GABA supplements do not cross the blood-brain barrier. This notion, that GABA is ineffectual, clearly originated from someone who had little or no actual clinical experience with GABA supplements. It is so effective that we actually have to caution our clients not to buy it at high doses (500 to 750 mg) unless they don't respond to trials of lower doses (100 to 250 mg). About one-third seem to need the higher doses. I, my colleagues, and the health professionals I've trained are all incredulous when we hear this rumor yet again. Early research raised the question, but more recent research confirms that supplementary GABA does cross the blood-brain barrier.[7]

A busy fifty-year-old mom, who had formerly been the hyper-stressed VP of several start-up companies, had, like so many women, been a mostly closet bulimic since she was eighteen. She still binged and purged almost daily, particularly when she felt stressed.

Her initial Type 4 Stressed Craver symptom scores were all high. She'd been feeling overwhelmed for many years even though, lately, her life had calmed down. So she kept on bingeing and she was afraid to stop purging, in spite of extensive dental damage, shame, and fear for her health, because of her even greater fear of weight gain.

Three minutes after her low-dose GABA supplement trial, she felt calm and free of cravings. When she redid her Craving Questionnaire four weeks later, after taking higher doses of GABA twice daily, her total Stressed Craver scores had gone down from 10s to 2s! More important, her binge and purge episodes had gone down to zeros. She had a few slips over the next few months, mostly because she'd forgotten to take her supplements. But overall she was a happy woman.

THE STRESS FIGHTER'S BACKUP: THEANINE

Although over 80 percent of our clients have thoroughly benefited from GABA supplementation, some have felt nothing from it, even when they've raised their dose. Happily, there are a few other calming aminos that can benefit Stressed Cravers. Taurine can be helpful, especially when *combined* with GABA, but over time we've found that *theanine*, a unique amino found only in the tea plant, is the most universally successful stand-in for GABA itself. Theanine's mechanism of action in the brain has not been as well identified as GABA's, but it clearly enhances the utilization of GABA. As with GABA, a little theanine typically goes a long way. All dosing particulars are provided in Chapter 12's section on Type 4 Stressed Cravers, page 184.

MORE GABA SUPPORT: SUPPLEMENTS, FOODS, AND LIFESTYLE CHANGES

For GABA repair and restoration you will be taking a few nutrient supplements that will include stress-reducing B vitamins and magnesium along with your GABA or theanine. These *support nutrients* are vital assets in the brain's recovery from stress burnout and stress-eating. Of course the Craving Cure's antistress diet will need to be put in place, as well. Getting enough traditional food regularly will make a big difference; undereating and skipping or delaying meals raises adrenaline and cortisol levels and lowers GABA levels. You don't want that!

Once your nutritional stress-reduction program is underway, you'll start breathing and sleeping better (GABA supplements can be a big help at bedtime). But other stress-protective steps will also be required: taking *time off* daily, taking regular *slow* vacations; getting enough exercise, stretching, and fun.

Don't hesitate to get counseling too if you come up against any particularly stubborn stressors or have PTSD (post-traumatic stress disorder responds well to GABA but typically requires other aminos too along with trauma counseling). We've had clients suddenly lose weight they'd been fighting for years after getting help in leaving a high-stress job or getting good marital counseling. With the improvements in your diet and lifestyle, you'll soon get to the point where you won't need your GABA supplements anymore, except under unusually stressful circumstances. Your brain's own calming functions will be restored.

ANOTHER GROWING CAUSE OF STRESS AND INSOMNIA: ADRENAL CORTISOL IMBALANCE

We've learned through our Type 4 clients that some more severe or chronic kinds of stress reactions require help beyond what the Type 4 aminos, alone, can provide. If your sense of overwhelmedness does not completely and quickly lift once you start taking the Type 4 aminos and support nutrients, are consistently eating well, and have been able to calm your lifestyle, your stress-fighting adrenal glands may well need some special attention. These two small but mighty glands produce both of our stress-coping hormones, adrenaline and cortisol. But they are also responsible for producing all of our sex hormones and a number of other vital hormones including some that help regulate blood sugar and blood pressure. With all this responsibility, not to mention having to respond to our endlessly stressful lives, the demand on them is heavy and constant.

Adrenal exhaustion often eventually sets in. That means cortisol (and other hormones, often) begin to be *under*-produced. This is especially common following a long period of particularly severe stress. A chronic state of fatigue and a general inability to face even minor strife ensues. "I can't go on, even with my most soothing snacks" becomes a real fact of life which sufferers assume will never change. But we've seen it lift nicely. There are many effective herbal cortisol elevators, like licorice, available alone and in blends, as well as medication that is composed of cortisol itself.

Others who've endured long periods of stress have found that their high cortisol levels can remain abnormally high (sometimes even years after the stress has passed) and cause chronic tension, high blood pressure, insomnia, and/or abdominal overweight. It's not unusual for cortisol levels to become abnormally low in the day and too high at night.

One of our clients could not lose her last ten pounds till she left her abusive husband. We'd tested her cortisol levels initially, and again a few months later, and her levels were too high. It was only after her separation that her cortisol levels finally went down into the normal range, along with her weight and all of her inner tension. She was also able to start sleeping through the night.

As I mentioned earlier, low-calorie dieting is another stressor that predictably elevates cortisol levels (starvation is our number one stressor), and those high cortisol levels can slow down thyroid function,[8] which helps account for how easily we can regain weight after a diet. We've seen chronically elevated cortisol levels result in chronic insomnia. This is a double whammy, as both insomnia and high cortisol can impede needed weight loss (as I mention in Chapter 6, page 114).

High cortisol levels can sometimes be subdued with the help of nighttime supplementation with GABA and/or other calming aminos like tryptophan or melatonin. The use of phospho serine (*not phosphatidyl* serine) can be very helpful, too. Visit cravingcure.com and my book *The Mood Cure* for more on these and other insomnia resources.

Note: The Type 1 amino 5-HTP *raises* cortisol somewhat, and should not be used if it worsens sleep, but that can be a good indicator that your cortisol is high, at least at night, and that you should test it.

The Best Stress Test: How to Measure Your Cortisol Levels at Home

We have found no accurate tests for GABA levels. Neither plasma nor urine testing correlates well with symptoms. Salivary cortisol testing, on the other hand, is the most reliable and accurate test I've ever run across. It can very accurately measure levels of *cortisol* throughout the day *and* night. It's also our favorite test because it's so convenient (you take it at home) and inexpensive, easy to order and interpret, and because test results effectively guide nutrient supplementation. See page 292 in Tracking and Testing Tools for the details.

Are You Using Tranquilizing Drugs to Deal with Low GABA or Cortisol Overdrive?

Too much stress can leave you permanently unable to sleep and unequipped to cope, even with the help of soothing foods. Drugs may seem to be your only recourse. Alcohol, pot, and benzodiazepines like Xanax, Ativan, Klonopin, and Valium can activate GABA and lower cortisol levels short term. But they all have side effects including, of course, addiction. Benzos are particularly addictive and have potentially deadly withdrawal effects for frequent users. The suggestions in this chapter can help reduce cravings and withdrawal symptoms for all of these "downer" substances, but if you're addicted to benzos, taper very slowly with the kinds of expert help I mention in the chapter on drug addiction in *The Mood Cure*.

10

Are You a Type 5 Fatigued Craver?

If you're craving an energy boost from caffeine, choco-late, or jelly beans, you're probably low in your own natural stimulants, the neurotransmitters I call the "Cats." No problem—you're about to discover the superior effects of the two amino acids I call the "Cat Foods."

WHEN THE NATURALLY ENLIVENING NEUROTRANSMITTERS, the catechol-amines, are functioning normally, we feel mentally alert, physically ener-gized, up for exercise, able to concentrate at will, enthusiastic about daily life, and more expressive and outgoing. We also have a sense of reward in life and the motivation to reach for our goals. As a result, we have no particular interest in artificial stimulation from stand-ins like caffeine, chocolate, or sugar.

If you're feeling the opposite of all this, you've come to the right place.

Type 5 Fatigued Cravers: A Short List of Symptoms

Here's an abbreviated list of the key symptoms of Type 5 Fatigued Cravers, based on the questionnaire you completed at the start of the book. If you are a Type 5 Craver, you:

- Crave foods, drinks, or other alternative substances for energy, focus, or the ability to exercise
- Lack energy
- Feel apathetic, flat
- Lack drive

- Lack focus, concentration
- Feel easily bored
- Have attention deficits

Fifty-four-year-old Wanda was prediabetic and a self-described "carb craver" who had been obese, fatigued, and in generally poor health for ten years before she dragged herself into our clinic. We didn't even need to look at her Craving-Type Questionnaire to see that she was a Type 5 Fatigued Craver.

She brightened up immediately after we trialed her on one capsule of tyrosine, the amino acid we typically use to restore normal levels of the activating neurotransmitters. Twice-daily doses of this supplement lifted her energy all day and she was able to start exercising again. She also felt up to preparing food for the first time in a long time, so she quit ordering fast food to go. And she didn't miss it. She liked her new, wholesome meals, and she was surprised that "all this healthy food" was actually resulting in weight loss.

THE THREE CATS: OUR NATURAL ACTIVATORS

The three neurotransmitters that comprise this family of brain- and body-energizers share the family name catecholamine. Their first names are *dopamine, norepinephrine*, and *adrenaline*. Between them, they have hundreds of vital jobs in the brain and body. The most well-known of these jobs is the programming of physical movement—the Cats are all about action. But they are mentally activating too, providing us with our own natural caffeine.

The first Cat, *dopamine*, helps us to move well, but it enhances our mental drive, arousal, and alertness too, and has many other functions throughout the body. It is of major interest to researchers in the addiction field because of its central involvement in what they call "natural reward-seeking behavior," which drives all addictions, whether to food or to other substances. Drugs that specifically target dopamine, like Ritalin or cocaine, can powerfully exaggerate sensations of mental and sensual arousal. Most neuroscientists are convinced that no pleasurable sensations, including the satisfaction of eating, can be experienced without adequate dopamine release. If we're dopamine-deficient Type 5 Cravers, we can't seek and experience the natural "rewards" in life. This is where the Techno-Karbz come in: sugar and certain other substances and activities can temporarily set off a dopamine surge that sets us up for a drug-like dependence.[1]

Norepinephrine is most notable for giving us mental energy and the ability to concentrate, a function that seems to be weaker for many of us now than ever before in history. Many drugs try to amplify this Cat effect: caffeine, ADD drugs like Dexedrine, and SNRIs (selective norepinephrine reuptake inhibitor antidepressants) like Wellbutrin, to name a few.

The notorious Cat *adrenaline* actually serves many positive functions as well as the better-known negative ones. For example, the pleasant energy we experience during and after exercise is a gift of moderate adrenaline signaling. We do not tend to run out of this Cat because it is required ensure our survival: it provides our first line response to stress. When we're in trouble, the fight-or-flight state it sets in motion can save our lives. Fear, panic, agitation, hypervigilance, aggression—these are survival responses along with elevated blood pressure, high blood sugar, and raised insulin levels.

WHEN CAT LEVELS DROP TOO LOW

I saw what it was like to be deeply "Cat" deficient when I met my first cocaine-addicted clients. One was a forty-three-year-old health professional I'll call Ben.

On cocaine, Ben's Cat function has been towering. He'd felt like a superhero. But when he'd run out of the drug, he'd feel crushed. When we met him, he was totally deflated: depressed, tired, and lifeless. He was sleeping twelve hours a day and gaining weight fast—he'd gained thirty pounds in his first thirty days off cocaine. He was having to load sugar and caffeine all day just to try to stay out of bed. He had relapsed because of his awful lethargy so many times that he was convinced he was worthless and hopeless. But we were able to explain to him that he was just Cat-less. When he started using the Cat-supportive amino acids and was able to shift his diet, he—and his family—could see that he really had been suffering from a severe, but curable, neuro-chemical disability.

THE AMINO SOLUTIONS FOR TYPE 5 FATIGUED CRAVERS

If your Type 5 Fatigued Craver score is high, it indicates that your brain's current supplies of dopamine, norepinephrine, and/or adrenaline are likely to be inadequate, and you need to know why. You might have inherited some dull

Cats, but it's more likely that you haven't been feeding them enough amino-rich fuel. Two amino acids that can only be found in abundance in dense proteins like meat are the only nutrients that can fuel Cat production. The first thing our protein-skimping Type 5 clients report when they start eating animal protein three times a day is: "I've got *energy*!" What they mean is "I've got Cats!"

There are two cat-fueling amino acids that can give you the natural energy and focus that will allow you to back off the coffee, decaf, caffeinated sodas, energy drinks, iced tea, chocolate, hard candy, and gum. Their names are *tyrosine* and *phenylalanine*. Both convert quickly into all three of the Cats, starting with dopamine. They can both also raise the levels of the potent appetite shut-off hormone cholecystokinin, which can reduce calorie intake by as much as 30 percent.[2] In one study, participants who were given phenylalanine ate 400 fewer calories at a buffet free-for-all.[3] This is the aminos' marvelous dual effect on Type 5s: more energy (including for exercise) and less appetite for junk food.

Tyrosine and phenylalanine were the first aminos ever to come to my attention. I started hearing about them in the 1980s, during the early years of the cocaine epidemic. Well-known East Coast addiction treatment leaders like Mark Gold, M.D., recommended phenylalanine, while West Coast experts favored tyrosine. My hero and the most successful cocaine fighter in the country, judging by his research studies, was Kenneth Blum, Ph.D., who used *both* aminos together. I describe the pioneering work by Blum that electrified the addiction field in Chapter 5, page 102. Let me just say briefly here that it improved cocaine treatment compliance by 800 percent! At a time that no cocaine treatment programs could hang on to their clients at all.

At my clinic, we, too, have experimented with both aminos. We typically now use tyrosine first. Its results tend to be more dramatic for more people. We usually reserve L-phenylalanine for children, for those who are sensitive to supplements, or for those who have felt tyrosine to be too stimulating. LPA, as we call it, converts only in part to tyrosine and thence to the other Cats, so it's a few steps less direct and potent.

During trials of these aminos, it's so much fun to see newly bright-eyed clients sit up, lean forward, and start chatting easily even before they are aware of the changes themselves! In terms of appetite, having better morning energy naturally means that our clients can forgo caffeine and eat a good breakfast, which is crucial for preventing cravings throughout the day. (Morning coffee is one of the little-known promoters of junk food eating.)

Janice, a fifty-year-old bookkeeper, called our virtual clinic after drinking at least four 12-ounce regular Cokes and two chocolate milk shakes a day for thirty-seven years. She had struggled with fatigue most of that time, in spite of all the stimulants, as well as with her weight. She had gone up as high as 185 pounds at times (she was only 5 feet 4). But she just couldn't stop drinking these high-calorie, brain-disrupting junk beverages. Janice's real problem was that her brain was not producing enough of its natural get-up-and-go. This tendency to lethargy ran in her family, but it got worse after she started to diet.

Janice had seen my earlier books and had scoffed at the idea that she, or anyone else, could actually kick a thirty-seven-year habit in twenty-four hours. But then she got desperate enough to try it. She started taking tyrosine on Monday. On Wednesday she wrote an ecstatic e-mail to her nutritionist to say that she had no cravings for colas or chocolate at all anymore. Without them she began sleeping well, her physical and mental energy increased (without the jitters), and her weight quickly began to drop. She also reported having no caffeine withdrawal symptoms! After about six weeks she was feeling a bit buzzy on the tyrosine so she switched to milder phenylalanine and did just fine, and was permanently able to get up and go on her own steam.

The Cats and the Phen-Fen Effect

Many overeaters are low in both dopamine and serotonin.[4] The most effective weight loss medication ever designed was a combination of two drugs, fenfluramine, a serotonin booster, and phentermine, which boosted dopamine as well as serotonin. Fenfluramine was eventually banned because of deadly side effects and millions went into deep mourning. But phentamine lives on as a not-as-effective, but still popular, diet aid. If you'd liked the effects of Phen-Fen or of phentermine by itself, especially if you have Type 1 as well as Type 5 cravings, you'll like a combination of Type 5 and Type 1 aminos.

Tyrosine and Exercise

So many exercisers use caffeine to force "better" weight loss workouts. The aminos can typically provide caffeine's positives without its negative side effects. I consulted with some golf professionals who wanted to add supplements to a line of golf-oriented products they were developing. I suggested that they take tyrosine during their next game and decide for themselves. They felt the difference in energy and performance right away!

The current "obesogenic" (obesity-promoting) American diet is known to lower dopamine levels. This seems to at least partially account for a type of inactivity unique to people with obesity, making them even more vulnerable to continued overeating and weight gain. Since tyrosine converts directly into dopamine we have found it to be very helpful in getting our clients of all weights into action.[5] One other direct benefit of tyrosine for physical energy and weight loss is that it is used directly by the thyroid to make all four of this gland's metabolically activating hormones.

Tyrosine and ADD

ADD can prevent our clients from remembering to take their aminos! Those who've used stimulant meds such as Dexedrine, Adderall, and Ritalin have often found effective alternative relief from their inattention from the amino acids that fuel the Cats. Tyrosine has been studied for ADD at 200 mg per dose. Not surprisingly, it showed little benefit. We get good results at 1,000-1,500 mg per dose. See my book *The Mood Cure* for more on this as well as, the book by pioneering clinician Charles Gant, M.D., *End Your Addiction Now,* on his successful use of these aminos and other alternative strategies for ADD (and for cocaine, methamphetamine, and ADD drug addictions).[6]

HOW YOUR FAVORITE FOODS AND DRINKS CAN CAUSE CAT PROBLEMS

Like most Americans, you've no doubt been relying on addictive stimulants to keep you going in the absence of your natural quota of Cats. In order to restore your *natural* vitality, you'll need to relieve your brain of the *over*stimulating substances now occupying it. Here is why getting rid of some of your favorite foods and drinks is so important for revitalizing your natural Cat function and for your total health:

CAFFEINE

I can hear you thinking, "I know I should give up the sweetened drinks, but I've heard that coffee and tea keep me from eating bad foods and that they don't contribute to weight gain or health problems—and don't they help my workouts?"

Here's why *caffeine* in all forms—in coffee, tea, sodas, and energy drinks—needs to go:

■ It temporarily ruins your appetite for real food. Not eating makes you prey to cravings. When the caffeine wears off, you realize your blood sugar has plunged and you grab the first Techno-Karb you run across. Skipping breakfast robs you of your a.m. "Cat Food," so you need more caffeine throughout the day. This can add up to over three cups a day, increasing your risk of premature death by 50 percent.[7]

■ Caffeine too often comes laced with sugar and chocolate, thus becoming a double or triple addictor that adds harmful calories.

■ Caffeine suppresses your calming neurotransmitters serotonin, GABA, and adenosine by overstimulating adrenaline. Too much adrenaline compromises cardiovascular function, adrenal function, and your overall sense of well-being. It also increases anxiety and interferes with sleep, which weakens health generally and contributes to weight gain (see page 114).

■ Caffeine reduces the levels of the Cat-fueling amino acids phenylalanine and tyrosine as well as energizing, calorie-burning thyroid hormones.[8]

■ It can accelerate your progression toward diabetes by suppressing the insulin response.[9]

■ Unlike coffee and tea, with their complex contents that moderate caffeine's effects, synthetic caffeine is more like straight amphetamine. Even Diet Coke, and certainly energy drinks, are associated with an increased risk of stroke.[10]

CHOCOLATE

Chocolate contains caffeine and at least three other stimulants, including one called PEA, which is known as "the chocolate amphetamine." It should actually be known as "the chocolate cocaine" because, like cocaine, it spikes both dopamine and norepinephrine levels. Forget the superfood hype. For many of us, chocolate is a super-drug and the darker it is, the more concentrated.[11] Cocoa is a complex plant that, like coffee, tea, cannabis, and tobacco, contains a mix of chemicals, some addictive, some harmful, some healthful. Of course, most chocolate is combined with milk, sugar, starch, and fat to create the great American weight-gain bombs, but unsweetened (dark) chocolate contains three times more caffeine and other stimulants and it, too, is linked with weight gain.[12, 13]

SUGAR

All by itself, sugar can have stimulating effects on some people. We regularly have clients looking for energy from their Skittles, mints, and gum. When we ask them why they tend to nibble these sugary treats all day, they say, "They keep me going."

Caffeine Withdrawal

Don't worry about caffeine withdrawal. Even the headaches are typically either mild or nonexistent once you start taking the Type 5 aminos. *The Caffeine Detox Protocol* in the Type 5 section of Chapter 12, page 191, spells it out.

A local health radio show host who regularly had me on as a guest admitted, on the air, that he was still drinking coffee because when he tried to quit, his detox headaches went on and on. I told him about the amino detox and, the next time I was on his show, he announced he'd been coffee-free for a year, painlessly, because of tyrosine. (He'd also lost weight because he was no longer consuming all the brown sugar he'd added to his coffee.)

Are You Taking a Cat-Activating Drug?

- ADD drugs such as Ritalin, Adderall, Dexedrine, or Concerta?
- Antidepressant drugs (SNRIs) that target norepinephrine, such as Wellbutrin and Effexor?
- Phentermine for weight loss?
- L-dopa drugs for Parkinson's?

Speak to your prescribing physician about whether combining the pro-Cat aminos with your medications for a brief trial period of a few days or weeks would be a good idea or not. Always take these aminos several hours *away* from the drugs that also target the "Cats." If your tyrosine or phenyl-alanine trial is a success, you may not need your drugs. On the other hand, there may be good reasons not to take these aminos at all while you are taking certain medications. Let your physician be your guide.

If you're getting cocaine, crack, or meth on the street, only trial the Type 5 aminos away from them. (If you're withdrawing from them you might need as much as 2,000 mg three or four times a day for a while; see *The Mood Cure* and Charles Gant, M.D.'s *End Your Addiction Now*.)

If your new amino-supplied vitality turns out not to be strong enough to drive you to the gym or the dance floor, see Chapter 16, page 253, Dodging Slips and Shooting Trouble, for suggestions regarding other causes of fatigue that you should investigate.

PART III

The Amino Breakthrough

11

Cracking the Craving Code: Prep Steps for all Craving Types

WELCOME TO THE CORE OF the Cure! This two-chapter appetite-repair manual will teach you how to use the right amino acids in the right amounts to propel your brain out of its current craving mode. This first chapter unveils the general steps that *any and all* Craving Types need to take. Read it all carefully and do what it asks. The second chapter provides more specific directions for each *individual Craving Type*. Study only the sections in it that pertain to your own Type or Types. Underline, highlight, annotate, or index both chapters so that you can easily refer back to their instructions while you're cracking codes and breaking through.

The steps that you'll find laid out in these chapters are the same steps that all the clients at my clinic follow. In fact, I've summarized here everything we've learned while supervising thousands of amino breakthroughs over more than thirty years. When you've read the whole book, giving special attention to the chapters in Part II that pertain to your personal Craving Type(s), plan to spend a few hours studying both of these chapters and filling out the indicated questionnaires. After that, you'll be ready to crack and break. You're going to enjoy this process, especially your amino trialing. After that, it will feel like you're living a miracle, which you will be.

PREPARING YOURSELF FOR BREAKTHROUGH

It won't matter that my staff nutritionists will not be by your side, although if you need help anywhere along the line, you can get some virtual coaching at cravingcure.com. You'll do well on your own because you'll be using tools similar to those our clients use, starting with the Craving-Type Questionnaire and Profile that I placed at the head of this book on page 12. If you haven't filled it out yet, stop now and do so. Your scores on this questionnaire are *gold*! It's the first in a set of invaluable questionnaires and forms—I call them Tracking Tools— that we've developed to help our clients navigate their amino breakthroughs. I'm about to introduce them to you and to train you in how to use them. You'll soon see why we rely on them so heavily.

STEP 1: GET SOME TRACKING TOOL TRAINING

> ## Where to Find Your Tracking Tools
>
> These tools can be found on page 267 in the Tracking Tools section. Photocopy the blank questionnaire and forms there or download copies at craving cure.com/trackingtools.
>
> *Start a binder or a computer file for each one and keep them in chronological order for comparison purposes.*

Set Your Course Using The 12-Week Craving Cure Timeline

After you've read the book, you'll need a map of where to go from there. That's when you'll pick up this first Tracking Tool. It's a two-page itinerary that lays out the whole Craving Cure process, week-by-week and step-by-step. Previewing the course you'll be taking will help get you on track. Referring back to it regularly over the next twelve weeks will help keep you on-track.

Establish Your Baselines Using Your Tracking Tools

Once the Timeline has helped you *set* your course, it will be time to *establish your baselines*. That will involve the next three Tracking Tools. Between them, they'll allow you to create an accurate record of your current, *pre-cure* craving symptoms and eating habits. Why is this so crucial? There is no other way for you to determine which Types of cravings you have, which aminos you'll need, or how well they work. Over the next twelve weeks, you will be able to compare the scores on these *pre-cure baselines* with your later scores to *precisely* gauge the effects of your aminos. You won't just vaguely think "I seem to be doing a lot better," you'll know *exactly* how much better you're doing and how much better yet you *could* be doing. So please fill them out right away, before you start your aminos or make any dietary changes.

The Craving-Type Questionnaire. As I said, your score on the Craving-Type Questionnaire and Profile on page 12 will establish your *craving* baseline. After your amino trials, when you've been taking the indicated aminos daily for a week, you'll switch to a "mini" version of this questionnaire. You'll score this shorter version *every week* and marvel at the changes you'll be documenting. These changes in your scores will inform you of the exact degree of your progress and guide any adjustments you'll need to make in your amino dosing going forward.

Let me give you an example. If your initial Craving-Type Questionnaire and Profile showed that your Type 1 symptom severity ratings were all 10s, I'd expect that, after you'd been taking your aminos daily for a week, your next Type 1 ratings (using the Mini Questionnaire) would be all in the 0 to 3 range. If your ratings instead were all 5s, that would indicate a 50 percent improvement—meaning that 50 percent of your cravings were still there. That constitutes progress, but *not* a cure. It does tell you where you stand (halfway there) and what your next week's scores should be (better). By that next week, after adjusting your aminos further upward (as per the directions in the next chapter), your scores on the Mini Questionnaire should be much closer to zero. Without the first Craving Type scores as a baseline, you wouldn't know what to aim for. You'd probably think a 50 percent improvement was a great achievement, and it is, but the remaining cravings would eventually have dragged you back into the toxic fudge.

Your Daily Log. This Tool will help you set a *dietary baseline,* a detailed record of three representative days of your *current* eating. Record each day's eating honestly and in good detail. (You'll find a sample log as well as a blank form in the Tracking Tools section. Use the Spark People app or website to add *baseline calorie estimates*.) You'll love being able to refer back to your early entries to remind yourself of exactly what your life was like *before the cure.* As soon as you start taking the aminos regularly, start recording your reactions to your aminos and new foods *daily.* But please don't dread it. I call the Daily Log your "Darling Diary." Unlike any of your former diet records, this will be neither a slag heap of shame and guilt nor a sterile list of starvation rations and grim reports from the scale. You're about to make dietary history! But you'll be surprised at how quickly you'll forget the exciting details if you don't record them daily. I know you're busy, but I promise that you will not have to keep daily records forever. For the next few months, though, use your log to record how the aminos *and* foods are making you feel. Most important, your log can keep you alerted if things start going wrong. You'll be able to use it for investigative purposes; backtracking through it to figure out when and how a problem started. This will tell you what you need to do to fix it. For example, after doing well for weeks, you might start craving again. You'll look back at the 24 hours of logs you'd kept prior to the start of those cravings to see if you'd missed a dose of aminos or a meal, started eating too few calories, or got really upset (or all three). Then you'll fill out a quick Mini Questionnaire. The results will indicate which extra aminos you'll need to take for a few days at least. This will stop the cravings quickly again and that will allow you to quickly get your eating back on track. Without your log, you wouldn't have been clear on what had triggered your cravings; you would literally have been clueless and headed back into the toxic fudge.

Our clients who do not keep their Food Logs do not do as well as those who do. I hope you can see now why.

After at least four weeks on your aminos and one of the anti-craving food plans from Part IV, feeling good and craving free, you can quit logging. After that you will only log again when you formally eliminate or reintroduce a food *or* if a craving, a slip, or any other problem suddenly crops up. (If the latter, your friendly Chapter 16, Dodging Slips and Shooting Trouble, will be there for you as well.)

The Trigger-Foods Rating Sheet. This tool actually does quadruple duty. It allows you to check off, from its list of the "most craved" foods, the ones that you crave *now* and rate them on a scale of 0 to 10. Then you'll use this baseline list to determine which foods to leave behind as you embark on your new food plan. A month later, you'll *re-score* the list to track your progress. (Do you still crave any of these foods and how much?) Lastly, you can use it to decide whether to reintroduce any of the formerly craved foods on the list, and in what order, to see if they'll reignite cravings or not. (But you don't have to.)

The Amino Trialing Record and the Amino Supplement Schedule. These two Tracking Tools will come into play when you *trial* your aminos. The Trialing Record will document your reactions to specific doses of specific aminos. Right after you've completed your trials, you'll fill out your *Supplement Schedule,* a list of the aminos that trialed well, when you should take them daily, and at what dose. You will revise the schedule when you raise, lower, or discontinue your amino doses.

Testing Guidelines. Testing is another way to track your progress. For example, you might like to get a lab test to measure some of your amino acid or neuro-transmitter levels before, during, or after your amino breakthrough process. All of the details about the lab and home tests that I mention in various parts of the book are located at the end of the Tracking Tools.

Your Tracking Tool Review

1. Your 12-Week Craving Cure Timeline (to get and keep you on track).

2. The initial Craving-Type Questionnaire and Profile (for you to complete once, *before* you start your aminos).

3. The Mini Craving-Type Questionnaire (for you to complete *weekly, after* you start your aminos).

4. Your Food Log (for you to keep for three days *before* you start your aminos and change your diet, and *daily afterwards*).

5. The Trigger Foods Rating Sheet (for you to complete *before* you start the aminos and *monthly* after that).

6. The Amino Trialing Record (to complete only when you trial an amino).

7. The Supplement Schedule (to complete only right after your amino trials, then to revise if you change your amino doses).

8. The Testing Guidelines (to help you explore any of the lab- and home-testing options I mention in various parts of the book).

STEP 2: MATCH YOUR CRAVING TYPE(S) TO THEIR AMINO SOLUTION(S)

Review your completed Craving-Type Questionnaire and Profile at the beginning of the book on page 12 to identify your craving repair priorities. Look at your Pro-file graph (page 19) to note which of your Craving Type scores were above the ideal range. After identifying your top-scoring Type, rank and match up any other above-ideal scores in order of severity in the middle column of the chart below. Then look to the right column to confirm which aminos you'll need for each re-pair job indicated.

MATCH EACH CRAVING TYPE WITH ITS CORRESPONDING AMINO ACID SOLUTION

CRAVING TYPE	REPAIR PRIORITY: RANK AND CIRCLE FOR EACH CRAVING TYPE	AMINO SOLUTIONS
Type 1: The Depressed Craver ____Yes	#1 #2 #3 #4 #5	5-HTP or Tryptophan
Type 2: The Crashed Craver ____Yes	#1 #2 #3 #4 #5	Glutamine
Type 3: The Comfort Craver ____Yes	#1 #2 #3 #4 #5	DLPA or DPA
Type 4: The Stressed Craver ____Yes	#1 #2 #3 #4 #5	GABA or Theanine
Type 5: The Fatigued Craver ____Yes	#1 #2 #3 #4 #5	Tyrosine or 1-Phenylalanine

Now you know which aminos are in your future and in what order you'll trial them. Chapter 12 provides the specifics on each amino solution, including factors for deciding which of two supplement options to try first, in the cases where you have a choice.

STEP 3: REVIEW GENERAL AMINO PRECAUTIONS

I know you're eager to get into action with the aminos, but do not skip this step. In the Amino Precautions Box opposite, you'll find some general cautionary considerations that apply to all the aminos. Please review it carefully. (You'll find some other precautions *specific* to the amino for your Craving Type(s) in the next chapter.) I want you to have a completely successful amino breakthrough. So let's be sure that you don't stub your toe on an amino that may not be right for you. We've only rarely encountered clients who have been unable to use *any* of the aminos, but some have had to avoid one or two.

Part of the reason our clients rarely have trouble with their aminos is that we look into possible amino contraindications early on, steering our clients away from potential problems. The doses of aminos that we suggest are very moderate and, because they are so well tailored to our clients' needs, they seldom cause problems.

First, based on previous experiences, are you sensitive to supplements in general?

While any of the amino supplements included in this book could disagree with some takers, over 90 percent of our clients tolerate all of their aminos very well. That includes children, who are typically only reactive to too high a dose. Less than 5 percent of our clients have been sensitive to one or more amino. They've usually had similar sensitivity problems with a variety of other supplements in the past. If you have frequently had adverse reactions to supplements you've tried, the aminos may not be for you. In these cases, we start trialing with a quarter of the lowest recommended starting dose. We also give our sensitive clients at least an hour to adjust to each amino before trialing another. If you're in this category, take the same slow approach to introducing not only the amino, but the supportive nutrients that are recommended, as well. That way, if you have an adverse reaction it won't be severe and you'll know exactly which supplement is causing it.

Second, for all readers, review the box below that lists other conditions that could disqualify you from taking *any* amino acids *at all*.

Before Taking *Any* Aminos: General Precautions to Rule Out

Please check off any items below that apply to you. Before taking any amino acids, consult a knowledgeable health practitioner about any items you check off here. If you decide to continue with a trial, start at half doses.

☐ Are you taking any medications on a regular basis? Discuss potential interactions between the aminos you might take and any medications you are taking with your prescribing doctor or a pharmacist.

☐ Are you regularly consuming alcohol, cannabis, or any other psychoactive nonprescription drug? If so, do not trial or use aminos while under the influence.

☐ Do you have a bipolar disorder, major depression, schizophrenia, or other mental illness? If so, the aminos can have negative or unpredictable effects. If these conditions are now stabilized on medication, however, the aminos can be helpful with any remaining mood or craving symptom (if approved by your prescriber and monitored by this or another knowledgeable professional).

☐ Do you have an ulcer? Amino acids are slightly acidic and have, though rarely, caused stomach pain.

☐ Do you have any serious physical illness? Your doctor may know about specific contraindications to the aminos related to your health problem or the medications used to treat it. Let the doctor know that the aminos can help you eat a healthier diet, lose weight, and improve your mood. Depression, for example, is very common in conditions like diabetes and stroke. (Feeling happier on the aminos improved a stroke victim's recovery dramatically in just one week!)

☐ Do you have liver or kidney disease (e.g., hepatitis, lupus)? Since the aminos are processed in these organs, their use *must* be discussed with your doctor (we've only had one lupus patient, but her kidneys could not tolerate any aminos).

☐ Are you pregnant or nursing? If you are, discuss the aminos with your OB/GYN before trialing them. We recommend a complete amino blend (which all OB/GYNs have liked) instead, e.g., *Total Amino Solution* by Genesa. It provides nice results. If a plasma amino acid test and/or plasma or platelet neurotransmitter tests (page 285) show deficiency, certain individual aminos may be warranted, (e.g., for insomnia, depression, or excessive weight gain). Otherwise, they're discouraged.

CAUTION: Even if your doctor agrees that you can try an amino acid (or any other nutrients), if you experience discomfort of any kind after taking any, stop immediately. If you aren't sure which supplement is causing the problem, stop all until the discomfort passes, then slowly reintroduce them one by one to find out. Additional contraindications may be identified that I am not now aware of (e.g., problems with particular brands or products). I will post any I discover on cravingcure.com/aminonews.

STEP 4: GO SUPPLEMENT SHOPPING

Where can you find the aminos you need? You may be surprised at how widely available they are. You can buy them at your nearest supplement supply outlets like health food stores, vitamin stores, drugstores, supermarkets, or stores like Costco. You can shop all over the Internet at sites like drbvitamins .com, PureFormulas.com, iHerb.com, and Amazon.com to name just a few. You can visit cravingcure.com/shop where all of the supplements that we use at our clinic are available, including a Trialing Kit with samples of all the aminos.

Look for aminos in capsules, unless otherwise recommended in Chapter 12. (Large tablets are often too big and can be harder to swallow; they take a while to dissolve, and contain more additives.) Before you buy anything, of course you'll need to study the section(s) in Chapter 12 on the specific amino acids your Craving Type(s) call for, and the section at the end of that chapter on the support nutrients you'll need.

Try to get aminos with no other added nutrients, for example no added vitamin B$_6$.

STEP 5: BEGIN YOUR AMINO TRIALS

Once you have your aminos in hand, start trying them out one by one, using the specific trialing suggestions for each that you'll find in Chapter 12. Set aside at least half an hour for each amino trialed (you may need to raise or lower your starting dose). Use your Trialing Record (on page 288 or cravingcure.com/tracking tools) to carefully report on your trialing experiences. Don't trust your memory, especially if you have to trial more than one amino.

Begin your trials with the amino identified as the solution to your highest-scoring Craving Type, as ranked in Step 2, page 155. *Note:* A stimulating Craving Type 5 amino would need to be trialed before 3 PM. *All the others can be trialed any time of the day or night.*

Caution: Do not take any aminos that your Craving-Type Questionnaire indicates you do *not* need. *Do not skip meals on any trialing day.*

If you can, have an observant friend or family member with you when you do your trials. It's more fun and an outside view of your responses is often very helpful. Let your trialing buddy see your completed Craving-Type Questionnaire and Profile first. He or she may surprise you with insightful feedback on your self-scoring (e.g., "you *are* irritable!"). Family members tend to notice even little post-amino responses right away, often before the trialer does! Include their observations before and during a trial in your Trialing Records.

Amino Trial Dosing

- Start with the lowest trial dose of your first amino. Note the exact recommended starting dose from Chapter 12. Factor in *age* and *sensitivity*: Most adults start at 500 mg, the usual amount found in amino supplement capsules. (Type 4s start with less, as you'll see in Chapter 12.)
- Toddlers and sensitive older children or adults: trial only a pinch. Open a capsule and put a pinch in the mouth (¼–½ capsule if they're not ultra-sensitive, mixed with a little water or mashed fruit).
- Nonsensitive child 5–13 years: ⅓–½ dose.
- Nonsensitive child over 13 years: 1 full adult dose.

- Increase dose until symptoms are gone. Increase very gradually for the very young or sensitive.
- Stop with any adverse reaction.

Open one capsule and empty the recommended amount of the powder into 2 to 3 tablespoons of water in a small cup. We use Dixie cups at the clinic. Stir the mixture as best you can and pour it into your mouth. Some aminos, particularly Type 1 Depressed Craver's tryptophan, can be hard to mix with water, and you'll end up having to suck some of the powder off of your stirring spoon. You could also mix the aminos with a spoonful of mashed banana, yam, or applesauce, especially for children. *Note:* If you or your child find any amino too unpleasant-tasting, just swallow the closed capsule. For a child, remember to empty out part of the capsule first.

Wait! Don't swallow it right away (unless you're taking a closed capsule). Swish it around in your mouth for at least a minute and then swallow. Be sure you get all the contents down, even if you do have to lick the spoon. Amino acids are fastest absorbed through the mucous lining of your mouth and reach your brain somewhat more quickly than when they're swallowed in sealed capsules or in compressed tablets. If this procedure is too unpleasant or complicated and you opt instead to take the whole, unopened capsule, just wait five to ten minutes instead of three for a reaction.

Be observant. Don't distract yourself with other activities while trialing (like watching TV, using your phone, or surfing the Internet).

If you get little or no benefit in fifteen minutes, raise your dose one notch, as indicated for your particular Craving Type in Chapter 12, until your cravings (and probably several negative mood symptoms) disappear. For adults this typically means taking a second capsule. (You can swallow this one whole if you hated the taste of the first one you emptied into the cup.) Maximum doses will be indicated for each Craving Type in Chapter 12. The basic rule is to *raise the amino dose until you get either a positive or a negative response.* Some people respond right away. Some even point to where they feel the aminos entering a particular part of their brain! If the positive response is faint or subtle, try another dose *(up to four).*

Variations in Response

Please do not get overzealous and start with the highest possible dose. More is *not* necessarily better. As you trial each of the aminos recommended for your Craving Type(s), go slowly. You don't want to risk unwanted side effects by starting at too high a dose. Some people are, as my senior nutritionist, Karla Maree, calls them, "pixie dust people." They are so responsive to even small doses that a single whole capsule of an amino can be too much. If you aren't sure what kind of a supplement responder you are, start any trial with half a capsule. Too low a dose might leave you feeling nothing, but you can always take the other half or more if nothing happens in fifteen minutes.

Genetic Variations

Native North Americans have been by far the quickest and most sensitive amino-responders, in my experience. A little of any kind of supplement seems to go a long way with this group. We have not noticed the same sensitivity in the Native South Americans, Asians, Africans, Europeans, or Middle Easterners we've worked with. Native (North) Americans have told me that, as hunter-gatherers, they have "the thrifty gene," which allows them to make the most of *anything* they ingest. This also accounts for their terrible sensitivity to toxic substances like sugar, alcohol, and drugs. Their quick response to aminos means that those in this group, the hardest hit by our current diet, often recover the fastest!

If a first dose, or a second, makes you feel nothing, try a third, all in the same period of thirty to sixty minutes. It's very unusual for a third dose to elicit no response. We typically stop trialing at three capsules if clients experience no effects, and begin trialing the alternative amino. This is why we are glad to have two amino options for most craving types. If one doesn't work, the other usually does. The rare instance of someone not responding to either amino option is addressed in Chapter 12, in each of the five Craving Type sections.

Wait at least fifteen minutes after a trial before you eat a meal, and ninety minutes after a meal to do a trial. Why? Because all of the aminos in the protein you eat at mealtime will compete with the targeted amino in your capsules for the limited entry slots into your brain.

For your second trial, and any subsequent trials, follow these guidelines:

Wait till you're sure you're clear on how you've been affected by trial number one and that you have recorded that first experience in the *Trialing Record*. Then take the starting trial dose of the amino acid indicated for your second highest Craving Type (of course, only if your second highest score is above the optimal range).

You'll trial your second, third, fourth, or fifth aminos, as you have time in the next few days, depending on how many Craving Types you've identified and how much free time you have. Usually you'll be able to identify your optimal dose in one day. But if, for any reason, it takes two days to identify the right dosing, no problem.

Neutralizing Any Adverse Reactions to Aminos

We've found that, in about one out of ten trialing sessions, a client has a negative reaction to an amino. They're usually mild reactions: a slight headache, a twitching eyelid, a feeling of edginess or fatigue. Usually there's no explanation, just individual biochemistry at work. Sometimes they just haven't read or scored their questionnaire properly and they trial something they don't really need. Or they took too much, not realizing they were sensitive responders. Adverse reactions later on are even more rare but can indicate that the amino is no longer needed, that the brain deficiency problem has been repaired! Like too much gas in the tank.

Whether an adverse reaction occurs during a trial or later:

- Immediately stop taking the amino acid that triggered your adverse reaction. If it's a sublingual tablet, spit it out. Rinse your mouth.

- If you're not sure which amino acid triggered your response, stop any of the amino acids you had taken most recently before it happened.

- Neutralize the adverse reaction by taking 1,000 to 2,000 mg of vitamin C powder dissolved in four ounces of water. The shopping directions for each Craving Type will remind you to purchase vitamin C as powder or in 1,000 mg capsules. If you have capsules, open and empty 1,000 to 2,000 mg into a glass of water. If you have some Emergen-C packets (the low-sugar version with MSM), that's even better for this purpose. (The Craving Cure Trialing Kits come with the packets included.) Your symptoms should clear in five to ten minutes.

Caution: Do not take more than 1,000 mg if loose bowels are a problem, as excessive amounts of vitamin C can cause bowels to loosen.

Does the vitamin C detox work for everyone? Almost. So far it has a 95 percent success rate with clients and trainees. Trialing aminos (which I started doing in 1996) has worked so well, for so many years in our clinic, that I began to add an amino trialing option to my weekend presentations for professionals. Out of a typical audience of 100 people, two or three would have a mild adverse reaction. In almost every case the neutralizing vitamin C took care of it in moments. When I've asked these participants about their negative reactions, it almost always turns out that they had trialed an amino acid that they did not need, just out of curiosity. In the very rare instances in which the vitamin C didn't have an immediate effect, the symptoms cleared within a few hours.

Notes for Craving Type 5 and children: For those who get overstimulated after trialing either of the Craving Type 5 amino, we usually suggest one 500-mg tryptophan capsule or 100–200 mg of GABA to neutralize the reaction.

For children: Use smaller doses per the dosing guidelines above.

STEP 6: SET UP YOUR DAILY SUPPLEMENT SCHEDULE

When you've discovered through trialing which and how many amino supplements to take in total, you'll create a daily schedule for taking them, using the Supplement Schedule, page 290. You'll notice that there are three primary times for taking your aminos: right before breakfast, right before lunch, and afternoon. Some aminos might also be taken later, if late-night eating or insomnia is a problem for you.

Here is an example of a daily supplement schedule of a craver with Types 1 and 3:

A Sample Amino Schedule of a Types 1 & 3 Craver

AMINO ACIDS	BEFORE BREAKFAST	BEFORE LUNCH	MIDAFTER-NOON	BEFORE DINNER	NIGHTTIME
Tryptophan 500 mg			2		2
DLPA 500 mg	2	2	1		

Your schedule will change as you adjust your amino doses, so keep extra blank copies around to update, downloaded and printed from cravingcure.com/trackingtools. Keep all copies of your schedules to refer back to.

Organizing Your Aminos

Once you have your aminos scheduled, assemble your supplements in a tidy pack for the next day or week so as to not miss a dose. One way to organize them is in small, labeled plastic zipper bags. Each one will contain a specific, scheduled dose for a specific time of the day. For the schedule charted above, for example, the zipper bag for the midafternoon would contain two 500-mg capsules of tryptophan and one of DLPA.

You can prepare on Sunday for the whole next week or the night before for the following day. It should only take a few minutes. You can then throw them in your purse/pocket/briefcase. For any before breakfast or nighttime doses taken at home, you can put supplement bottles with a glass of water on your nightstand as a reminder to take them when you wake up or go to bed. Of course, if you're at home a lot you can just use the bottles all the time. (Some clients keep a set of bottles at work, as well.)

You can also find a stacking or other supplement container that has several compartments that you can label. You can take the whole thing or individual compartments with you.

How Not to Forget Your Aminos

Remembering to take your supplements can be hard to do, *especially if you need to take afternoon doses*. Since most relapses occur sometime in the late afternoon to early evening, we recommend that our clients set alarms on their cell phones or computers to remind them to take those critical afternoon supplements, and any others they tend to forget.

STEP 7: CLEAR YOUR BRAIN FIELD: EXPEL THOSE BRAIN-DISRUPTIVE TECHNO-KARBZ

During week one, as soon as you have trialed your aminos and begun following your supplement schedule, begin making your dietary changes. (Review Part IV, Craving-Free Eating, beforehand, of course.) On the aminos, your cravings will be subsiding, so now is the time to make your dietary move. The Techno-Karbz you're now eating are compromising the areas in your brain that your aminos will be working to repair. When you replace them with lots of amino-rich protein, vital vegetables, and friendly fats, you will be even more immune to cravings than the amino acids, alone, can make you.

STEP 8: FINE-TUNE YOUR AMINOS: MONITOR YOUR CRAVING TYPE SCORES AND ADJUST YOUR DOSES

Each week, you'll fill out a new Mini Craving-Type Questionnaire and compare those new scores to prior scores to make sure that they are actually dropping, and by how much.

If any of your scores stop dropping before they get down to zero, raise the indicated amino doses one notch, or more, as needed. Trial the new doses for two full days before deciding whether to raise it further at one or more of the scheduled times.

If any of your Craving Types' symptoms aren't lessening fast enough, review the specific instructions in Chapter 12 for that Craving Type whose symptoms persist. Look for suggestions you might have missed about how to further maximize your benefits.

Record any new dosing changes, with the date, on your Supplement Schedule and in your Daily Log to help track its effects.

CAN YOU TAKE TOO MUCH OF AN AMINO?

Anyone *could* take too much of *any* nutrient for their particular system. We've even seen people overdose on carrots: the beta-carotene turned their skins orange!

With the aminos, if we see any adverse reaction after our client has been taking an amino for several months with benefit, it's usually due to something called the Reverse Effect: *too much* of any nutrient can cause the same symptoms as *too little* of that same nutrient. That means that if you take too much of a calming amino, for example, you could experience deficiency symptoms like anxiety or fatigue. That's why we begin with low starting doses and find the right dose by raising the dose (or lowering it in some cases), as needed. That's also the reason for reevaluating your craving symptoms weekly with your Mini Craving-Type Questionnaire, to make sure that any negative effects go away and don't come back.

Truthfully this rarely happens. Because of our amino tailoring process, the Reverse Effect is a very uncommon occurrence among our clients. We almost never see it during trialing, but clients have sometimes raised their doses too high later and encountered it. When this has happened, we've suggested lowering or stopping all doses of that amino, neutralizing the adverse effect with vitamin C powder, and watching the symptoms for that Craving Type over the next week to see if they will need to resume taking it at a lower dose or not.

The comforting thing about an amino "overdose" is that any negative reaction typically stops within an hour after the last dose of the offending nutrient. Even better, the vitamin C detox detailed on (page 162) can stop most any discomfort in minutes.

If you're taking more than one kind of amino at the same time, how would you know which nutrient was the offender? If you're not sure, stop taking all of the aminos you'd taken most recently before the reaction and, as soon as the negative symptoms are gone, retrial those aminos, one at a time, until you isolate the culprit. Here are some tips:

Possible Mild Adverse Reactions to Particular Aminos

IF YOU START TO HAVE:	LOWER OR STOP THE FOLLOWING:
LOOSE BOWELS	5-HTP (or vitamin C or magnesium)
NAUSEA	5-HTP
BLOOD PRESSURE UP	Tyrosine, LPA, DLPA
BLOOD PRESSURE DOWN	GABA, Theanine
TIRED/LETHARGIC	Tryptophan, GABA, Theanine
HEADACHE	Tyrosine, LPA, DLPA
JITTERYNESS	Tyrosine, LPA, DLPA
POOR SLEEP	Tyrosine, LPA, DLPA, 5-HTP, melatonin

Fortunately only very rarely, for no reason that we can understand, someone who has high scores for a particular Craving Type and typically tolerates supplements well, will not tolerate the indicated amino well. Usually the person has started at too high a dose or has not carefully reviewed the general precautions here in Step 3 page 156 or the specific ones for each Craving Type in Chapter 12.

You can almost always neutralize any adverse reactions by following the simple directions on page 192. If not, it will typically fade out on its own within a few hours. We have seen discomfort that lasted longer and did not respond to vitamin C in only three cases over a period of thirty years.

STEP 9: TERMINATE YOUR AMINOS

How do you know when you no longer need an amino? There should be no hurry to terminate. Even if the expense is weighing on you, you can't rush your brain. Look for other ways to save. And don't worry about becoming dependent on aminos for life—you won't get "hooked." Be assured that aminos are absolutely not addictive.

If you take too many aminos, or take them for too long, you can actually start *disliking* their effects. You'll need to stop using them immediately if that happens. Typically you'll find that your original craving symptoms don't come back. Many clients quit taking their aminos by accident: They run out of them or forget them at home when they go away for the weekend. When they do this in the first month or two they usually regret it and get right back on them. Eventually, though, they don't miss them when they forget to take them and they realize that they just don't need them regularly anymore. It's one of the reasons, as an addiction specialist, that I love the aminos. They are healing, not addictive. No tapering is required and there are no withdrawal symptoms.

Most of our *adult* clients have needed to stay on all of their aminos for at least three months, some for a year, some older clients for longer. *Children* vary from one week to three months. *Teens* vary from three to six months. Those with long years of severe bingeing or bulimia, or with a family history (a genetic legacy) of food, alcohol, or other addiction tend to need them longer (especially if they, themselves, have had more than one addiction). In these cases, at least one year is usually required. But amino termination is a very individual process. Out best guide is the following:

- Most *adult* clients do best waiting until the cravings and other negative symptoms of a Craving Type have been gone for two months and their Mini Questionnaire scores are consistently 0–2. *Children* and *teens* can try quitting after one week or one month, respectively.

- Remove aminos from your Supplement Schedule one by one.

- Live without that amino for forty-eight hours. If your cravings or other symptoms return, retrial that amino, starting at the lowest dose. You may be ready to lower, but not yet eliminate, your dose. If not, go back up to your most recent dose for another month or two and lower your dose in stages before you try stopping altogether again.

If your cravings and other symptoms do *not* come back, do a samba around the house—you've cured a supposedly incurable brain defect.

Rescore your Mini Craving-Type Questionnaire once a month for a year to monitor your symptoms while you focus on consuming lots of protein as well as traditional fats and carbohydrates to keep your brain's neurotransmitter and blood sugar levels strong.

A Type 2 Termination Story

Here's an example: A prediabetic Type 2 Crashed Craver, after four months on the program, finds her symptom scores close to zero for two months. Her glucose and insulin levels have also been in the solidly normal range for two months. She stops all of her glutamine for twenty-four hours. Meanwhile, she keeps taking all of her other aminos and her support nutrients. She gets a return of Type 2 cravings after four days, so she takes two glutamine, at the times that she was taking three glutamine before, to see if her cravings totally disappear again. They don't, so she goes back to three throughout the day, just as before. She tries quitting entirely again three months later. This time her cravings do not come back. She does the samba, but leaves some glutamine in the fridge, in case.

Now that you have a good idea of how the breakthrough process will work, Chapter 12 will give you the specific details. You won't have to read the whole chapter. You'll only have to read about *your* own Craving Types.

12

Your Personal Breakthrough: Specific Directions for Each Craving Type

N**OW THAT YOU HAVE THE** breakthrough basics, it's time for amino action. Here you'll find directions for eliminating your own particular type (or types) of craving. These directions have been defined, refined, and streamlined by my staff over the past thirty years in more than twenty thousand individual sessions with our clients. This is the most important chapter in the book, but you won't have to read all of it, unless you have all five types of craving, because the chapter is divided into five sections, one for each of the five Craving Types. To make it easy for you to locate your target sections, we've put the page number for each of the five sections in the book's Contents. Each section will contain the following amino action steps, as they pertain to particular Craving Types: *taking precautions, shopping, trialing, dosing,* and *terminating.*

The chapter concludes with two topics pertinent to every Craving Type: The first is the story of how a client with *all five* Craving Types won her Craving Cure. The second has to do with the *Support Nutrient* supplements that all types need to take to optimize the aminos' effects. The very last page of the chapter consists of a Cheat Sheet, a chart of all the aminos and support nutrients mentioned in the entire chapter, along with their dosing ranges and typical times to take them.

TYPE 1: CRAVING ELIMINATION FOR THE DEPRESSED CRAVER

TYPE 1 AMINOS AND CO-NUTRIENTS

Type 1 Amino Acids and Their Expected Benefits

AMINOS NEEDED BY TYPE 1s:	BENEFITS PROVIDED:
5-HTP	No cravings in the afternoon, evening, or winter
or	Positive outlook
Tryptophan	Emotionªl flexibility
or	Self-confidence
Melatonin (for sleeping)	Sense of humor
	Healthy sleep

Type 1 Aminos

Tryptophan and *5-HTP (5-hydroxy-tryptophan).* Types 1s are the most common of all cravers and their deficiency symptoms the most extensive, so it's fortunate that there are not one, but two forms of the amino acid tryptophan available for using as Type 1 brain fuels. In our experience, 5-HTP and tryptophan convert equally well and equally quickly into sunny, craving-eliminating serotonin for about 80 percent of Type 1 cravers. About 20 percent of our Type 1 clients do better on one amino than the other. Use the chart below to help you decide which to try first. If the form you choose disagrees with you or disappoints you in any way, you'll have a great alternative. Some clients take both: the somewhat more-energizing 5-HTP in the day, and the mellower tryptophan in the evening or at bedtime.

Comparison of 5-HTP and Tryptophan

5-HTP	TRYPTOPHAN
Somewhat more energizing.	More sleep-promoting.
Smaller dose is easier to swallow.	Provides broader nutritional benefits so preferred for those who are most nutritionally depleted, and for children.
Easier to find and less expensive.	Online sources and many health stores now carry it. Prices are dropping.
Consistent effectiveness between brands.	More variation in results between brands (see Shopping Suggestions).
Occasionally causes *insomnia* if taken at night or *nausea* or *diarrhea* (especially if capsules also contain vitamin B_6).	Does not cause sleep or GI problems.

Whether you start with 5-HTP or tryptophan, if your first choice does not eliminate your Type 1 symptoms after a trial of up to three doses, you should try the alternate choice.

Melatonin. Are you a late-night or middle-of-the-night craver? Are you unable to fall asleep or stay asleep without your "midnight snack" (or even with it)? Do you worry and ruminate instead of getting to sleep? If neither tryptophan nor 5-HTP reliably get you to sleep by ten PM, try adding melatonin.

Melatonin, a hormone made out of serotonin in your brain's pineal gland, is specifically intended to get you to sleep at the right time. Tryptophan and 5-HTP supplements are both converted into serotonin, and serotonin is supposed to convert, in part, into melatonin—starting in the afternoon. But you may be so low in serotonin that it will take a while before your tryptophan or 5-HTP supplements can provide enough serotonin to take care of both your daytime craving and mood needs and your nighttime, melatonin-building needs. A dose of melatonin by ten PM, if you are a night owl, and/or in the night if you wake up between two and four AM, or too early, can help you get the sleep you need and free up some of your serotonin to do other important jobs, like stopping bedtime snacking. An added bonus is that melatonin is also a potent antioxidant that will help you get your health back.

Note: If 5-HTP causes worse insomnia and tryptophan and melatonin don't help much either, read about GABA deficiency and adrenal cortisol excess, the other common causes of chronic sleeplessness, in Chapter 9, page 133.

TYPE 1 PRECAUTIONS

There are certain medications and health conditions that warrant caution when contemplating using the Type 1 aminos. I have marked with **Xs** which supplements might have what adverse effects.

POSSIBLE CONTRAINDICATIONS	5-HTP	TRYPTOPHAN	MELATONIN	RISK LEVEL
If you take a serotonin-targeted SSRI antidepressant (including Zoloft, Lexapro, Prozac, Paxil), a tricyclic (including Pamelor, Norpramin), or an MAOI antidepressant, check with your pharmacist or prescriber to get information	X	X		**Moderate to severe** DO NOT USE TYPE 1 AMINOS IF YOU ARE ON AN MAOI. IF YOU ARE TAKING A TRICYCLIC OR SSRI, CHECK WITH YOUR PRESCRIBER. DO NOT TAKE IN

on possible adverse interactions				ANY CASE IF YOU ARE TAKING MORE THAN ONE SSRI. (If you're on only one SSRI, see box below and check with your prescriber.)
You regularly take anti-migraine, antimicrobial, or other serotonin-targeted drugs (e.g., Imitrex, linezolid, ecstasy)	X	X		**Moderate to severe** Check with your prescriber or pharmacist
Asthma	X	X	X	**Mild to moderate, but rare***
A carcinoid tumor	X	X		DO NOT USE**

* Asthma We've seen five clients in thirty years who've had this reaction to Type 1 aminos.
** We've never seen anyone who has been diagnosed with one.

For Type 1 Cravers on Antidepressant Medications

Up to 13 percent of Americans, including many of our incoming clients, are using a serotonin reuptake inhibiting antidepressant (SSRI). If you are using *one* such medication (but *not two or more*—as per the Precautions chart above), and would like to trial one of the Type 1 aminos for a few weeks *without going off of your meds,* consider the following process that has worked *so well* for so many of our clients. *Note*: I have written a whole chapter in my book *The Mood Cure,* and more on moodcure.com, about this process:

Caution: *We have found that taking a Type 1 amino, even short term, with two or more serotonin-boosting medications does not work well. We have known symptoms of the serotonin syndrome to result, especially if the Type 1 amino was taken too close to the medication. We now ask our clients to work with their doctor to go down to one SSRI before trying a Type 1 amino. (The other aminos are fine to take at any time.)*

Caution: *In our experience, Type 1 aminos do* not *help much with major (unipolar) depression, bipolar depression, or other severe or suicidal kinds of depression.*

- Ask your prescribing physician about your interest in trialing 5-HTP or tryptophan. Explain that you will not take it within five hours of the time(s) you take your SSRI medication. Hopefully you can take your meds in the morning, since the Type 1 aminos are needed most in the afternoon and evening. We have found this to be a safe and effective way for hundreds of our clients to test out the value of tryptophan or 5-HTP, without risking the loss of the benefits of their medication.

■ With your physician's okay (they don't usually object), trial and take your Type 1 amino for two weeks *five hours away from the time you take your medication*. If it works well for your cravings and improves your mood (as it usually does), you and your doctor can decide whether you should stay on the amino acid and taper off your medication or stop any Type 1 amino. We do not know if prolonged use of *an amino and your medication together* would be safe, so we have never recommended it. Most of our clients on antidepressants have opted to try going off their medications and it has worked very well for almost all of them. We always have them read the chapter called Alternatives to Antidepressants in *The Mood Cure,* and work with their doctors to develop a taper-off plan first. Because they are on the aminos while they taper their medications, they have little or no withdrawal discomfort and they typically continue to feel much better than they had felt on their meds, with no side effects!

TYPE 1 SHOPPING, BRANDS, AND FORMULATIONS

Remember that you can order Amino Trialing Kits and full supplies online at cravingcure.com/shop or by phone (415) 383–3611.

5-HTP. This amino came out in 1997. At first, there were inconsistencies in the effects between brands. Since 2010, though, we have run into no inconsistencies between brands, so any brand should do. *Avoid 5-HTP products that also contain vitamin B$_6$ (or P5P, another form of B$_6$), which can result in nausea.*

Use 50 mg 5-HTP products instead of higher dose products to give you more low-dosing flexibility. Or, for kids, 2.5 mg flavorless tabs by Life-link.

Tryptophan. Look for at least 98 percent purity or better from any product. There is some variation in purity and effectiveness between products. The consistently effective products we use are sold on our website: cravingcure.com/shop.

Among the products available in stores, Ajinomoto's (as AjiPure or tryptopure) tryptophan is made to a high standard and many products contain it. This Japanese company, which now has huge worldwide distribution, was a pioneer in amino acid development and the purity of its tryptophan has never been questioned. Jarrow's Tryptophan Peptide product may be the most potent, at 650 mg per tablet, but it is made from milk, not yeasts, so it is more allergenic. (Remember, the yeasts that aminos are made from are not the living, invasive yeast strain called *Candida albicans*.)

Use 500-mg tryptophan products. This is the lowest standard dose available. (It is comparable in anti-craving effect to 50 mg of 5-HTP.)

Melatonin

This is a very popular product in our era of insomnia, so you can find it everywhere that supplements are sold. At least initially, choose a brand that has no added herbs or nutrients. The typical range is from .5 to 3 mg. Try .5 or 1 mg first. Low doses can be surprisingly effective. If you find you need to raise your dose significantly, you can buy a higher dose product later.

There are two types of melatonin to choose from:

1. Instant release (.5–5.0 mg)
2. Extended release (1–3 mg)

Most instant-release products seem equally effective and work well if you have trouble falling asleep. Extended-release supplements are ideal if you wake up in the middle of the night and aren't able to fall back to sleep without a struggle. The most effective time-release product we've found is NOW Foods' Two-Stage Melatonin (1 mg). Clients with *both* kinds of sleep problems often benefit from a combination of these two melatonin formulations, one of each by ten PM, to start.

TYPE 1 TRIALING

Follow the general directions for trialing in Chapter 11. (The Trialing Kit at cravingcure.com/shop contains both tryptophan and 5-HTP.) Watch for the emergence of sunny feelings that dispel Type 1 cravings. Some people even report that, for them, colors get brighter during these trials!

5-HTP:

Start with a 50-mg capsule, the standard starting dose.

or

Tryptophan:

Start with a 500-mg capsule, the standard starting dose.

If *sleep* is a problem that is not resolved by the above two aminos:

Melatonin:

For trouble falling asleep, try instant-release melatonin (.5 to 6 mg). For those of you who can fall asleep but don't *stay* asleep, try time-release melatonin (1 to 3 mg). If you have both types of insomnia, try both types of melatonin. See the dosing instructions that follow, as this is an unusual trial. (The Trialing Kit, available on cravingcure.com/shop, can include both types of melatonin on request.)

TYPE 1 DOSING AND SCHEDULE

5-HTP. A dose ranges from 50 to 200 mg (meaning one to four 50-mg capsules) per dose. An average ongoing dose is 100 mg, meaning two 50-mg capsules twice a day, with optional additional doses morning or bedtime if needed for mood, craving, or sleeplessness. We have never needed to go over 200 mg three to four times a day.

5-HTP Dosing Example for a Type 1 Craver

	BEFORE BREAKFAST*	BEFORE LUNCH*	MIDAFTER-NOON	BEFORE DINNER	NIGHT-TIME
5-HTP 50-mg caps		1–4	1–4	1–4	

*Optional for unusual cravings, mood, or sleep needs in the mornings or middle of night.

Tryptophan. A dose can range from 500 to 2,000 mg, that is, one to four 500-mg capsules. An average ongoing dose is 1,000 mg twice a day. Occasionally someone will need as much as 2,000 mg (four 500-mg capsules) per dose, two or three times a day, for a total of 4,000 to 6,000 mg, but usually not for more than a few months.

Tryptophan Dosing Example for a Sleepless Type 1 Craver

	BEFORE BREAKFAST*	BEFORE LUNCH*	MIDAFTER-NOON	BEFORE DINNER	NIGHT-TIME*
Tryptophan 500-mg caps		1–4	1–4	1–4	

* Optional for unusual cravings, mood, or sleep needs in the mornings or middle of night.

Melatonin for Sleep Trouble. If neither tryptophan nor 5-HTP at bedtime get you all the way to deep sleep, you can add melatonin to them.

If you *have trouble falling asleep,* start with a dose of .5 to 1 mg 15–30 minutes before you should go to sleep. If you're not asleep in 30 minutes, take another dose of melatonin. Trial up to 6 mg if needed.

If you *wake up in the night* and can't get back to sleep, take a time-release product (1–3 mg) at ten PM or bedtime, whichever is earlier (nine hours before you need to wake up). The average dose of NOW Foods Two-Stage melatonin is 1 mg. Others are usually 3 mg. Increase the dose the next night, if needed. (Those with digestive problems may prefer time-release skin patches.) If necessary, try adding 1–3 mg instant-release melatonin if you still wake up in the night.

If you *have trouble both falling asleep <u>and</u> staying asleep*, take both an instant- *and* a time-release at bedtime, typically not more than a total of 6 mg.

After using melatonin, if you wake up groggy or have disturbed dreams, you'll know that your dose was too high. Adjust your dose downward the next night. If your sleep problems don't resolve in a few nights, discontinue the melatonin and consider the sleep suggestions in Chapter 9, page 137.

Melatonin Dosing Guidelines

	BEDTIME
Instant-release melatonin .5–6 mg For those who **can't get to sleep**	X
Two-stage melatonin 1–3 mg for those who wake up in the night.	X

TYPE 1 TERMINATION

When your Type 1 craving scores are consistently under 2 on the mini questionnaire's scale of 0 to 10 and you've been feeling optimistic and sleeping well for at least two months, you may be ready to try lowering or discontinuing your 5-HTP or tryptophan. If you stop any Type 1 amino and find that you still need it, try terminating again every month or so. Most of our clients need it for six months, some longer.

Since stress can suppress serotonin and melatonin levels, keep your favorite Type 1 aminos on hand to take during stressful times, as needed, in the future.

Regarding melatonin, keep in mind that melatonin levels tend to drop over the years, so you might need to take this supplement longer.

TYPE 2: CRAVING ELIMINATION FOR THE CRASHED CRAVER

TYPE 2 AMINOS AND CO-NUTRIENTS

Glutamine. This remarkable blood-sugar regulator and craving eradicator gives a sense of evenness and groundedness. It takes effect in seconds if dissolved in the mouth (it has a pleasant taste).

Chromium and Biotin. As additional supports, specifically for Type 2 Cravers, this mineral and vitamin can further stabilize blood sugar levels and insulin function. These two nutrients are included in the True Balance multi we recommend for all Type 2s. These nutrients are included in some other multivitamin/minerals but not in all, and not typically at the same doses.

TYPE 2 PRECAUTIONS

We have seen or heard of very few adverse reactions to this much researched and lauded amino supplement, but here are two that we *have* seen a handful of times.

POSSIBLE CONTRAINDICATIONS	GLUTAMINE	RISK LEVEL
Rise in a Diabetic's blood sugar: Typically diabetics get wonderful blood sugar stabilization from glutamine, but on rare occasions they find that it *raises blood sugar slightly. Monitor your blood glucose levels while you take this supplement, if you are diabetic.* We have seen this ourselves only once.	X	Mild
In the brain, glutamine regularly converts into the excitatory neurotransmitter glutamate, and vice versa. The two keep in proper balance that way, but if too much glutamate is made, an agitated	X	Mild to Severe

POSSIBLE CONTRAINDICATIONS	GLUTAMINE	RISK LEVEL
reaction can take place in those who are on the bipolar spectrum (whether they've been diagnosed or not). They might get depression relief, they might get an energy surge, or they might become manic. We have seen this perhaps 10 times.		

TYPE 2 SHOPPING, BRANDS, AND FORMULATIONS

Glutamine. Shopping for this Type 2 amino is straightforward. Glutamine is easy to find and buy. Our clients have reported identical success with every brand of 500-mg glutamine capsules they've tried.

This is the only amino also readily available as loose powder. We prefer to use capsules instead. Powder (which you will find everywhere because it is popular with body builders) is less convenient to take and less precise to measure, especially while you need doses 2–4 times a day.

TYPE 2 TRIALING

Glutamine's mildly sweet flavor makes it pleasant to trial. Follow the general directions for trialing in Chapter 11.

This trial must be done between meals and away from snacks. If you're in a "crash and crave" state when you trial, all the better! Those unpleasant symptoms should fade within minutes after taking some glutamine. You should notice feeling "even," "balanced," as well.

TYPE 2 DOSING AND SCHEDULE

Glutamine. A dose ranges from 500 to 2,000 mg (meaning one to four 500-mg capsules). An average ongoing dose is 1,000 mg, meaning two 500-mg capsules.

Timing. Because between-meal blood sugar control is so critical to Type 2s, the timing is a bit different from other aminos. Take your dose of glutamine at the following times: before breakfast, ideally upon waking, at midmorning a few hours after breakfast, and midafternoon a few hours after lunch. *If you take other aminos, it is fine to take them at the same time as your glutamine.*

If you wake up hungry for sweets or starches in the night (or have Type 2 cravings at any other time), try an extra dose: one capsule opened under your tongue at the moment the craving hits is amazingly fast-acting.

Avoid skipping meals or undereating. If you tend to undereat or skip meals, snacks, or your glutamine, your Type 2 symptoms will come back. They will respond almost instantly, though, to an "emergency" dose of a glutamine capsule opened under your tongue (they taste good). Keep some capsules handy at all times, if you can, for this purpose.

Glutamine Dosing Guidelines

	BEFORE BREAKFAST	BEFORE LUNCH	MIDAFTER- NOON	NIGHT- TIME*
Glutamine 500-mg caps	1–4	1–4	1–4	(1–4)

*Optional—if your blood sugar tends to drop late in the evening, or during the night, or you want bedtime Techno-Karbz.

TYPE 2 AMINO TERMINATION

After a few months of mostly zero Type 2 symptoms and regular, anti-craving meals (and snacks, as needed), stop your glutamine following the general directions in the previous chapter. If you have a family history of hypoglycemia, diabetes, or alcoholism, you may need to continue for a year, or even longer, as needed, before you can say good-bye to glutamine.

Special Supplement Support for Diabetics

We've been using diabetes-targeted foods and nutrients at our clinic for years. Now, though, there is much exciting and solid research on the use of additional nutrient supplements. Learn about it here. You can also pursue it through the references in the Notes section on page 375.

- Take any of the amino acids that your Craving-Type Profile indicates, always including glutamine, of course!

- Take all of the Support Nutrients recommended at the end of this chapter. The particular multivitamin-mineral I recommend provides extra doses of diabetes-healing chromium and biotin, along with zinc and the B vitamins. (*Note:* Don't use selenium beyond the small dose in this multiple. Higher levels can *contribute* to insulin resistance.)

- It's very important to get the vitamin D test described in Tracking and Testing Tools, page 267 and take this vitamin as indicated there to keep your levels between 35 and 70.

Also consider the nutritional suggestions that follow:

- *If, like 70 percent of diabetics, you have nonalcoholic fatty liver disease* (NAFLD), 2 tablespoons of lecithin granules (soy only) contain phosphatidylcholine, which is specifically required for the healing of fatty liver.[1,2] Swallow with water (do not chew or it will stick in your teeth).

- For the prevention and reversal of *glycation*, which affects most type 2 diabetics and pre-diabetics, take a methylated multi B-complex that gives extra vitamin B_1 and B_6 (*in the P5P form*), twice a day.[3] Also take the amino carnosine daily [4,5] (500 mg per meal) at or right after meals (especially any that include seared, browned, and sweetened foods). Adding the amino taurine (500–1,000 mg) twice a day (before or between meals) is also recommended.

Note: Two tablespoons of lecithin a day provide phospholipids to help with *both* fatty liver and glycation. *We've also found it helps emulsify fat, for those with no gallbladder, along with 300–500 mg Ox Bile.*

- Diabetics may also benefit from specific herbs and nutrients to further address compromised kidney, pancreas, liver, or heart function. (We have used herbal supplements by Systemic Formulas with early stage diabetics.) More progressed clients need acupuncturists or others experienced with more progressed diabetes, who can collaborate with their medical doctors.

- For those who need an alternative to Metformin (which can cause digestive problems and may contribute to Alzheimer's), the herb berberine can provide similar benefits.[6] Both are known to help with the fatigue and carb cravings that can hit diabetics during and after meals, if the Craving Cure's approach does not entirely eliminate them.

Are you taking any diabetes medication? If so, *plan ahead* with your prescriber. A medication adjustment may be needed when you start taking your glutamine and have your first Techno-Karbz-free days, to prevent your blood sugar from dropping *too* low! Run all of the supplements mentioned in this chapter by your physician. Be sure to show him/her the references in the Notes section in Chapter 7 that so strongly support their use.

TYPE 3: CRAVING ELIMINATION FOR THE COMFORT CRAVER

TYPE 3 AMINOS AND ADDITIONAL NUTRIENTS

DLPA (DL-phenylalanine) or DPA (D-phenylalanine).

Either of these two aminos can stop comfort-food cravings cold because both contain D-phenylalanine, an unusual amino that can immediately raise the endorphin level by slowing down the rate at which your body automatically destroys endorphin (the body has enzymes that destroy each of our neurotransmitters).

DLPA is a blend of two different forms of the amino acid phenylalanine: 250 mg DPA and 250 mg LPA. Some LPA converts into one of the most potent endorphin sub-types called enkephalin. Some LPA is also converted into the energizing amino acid tyrosine and to an appetite regulator called cholecystokinin, and serves many other useful purposes in the body.

Some people use the more energizing DLPA during the day, and DPA at night (for example, if they have late-night Type 3 cravings, or physical pain that's worse when they lie down).

Most people with anxiety or sleep problems should automatically start with DPA. If you are trying to reduce your use of a painkilling drug, DPA should be your first choice and you will probably need doses in the higher range.

In a very few cases, DPA has converted to some energizing LPA and been uncomfortably energizing for sensitive people. If you're sensitive or easily agitated, trial DPA by opening the capsule and taking just a quarter of it to start with.

Comparison of DLPA and DPA

ADVANTAGES OF DLPA	ADVANTAGES OF DPA
Kills comfort-food cravings better for some.	Almost twice as strong. (Typically better if pain relief is needed as well as craving relief.)
Is somewhat energizing.	Not energizing, typically more soothing and better for people who tend to be nervous, tense, or sleepless.
Very easy to find online or in stores.	Fewer sources, mostly online.
Less expensive.	More expensive, though the prices are dropping.

Complete Amino Blend. Endorphins are made from not one amino, but from three to nineteen aminos! If you don't eat lots of complete (i.e., animal-source) protein at least three times a day, starting now (as per Chapter 13), you won't be able to take in enough aminos from food to rebuild adequate endorphin levels. That means that your response to the Type 3 aminos will be weaker. If you're *vegetarian or vegan, or otherwise unable to consume dense protein*, please add a complete "free form" (predigested, easy to absorb) amino acid *blend* containing all twenty amino acids. Our pregnant clients who can't use individual aminos, for example, generally report feeling much better and craving less on this product alone. Any Type 3 should try it if cravings don't completely stop on DPA or DLPA.

TYPE 3 PRECAUTIONS

As you can see in the box below, there are several conditions that might warrant caution or preclude the use of DLPA. One of the two aminos in DLPA, L-phenylalanine, has mildly stimulating properties so we occasionally see some jitteriness in reaction to a trial of DLPA. Any such reaction during your trial would let you know to take DPA instead. But I need to alert you to some more serious possibilities. The most common is raised blood pressure, especially if you have ever had a problem with elevated blood pressure. Keep track of your blood pressure if you decide to trial DLPA in that case.

POSSIBLE CONTRAINDICATIONS	DLPA	DPA*	RISK LEVEL
Hyperthyroidism (Grave's Disease)	X		DO NOT USE
Melanoma	X		DO NOT USE
Manic Tendencies	X		DO NOT USE
High Blood Pressure	X		DO NOT USE without a blood pressure cuff and start at half dose if blood pressure is currently low.
Headaches, Including Migraines	X		Mild—start at half dose.
Hashimoto's Autoimmune Thyroiditis	X		Mild—start at half dose.

*DPA has not caused any of the above problems, so far, though it can in, rare instances, convert to some LPA. If you have any of the above conditions, stop taking DPA if you find it energizing.

Are you on any endorphin-targeted drugs such as marijuana, alcohol, Vicodin, or Suboxone? If so, take Type 3 aminos a few hours before or after using such substances, when they are wearing off. This will allow you to see the specific benefits of the aminos clearly. After some "endorphin rehab," you might not feel as much need for your endorphin-targeted drugs. After all, DPA was tested for use in hospital settings to reduce the need for high-dose painkillers like morphine. See Charles Gant, M.D.'s book *End Your Addiction Now* and go to allianceforaddictionsolutions.org for more on nutritional recovery from pain-killing drugs.

TYPE 3 SHOPPING, BRANDS, AND FORMULATIONS

DLPA. This is readily available and seems to be uniformly good across all brands.

DPA. It is not as easy to find as DLPA. Look for it online by Doctor's Best, Montiff, or Lidtke. You can also order trialing samples of both DPA and DLPA as well as full bottles on cravingcure.com/shop.

Complete Amino Blend. There are few amino blends that supply adequate amounts of all of the aminos in the free form and in the ratio and quantity found in animal protein. Total Amino Solution by Genesa is the best we've used. (I helped design it, but do not profit from its sales.) Montiff, specializing in amino acid supplementation, has a good one, too, and they are famous for their products' purity. (Be sure whatever blend you choose contains tryptophan, as these do.)

TYPE 3 TRIALING

Follow the directions for trialing in Chapter 12 starting with the basic 500-mg standard capsule dose of either DLPA or DPA.

DLPA. Expect to feel pleased, and without cravings for comfort foods within 5–10 minutes of the first trial dose, or whenever your trial dose increases enough to "hit the spot." You might also feel slightly more energized, or a reduction in physical pain.

DPA. Many people report experiencing a dreamier state than with DLPA, especially in the first few minutes, along with comforted and craving-free effects. It can also immediately deliver stronger physical pain relief.

Complete Amino Blend. The response to this is subtler. It can take a full day or two to show results. Start with two capsules, not the usual one, and go up to four if needed to get an effect.

TYPE 3 DOSING AND SCHEDULE

DLPA. A dose ranges from one to four 500-mg capsules. The average dose is 1,000 mg per dose, meaning two capsules. If you have sleep problems, be careful about using DLPA after three PM. We do not usually recommend more than two capsules for an afternoon dose, in any case.

DLPA Dosing Guidelines

	BEFORE BREAKFAST	BEFORE LUNCH	MIDAFTER-NOON
DLPA, 500-mg caps	1–4	1–4	1–2

DPA. A dose ranges from one to two 500-mg capsules. The average dose is 1,000 mg, and we rarely need three capsules, because even a single dose of DPA is so effective for so many.

DPA Dosing Guidelines

	BEFORE BREAKFAST*	BEFORE LUNCH	MIDAFTER-NOON	NIGHT-TIME*
DPA, 500-mg caps	1–2	1–2	1–2	(1–2)

*Nighttime doses can be added if your Type 3 cravings or other symptoms, like pain, hit you in the evening.

Mix and Match. One of our clients did well on DLPA until she lost her beloved dog. Her emotional pain level rose instantly and some of her comfort-food cravings returned. We suggested she try adding one DPA capsule to each DLPA dose. That helped her greatly. After one month, she no longer needed the extra DPA.

Complete Amino Blend. Optional, if you are eating recommended amounts of animal protein. If not, take three to four 750-mg capsules *before* meals, three times a day.

TYPE 3 TERMINATION

When you no longer crave your comfort foods or cry over sappy TV commercials and you find that life, even without Techno-Karbz, is plenty rewarding enough and your Type 3 symptom scores are consistently below 3, wait one month and try eliminating these aminos (as per Chapter 11).

TYPE 4: CRAVING ELIMINATION FOR THE STRESSED CRAVER

TYPE 4 AMINOS AND ADDITIONAL NUTRIENTS

GABA. The amino acid GABA, we have found, turns off stress-stimulated cravings for about 90 percent of our clients who are Type 4 Cravers in very short order. Because everyone who comes to our office is stressed, GABA wins the instant-relief-amino-acid popularity contest at our clinic: "My neck feels so relaxed!" "I don't feel stressed anymore!" "I don't feel like nibbling on chips or gum!"

GABA is both an amino acid *and* a neurotransmitter! It is not one of the nine essential aminos found in food, but it can be made by our bodies out of several other aminos. But our protein-poor diets plus chronic stress seem to be wiping out our GABA stores so rapidly that GABA supplements are nothing less than twenty-first-century godsends. Because our clinic uses chewables that dissolve in the mouth for trialing, the results arrive in seconds.

Theanine. Of our few clients who don't get benefit from GABA, almost all love the alternate amino, *theanine.* This amino is just as easy to find for purchase as GABA and it comes in similar doses (100–200 mg). It is an unusual amino, not found in any food but the tea plant. We're not quite sure yet exactly *how* it supports GABA in calming the brain and neutralizing adrenaline, but it clearly does!

TYPE 4 PRECAUTIONS

There are certain medications and medical conditions that warrant caution when contemplating the use of GABA or theanine. *Note: Infants should not use GABA.*

POSSIBLE CONTRAINDICATIONS	GABA	THEANINE	RISK LEVEL
It could cause too much sedation if taken at the same time that you take a GABA-targeted medication, e.g., Neurontin (gabapentin), or benzodiazepines like Klonapin, Ativan, Xanax, or Valium.	X	X	*Moderate* Check with your pharmacists and get your prescriber's okay, trial 4 hours away from such medication.
If your natural blood pressure is really low (under 105/65)* or if you are on blood pressure–lowering medication**	X	X	*Moderate to severe* Type 4 aminos can lower blood pressure further and make you light-headed.

* If your blood pressure is low but you decide to trial GABA anyway, bite off one-quarter of a 125-mg chewable GABA Calm tablet (see Shopping, Brands, Formulations, below), chew it, and see if a trial of this tiny dose or more, gradually increased, makes you light-headed. (Do not ever trial while driving!) One of GABA Calm's minor constituents is tyrosine, which can slightly raise blood pressure and almost always keeps our client's blood pressures from dropping too low. Monitor your own blood pressure for a few weeks and discuss your medication dosage needs with your prescriber once you see how GABA Calm affects you. Other GABA products do not contain tyrosine and may be better for you *after* you're off blood pressure–lowering medication.

TYPE 4 SHOPPING, BRANDS, AND FORMULATIONS

GABA. This amino comes in many strengths and formulations and is more potent in smaller doses than other aminos, which is why we trial it at low doses. We recommend that our clients start with 100- or 125-mg capsules or chewables. In contrast, we trial most other aminos at 500 mg. Our favorite low-dose option is the 125-mg chewable GABA Calm by Source Naturals.

If you find that you need a stronger dose of GABA, or would prefer to avoid the flavoring of the GABA Calm, choose one of these client favorites:

- 100- to 500-mg plain GABA capsules
- NOW True Calm capsule (200 mg GABA mixed with the also-calming aminos taurine and glycine)
- NOW Chewable GABA (250 mg GABA with small amounts of theanine and taurine)

Theanine. There are two doses available: 100 mg and 200 mg. Half of our clients need the 200-mg dose. Suntheanine is a proprietary form of theanine and therefore more expensive. We've seen consistent effects between brands, so any brand should do. Do not buy a blend that includes other nutrients, at least at first.

TYPE 4 TRIALING

Follow the general directions for trialing in Chapter 11. You might need to experiment with a range of doses to find the right match for your needs.

GABA. Start with a 100-mg capsule or the 125-mg GABA Calm chewable. If you want to trial less than 100 mg (e.g., with children or "sensitives"), break up a GABA chewable, or just bite off one-quarter or half of it. You can swallow it rather than chew it, if you prefer, but the absorption is much faster while chewing. Chew slowly, allow it to absorb throughout your mouth, then swallow. You can also empty out part of a capsule rather than use the chewable tablets.

A trial with 125-mg chewable GABA Calm typically takes a record three seconds to have an effect. Have a friend or family member with you to witness the experience.

If the lower doses don't help and you need a larger dose, you could trial two to three of these low-dose products. That will tell you how much you need going forward and then you can switch to a stronger GABA capsule of 250 mg to 500 mg, whichever strength your gradually increasing trials show you to respond to best. Do not take more than three of the sorbitol-sweetened GABA Calm products a day on a regular basis. If you need more, switch to unsweetened capsules. If you start craving them, switch to unsweetened capsules. (We have not had much trouble with this, but better to be prepared.)

Reverse Effect*: If you don't feel quite relaxed enough on a lower dose of GABA, but feel more stressed than usual on a higher dose, find a happy medium. *Do* not *give to infants.*

Theanine. If GABA, at any dose, does not help, open a 100-mg theanine capsule and follow the general trialing directions in Chapter 11. If it is not enough, trial 1½ to 2 capsules. We very rarely see the Reverse Effect.

TYPE 4 DOSING AND SCHEDULE

GABA. A dose can range from 100 to 500 mg. There is no "typical dose," but about *half* of our Type 4s need more than 125 mg. All need it by midafternoon daily.

We've had to be careful of doses over 250 mg because too much GABA can make some people anxious or even briefly short of breath (Reverse Syndrome).

Note: Our clients have run into trouble with some, though not all, brands of 750-mg GABA products, so we don't encourage that dose.

Theanine. Many clients do well on 100 mg, but others do better on 200 mg per dose.

GABA or Theanine Dosing Guidelines**

	BEFORE BREAKFAST*	BEFORE LUNCH*	MID AFTERNOON	BEFORE DINNER*	BEDTIME*
GABA, 100–500 mg	1–2	1–2	1–2	1–2	1–2
Theanine, 100–200 mg	1–2	1–2	1–2	1–2	1–2

** Take either GABA or theanine as needed, whenever you're feeling stressed, especially if the stress is causing cravings, at any time of day. At nighttime, either can help with sleep. Add in extra doses before breakfast, before dinner, or at bedtime either *daily*, if needed, for *chronic* tension- or stress-related craving, or as needed, for *temporary* stress, for example, if you wake up with stress cravings, before, during, or after a crisis, to unwind in the evening, or to get to sleep more easily,

*The maximum GABA dose we recommend is usually one 500-mg capsule (after we've trialed lower doses), but a few GABA "sponges" seem to need more than one 500-mg capsule at a time, at least for a while. (That's particularly true if they're trying to quit taking drugs like Xanax at the same time!)

TYPE 4 TERMINATION

Try going off of GABA (or theanine) after you've been freed of Type 4 symptoms for a while, according to the general directions in Chapter 11 (e.g., sooner for children). Because unexpected stressors can come up at any point, always have some GABA (or theanine) in the fridge to keep stress from getting out of control and retriggering your cravings.

TYPE 5: CRAVING ELIMINATION FOR THE FATIGUED CRAVER

TYPE 5 AMINOS

Tyrosine. Tyrosine, or its backup amino, **L-phenylalanine** (LPA), can raise your brain's levels of its naturally stimulating catecholamines (the Cats).

Comparison of Tyrosine and LPA

TYROSINE 500 MG	LPA 500 MG
Stronger effects on energy and concentration.	Gentler and more broadly nutritious than tyrosine. Better for children and sensitives.
More likely to give headaches, high blood pressure, or other unwanted-reactions.	Less likely to give such unwanted or uncomfortable reactions.

How to Choose between Tyrosine and LPA

Having worked with Type 5 Cravers for over thirty years, I've seen that, overall, the majority have done best with tyrosine. At identical 500-mg doses, it is the stronger of these two Cat-fueling aminos and typically elicits more mental alertness, physical energy, overall vitality, and relief from the desire for a pick-me-up from gumdrops, lattes, or energy drinks.

If you're like a number of our Type 5 Cravers and have ADD/ADHD you may prefer a combination of tyrosine and LPA (plus GABA as a mental spam blocker and SAMe to prime the brain even more fully to produce natural energy and concentration, as I describe in *The Mood Cure*). The amino acid L-phenylalanine (LPA for short) is less potent as an energizer, because only a part of it converts into tyrosine (and from that into the Cats). The rest goes for jobs like painkilling, appetite regulation, and more, so it can't always fully stop Type 5 cravings and fatigue. It's best for children, sensitives, and for any of those who find tyrosine too stimulating, e.g., those with high anxiety or migraines.

TYPE 5 PRECAUTIONS

Here are some conditions that might give you pause or prevent you from using Type 5 aminos.

POSSIBLE CONTRAINDICATIONS	TYROSINE	LPA	RISK LEVEL
Grave's Disease or Hyper-thyroidism (Tyrosine is the central component of all thyroid hormones.)	X	X	DO NOT USE Never use Type 5 aminos if your illness is active. If your thyroid has been removed or its output of hormones reduced by medications or surgery, ask your doctor's advice.
Melanoma	X	X	DO NOT USE even in remission without M.D. advice.
Bipolar spectrum tendencies: if mania or hypomania is a problem, these aminos can be too stimulating. (And we have *not* seen them lift bipolar or unipolar depressions.)*	X	X	DO NOT USE
High Blood Pressure (on or off medication)**	Moderate to severe X	Mild to moderate X	If you closely monitor your blood pressure, you might use with your doctors' okay. Start with a trial of LPA. DO NOT USE if even low doses cause blood pressure elevation.
Headaches,*** especially migraines: If you get relief from Imitrex (or any other serotonin-targeted migraine medication) you are more likely to be adversely affected by Type 5 aminos.	Moderate to severe X	Mild to moderate X	Tyrosine is more likely to trigger this, so trial LPA first at ½ dose.
Hashimoto's Autoimmune Thyroiditis****	Moderate to severe X	Mild to moderate X	These aminos cause jitteriness in 15% of our clients with this condition. (Trial at a half dose, starting with LPA.)

POSSIBLE CONTRAINDICATIONS	TYROSINE	LPA	RISK LEVEL
Use of stimulating drugs such as caffeine, Adderall, Dexedrine, meth, diet pills, energy drinks, cocaine	X	X	Overstimulating if Type 5 aminos are used *at the same time* as these meds. (Good for withdrawing from such meds.)

*If you, like many who have more subtle bipolar-spectrum symptoms (as distinct from manic-depression) don't know that it may be a factor for you, research "the spectrum" and fill out a symptom questionnaire like ours on moodcure.com/findapractitioner.html.

**As our clients' diet and weight improve, their blood pressure often goes down naturally, and they can increase the LPA dose or switch to tyrosine, if needed.

***Occasionally, tyrosine has caused nonmigraine headaches at first. In several cases, our clients stopped it for a week, then retrialed it later with no problem and much benefit. This does not work with migraines, typically.

****If you get uncomfortable on these aminos, though you have Type 5 symptoms, get your thyroid antibodies tested (anti-TPO and anti-thyroglobulin). You may be an undiagnosed thyroiditis sufferer. To read more, see the two chapters on thyroid in *The Diet Cure*.

TYPE 5 SHOPPING, BRANDS, AND FORMULATIONS

Tyrosine and LPA. All brands seem to be uniformly good, so purchase any brand of capsules at the base dose of 500 mg.

TYPE 5 TRIALING

Trial tyrosine (or LPA) at least two hours away from caffeine or any other stimulant (e.g., ADD/ADHD medication).

Do not trial after two PM.

The starting *adult* trial dose of both tyrosine and LPA is 500 mg. Choose the Type 5 amino you'd like to start with and follow the general trialing directions in Chapter 11. Look for a "lift" in energy and alertness within the next 5 to 10 minutes and, of course, the disappearance of your yen for a double espresso. If nothing happens, trial a second capsule. Even a third is sometimes needed for caffeine-jaded brains to start firing normally.

Tyrosine. Start with a single 500-mg dose. That's often enough to start giving enlivening results. Go up to two capsules if results are good but mild, if needed. If you still get no response, try three or even four, three times a day. If there are still no results, stop the trial. See Chapter 16, page 253 for suggestions on what else could be causing your need for energy, since it does not seem to be a Cat problem. (Low thyroid is the most common cause we've found.)

LPA. If you decide to start with LPA but a trial of up to three capsules doesn't do much, switch to a trial of tyrosine a few hours later or the next morning.

TYPE 5 DOSING AND SCHEDULE

Tyrosine or L-phenylalanine (LPA). Doses for either could range from one to four 500-mg capsules, depending on the results of the trial. The average dose for either amino is two 500-mg capsules before breakfast and lunch. Clients rarely need more than three capsules at a time (unless they are withdrawing from a stimulant drug, when they often need four capsules at a time). We do not usually recommend more than two capsules for an afternoon (before three PM) dose, especially if a client has sleep issues. If, after a few days or weeks, you find that your starting dose seems too low (your Type 5 symptoms stop dropping or return), raise your dose one capsule at a time. Watch your sleep to see that the afternoon dose doesn't get too high. If your starting dose seems to be too high (you get to feeling jittery, edgy, or headachy, or your blood pressure rises), stop. If you retrial it, after these symptoms are gone, start at a low dose.

Tyrosine and LPA Dosing Guidelines

	BEFORE BREAKFAST	BEFORE LUNCH	MIDAFTER- NOON*
Tyrosine or LPA, 500-mg caps	1–4	1–3	1–2

*Optional. If needed. Best taken by 3 PM. OK to take 3 caps midafternoon if sleep is not disturbed by it.

CAFFEINE WITHDRAWAL SUPPORT

Type 5s usually depend heavily on caffeine to stimulate their brains' sluggishness. Few of them have been happy about the idea of quitting. But unless they quit, they can't repair the parts of their brains that the caffeine is operating in. The following plan has worked wonderfully, even for the eight-cups-a-day types! Some of our clients report a few mild headaches or mild fatigue as their bodies detox from years of caffeine. But they do not report cravings or severe discomfort.

The Caffeine Detox Protocol

Once you've established your dose of tyrosine or LPA, the night before you quit, place that dose on your bedside table. When your alarm goes off, take the aminos, hit snooze, and go back to sleep; when it goes off again—you should be ready to get up without coffee! If you typically get up after one alarm, take your first aminos then. Add more if you crave it after 10 minutes, either way take extra doses if you slump before your pre-lunch dose or any other time on the first day, and as long as needed (typically when you would usually have had a caffeinated drink).

Take 1,000 to 3,000 mg of vitamin C with each meal for at least day one. If your bowels get loose, cut the vitamin C to 500 mg. Stop the vitamin C altogether if the loose bowels persist. Feel free to also take an anti-inflammatory of your choice for the first few days, if needed (it usually isn't), for headaches. (Take it with 600 mg of gut-protective NAC, N-acetyl-cysteine.)

TYPE 5 TERMINATION

Follow the general guidelines in Chapter 11. You will eventually find that you need fewer and fewer of either of the Type 5 aminos. They may even begin to make you a little edgy or make it hard for you to get to sleep. That's a good sign—that your brain is producing more of its own Cats and that it's probably time to drop or stop the aminos! If you stop and fatigue or cravings for chocolate, sugar, or caffeine come back, resume taking the aminos at whatever dose returns you to zero on Part 5 of the Mini Craving-Type Questionnaire. Try to reduce or stop a month later.

Jamie's Five-Part Amino Breakthrough Process

To get a personal perspective on the amino breakthrough process, follow Jamie's course as she eliminated all five types of cravings. I picked her story because her process was especially easy to track. As you'll see, she chose to do her trials and start each supplement several days apart, which made her responses especially clear.

As you might imagine, when Jamie first came to consult with us, she was burdened not just by weight gain and five types of cravings but by five types of negative mood, plus fatigue and insomnia. Since half of our clients have all five Craving Types and could be described almost exactly this way, we thought nothing of it; but, like most of our new clients, Jamie was understandably skeptical and afraid to hope. We understood that too and didn't take it personally. We were working with her virtually so we'd e-mailed her the Tracking Tools and shipped her an Amino Acid Trialing Kit. She'd filled out the first three tools—the Craving-Type Questionnaire, the Trigger Foods Rating Sheet, and the Daily Food Log—and sent them back to us before her Skype trialing session.

Jamie's Trials: Which Amino to Start With?

Then it was time to trial the aminos indicated by the results of her Craving-Type Questionnaire and profile. In other words, all of them. When multiple aminos are indicated, we usually ask our clients which Craving Type they'd like to get rid of first. Even though she had higher scores on Types 1 and 2, Jamie chose to start with Type 5, Fatigued Cravings. She said she needed energy, which she was currently out of, to organize and carry out the rest of her five-part amino project. Her proposal: "Let's trial those aminos that help with energy and focus first. If it works, I'll know I can manage all the rest."

We reviewed each of the general and specific causes for caution before her first trial. Since we were meeting in the morning, we knew there was little danger of her trying something that could be too stimulating or interfere with her sleep. She reassured us on that point, saying, "I tolerate lots of coffee every day and I've even taken diet pills with it in the past with no sleep problems!" Based on how high all her Type 5 scores were (7 to 10), we decided to start her trial with the stronger of the two possible aminos for Type 5 cravings: tyrosine. We asked her to fill her Dixie cup one-third full of water and to empty one capsule of tyrosine into it. She stirred it around with a spoon and emptied it all into her mouth, swishing it around so she could absorb as much of it as possible through those porous mucus membranes. Then she swallowed (it didn't taste good so she was glad to).

Jamie was in the midst of telling us how fatigued she typically was when her eyes suddenly got brighter, her speech more animated, and her posture straighter. We asked her to stop talking and notice how she was feeling. "Definitely more energized," she answered after a pause. Then we asked, "On a scale of 1 to 10, how has the fatigue changed?" She replied, "I was about an eight before we started, now I'm a four!"

We asked her to record the experience she'd just had in her Amino Trialing Record. Then we had her fill out her Supplement Schedule, adding one to two 500-mg tyrosine capsules before breakfast, before lunch, and in midafternoon. It sounded like she might need a two-capsule dose to get her energy to a zero, but one capsule was having a strong impact, so we started her on one capsule three times a day, but encouraged her to go up to two cap doses on day two if she wasn't perky and craving-free enough.

Jamie did not experience any adverse reactions to 500 mg of tyrosine during her one-capsule trial or during her first two days on this dose, three times a day. But her Type 5 scores did not drop to zero. Though she did feel generally more energized, her scores were still fours or fives. So she started on two tyrosine and her Type 5 scores all went way down. After her afternoon dose, however, she realized she was feeling a little edgy. So she dropped the afternoon dose back to one, but continued at two before breakfast and before lunch. This kept her Type 5 scores close to zero consistently. She noted these adjustments on her Supplement Schedule and her reactions in her Daily Log.

__Trial Two:__ Twenty minutes after her tyrosine trial, Jamie trialed one of the aminos indicated for Type 1, which was actually her highest-scoring Craving Type. Since she'd done so well on the Type 5 amino, I suggested she start her second trial using 5-HTP, the more energizing form of the amino acid needed by Type 1 Cravers. That was an instant hit. Jamie only needed one capsule's worth in a Dixie cup to neutralize most of her Type 1 symptoms. On a scale of 1 to 10, 5-HTP took her from fives and tens down to twos and fours. A second dose, swallowed in the capsule this time, ten minutes later lowered her scores to ones and twos.

She had been having some cravings and bedtime trouble getting to sleep; 5-HTP can occasionally make sleep worse, so we suggested she take an afternoon dose but not take a bedtime dose the first night. The plan was for her to try a 5-HTP the __second__ night if that afternoon dose did not keep her awake. Then, if she didn't like the 5-HTP at night, she could try the less energizing Type 1 amino, tryptophan, at bedtime the third night. We reminded her to record her responses carefully in her log. Before we next met, she e-mailed her log, which reported that she was happy on two 5-HTP before lunch and two before dinner, but because she'd still had a hard time getting to sleep, she'd taken one 5-HTP the second night and had gotten to sleep in ten minutes! At that point she added one 5-HTP at bedtime to her Supplement Schedule.

How about her cravings? She was eating well for the first time in years because she no longer craved chocolate and caffeine for energy or cookies at bedtime, but her afternoon cravings for chips and noncaffeinated soda were only cut in half. (She was eating a healthier snack instead, but was having some struggle.) To help relieve that, we said it was time for a third trial.

__Trial Three:__ Her first Mini Craving-Type Questionnaire showed that her Type 2 score was still above normal.

So Jamie's third trial was with the amino acid glutamine. She didn't notice much after the first one (though she was relieved that it tasted so good), but the second glutamine completely eliminated the last stubborn afternoon craving. We suggested that she take two capsules midafternoon, along with her 5-HTP and tyrosine, and add it before breakfast and lunch too if cravings and other low blood sugar symptoms were still there. Then we looked at her Mini Questionnaire again and saw that Jamie's two last-remaining high Craving Type scores, for Types 3 and 4, had dropped down into the normal range! We do see with some clients that, by eliminating __some__ of their Craving Types with aminos and diet, the symptoms of other Craving Types not as yet directly addressed may disappear, too. This is one of the advantages of introducing the aminos more slowly, one at a time. However, most of our clients have such severe cravings that they need to address all of their Craving Types at once.

We reminded Jamie to rescore her Mini Craving-Type Questionnaire in the week before our next meeting to confirm that she really did not need any other aminos. When we met that following week, most of her scores were down below three. The next week, after five weeks on the same aminos, at the same doses, all her scores were zero to two. Two months later, she was still happy on this same amino protocol, still scoring zeros mostly and about to try reducing her doses "just to see." She later reported that she was unable to cut back much for another two months (till six months from the time she started). After that, though, she stopped taking all but one capsule of 5-HTP at bedtime for sleep and her Support Nutrients.

Amino breakthrough completed.

SUPPORT NUTRIENTS FOR ALL CRAVING TYPES

All amino-takers need supplementary amounts of a variety of vitamins and minerals to facilitate the marvelous transformation of amino acids into neurotransmitters and to fill up on the nutrients that their pre-cure diets had deprived them of. Plan to take the lovely array of supplemental nutrients listed below for at least the first six months of your Craving Cure. We actually recommend that our clients take some version of them permanently, even when their diet has been splendid for years (but especially if it's *not* been). Of course, you may need to or want to take additional nutrients of your own choosing. For example, if you are diabetic, I hope you'll try and benefit from some of the additional nutrients I mentioned in Chapter 7 and earlier in this chapter specifically for you.

YOUR MULTIVITAMIN/MINERAL

After trying many formulations over the years, we've learned which ones work best for our clients. We designed True Balance (produced by NOW Foods) based on what we'd learned. It was reformulated at our request in 2016 to be even better. If you have Type 2 cravings (like the majority of our clients) it's a particularly effective formulation. Feel free to use any other multivitamin-mineral with similar types and amounts of most nutrients. Here is a list of the contents of two capsules of True Balance. We recommend that our teens and adult clients take *two twice a day* with meals (see contents below).

True Balance Contents

Vitamin A (Fish Oil) 1,250 IU	Magnesium (Amino Acid Chelate/Citrate) 40 mg
Vitamin C (from Calcium Ascorbate) 120 mg	Zinc (Gluconate) 15 mg
Vitamin D_3 (as Cholecalciferol) 500 IU	Selenium (from L-Selenomethionine) 62.5 mcg
Vitamin E (as d-alpha Tocopheryl Succinate) 200 IU	Manganese (from Manganese Bisglycinate) (TRAACS) 2.5 mg
Thiamin (from Thiamin HCl) 20 mg	Chromium (Chelvite and GTF) 450 mcg
Riboflavin 15 mg	Potassium (from Chloride and Citrate) 50 mg
Niacin (as Niacinamide and Niacin) 70 mg	Gymnema Sylvestre Extract (Leaves) 50 mg
Vitamin B_6 (from Pyridoxine HCl) 16.5 mg	Vitamin K_2 (MK-7) 50 mcg
5-MTHF (5-Methyltetrahdroxyfolate) 200 mcg	L-Carnitine (from L-Carnitine Tartrate) (Carnipure) 20 mg
Vitamin B_{12} (as Methylcobalamin) 40 mcg	Choline (from Choline Bitartrate) 15 mg
Biotin 1.6 mg	Inositol 15 mg
Pantothenic Acid (from Calcium Pantothenate) 60 mg	Vanadium (from AAC) 9 mcg
Calcium (from Citrate and Ascorbate) 93 mg	

Vitamin C: Because few multis contain adequate amounts of vitamin C and it is one of the handful of nutrients whose depletion is known to contribute to the development of weight gain and diabetes, we recommend 1,000-mg capsules, preferably with bioflavonoids, *twice a day.* The current average intake of fresh vegetables and fruits does not provide nearly enough of this vital nutrient which we, uniquely among animals, cannot produce ourselves. So we have a lot of catching up to do.

Vitamin D: Test first, then dose as needed, as per Tracking and Testing Tools, page 267. Widespread vitamin D deficiency in the United States is contributing to many problems including rapid increase in insulin resistance (even in children under age five) that sets us up for obesity and diabetes.[7] We've especially liked emulsified vitamin D drops and cod liver oil, which also contains vitamin A and omega 3s.)

Fatty Acid Rebalancers: Flush out years or a lifetime of damaged hydrogenated and liquid omega-6 fat. Because fish (as listed in Chapter 13, page 210) can be so rich in the omega-3 fats that counterbalance omega-6 overdoses, eat it at least twice a week.

Eat one egg yolk or some liver daily because they are rich in the phospholipids that compose the fatty cell walls where the omega-6 expulsions will take place. If not, take *1 tablespoon* of lecithin granules (soy only) as a supplement.

Especially if you don't eat fish in this amount regularly, start taking omega-3 fish or algae oil supplements: 1,000–2,000 mg equal EPA to DHA (or more DHA) or 1 tablespoon Carlson's Cod liver oil (the only brand that safely limits vitamin A content).

Notes:

1) Do test your fatty acid levels if possible now and again in six months (as per Tracking and Testing Tools, page 286), then tailor your omega-3 oil supplements as indicated. There may be other deficiencies you should be aware of. Especially if you are pyroluric, your GLA levels may be low, for example. GLA is a beneficial anti-inflammatory omega-6 fat whose levels can be raised using Evening Primrose oil.

2) Keep fish oil or cod liver oil in the freezer to prevent burping and to best preserve freshness (it won't liquefy).

3) Don't chew the lecithin granules (they'll get in your teeth). Just swallow with water.

4) If you have no gall bladder, take 300–500mg Ox Bile with fatty meals and supplements.

THE ENTIRE AMINO BREAKTHROUGH AT-A-GLANCE

Here is the cheat sheet that summarizes this whole chapter: the aminos for each Craving Type, and their dose ranges and average times taken along with the Support Nutrients for all types.

Adult Averages for All Aminos and Support Nutrients Recommended

	BEFORE BREAKFAST	BEFORE LUNCH	MIDAFTERNOON	BEFORE DINNER	NIGHTTIME
Amino Acids					
5-HTP 50 mg *or* Tryptophan 500 mg		1–3	1–3	1–3	
Glutamine 500 mg	1–4	1–4	1–4	1–4	
DLPA 500 mg *or* DPA 500 mg	1–4 DLPA	1–4 DLPA or 1–2 DPA	1–4 DLPA or 1–2 DPA	1–2 DPA	

	BEFORE BREAKFAST	BEFORE LUNCH	MIDAFTER-NOON	BEFORE DINNER	NIGHT-TIME
GABA 125–500 mg *or* Theanine 100–200 mg		1–2	1–2	1–2	
Tyrosine *or* Phenylalanine 500 mg	1–4	1–4	1–3		
Support Nutrients					
Multivitamin-mineral	2			2	
Vitamin C, 1,000 mg	1			1	
Vitamin D, *as needed after testing*					
Fish Oil, 1,000 mg (equal amounts DHA and EPA or higher DHA) gel caps or Carlson cod liver oil*	2 1 Tb				
Soy Lecithin, rounded Tb**	1–2 Tb				
Add-Ons for Diabetics and others	as needed				

*Especially if fish is not consumed twice a week or more.
**If eggs (or liver) are not consumed most days.

PART IV

Craving-Free Eating

13

Finding Your Way Back to the Primal Plate: What, When, and How Much to Eat

THE CRAVING CURE IS A two-step process. It doesn't end with the amino acids and the elimination of your cravings. That's actually the beginning. By breaking the spell of addictive foods, the aminos give you a flying start. But you can't rely on them, *alone,* to keep your cravings at bay long term. A complete Craving Cure requires that you to take a second step. That step is presented here in Part IV, Craving-Free Eating. This is where you'll learn how to incorporate anti-craving foods and eating patterns into your daily life, so that you can stay *permanently* craving free. The aminos will shore up your crumbling defenses; healing foods will rebuild them in stone. Once you start your aminos, you'll be able to take this second step very quickly. Most of our clients start on their new foods the day after their first amino trialing session.

I've written the first three chapters of Part IV to describe the eating recommendations we make to the clients at our clinic and how they evolved. There are so many dietary theories in circulation and our clients have tried applying all of them before coming to us. They'd had one thing in common, though: none of them had historically proven themselves. On the contrary, their proponents were all convinced that only something new and *untried* could work! I fell for this questionable concept myself, so I know how exciting and convincing it can be. Now our goal is to help all of our clients discover their own versions of traditional nourishment.

If the prevailing diet winds of the last few decades have swept you far from the forgotten fundamentals of human nutrition, you may need some reorientation. To that end, I'll pass on some basics in this chapter: how much and what kinds of fat, protein, and carbohydrate? How many meals, snacks, *and* calories? And why? These are things that our clients have needed. In the following chapter, you can choose from the two start-up eating plans that my clinic has recommended. In the third chapter, you'll personalize that plan to your own specific needs and tastes. Then will come some delicious recipes and fresh meal ideas.

BACK TO THE BASICS: REPROPORTIONING YOUR PLATE

Nature's bounty really only comes in three forms. The world's traditional cuisines are composed of innumerable variations on a three-food theme. Until the 1970s,

AN AVERAGE PRE-1970S DAY	AN AVERAGE POST-2000 DAY
Meals: three	*Meals:* one or two
Snacks: 1–3 *(mostly whole food)*	*Snacks*: 3–6 *(mostly toxic)*
Proportions and calories:	*Proportions and calories:*
Protein: 30%, 700 calories	*Protein*: 20%, 500 calories
Fat: 40% (mostly animal), 800 calories	*Fat*: 30% (mostly vegetable oil), 850 calories
Carbohydrate: 30%, 700 calories	*Carbohydrate*: 50%, 1,200 calories
Sugar 200 calories	Sugar 550 calories
Starch 250 calories	Starch 650 calories
Vegetable & fruit 250 calories	Vegetable & fruit 100 calories
Total calorie average: 2,100, females; 2,500, males	*Total calorie average:* 2,600, females; 3,000, males

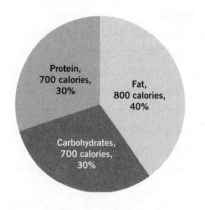

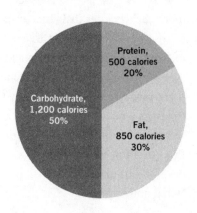

relatively unadulterated types of proteins, fats, and carbohydrates had been our sustenance and our delight for about two million years. Up to the 1970s, we'd been tremendously adaptable, sustaining ourselves on whatever amounts and proportions of these three fundamental foods we'd had access to.

How can we reaccess the diet of our forebears? Start by looking closely at what was on the average American plate right before the disaster decade started and compare it to what's on our plate now. Then take a look at the traditional, Techno-Karbz-free plate I'm recommending for your consumption. The serving and calorie amounts I've used here are averages. *Some of us need more and some less.* The figures that these pre- and post-1970s food averages are based on are estimates that have primarily been gathered from the USDA. But all reliable sources agree that both our calorie intake and our Techno-Karb intake have increased alarmingly over this time span. They differ in the exact numbers, so these are composite pictures.

A TRADITIONAL, TWENTY-FIRST-CENTURY DAY, FREE OF TECHNO-KARBZ

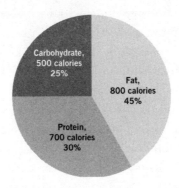

CHOOSING THE FOOD PROPORTIONS AND QUALITY WE NEED

Re Protein: Our consumption today is 10 percent lower than it was before 1970. We must raise that consumption back up to the pre-1970s levels to get the three foundational foods back into traditional proportions.

Re Fat: Our fat consumption has increased by only about fifty calories a day since 1970 (though the types of fats we're eating have changed dramatically). We're now eating so much *more* sugar and starch than we were then that the traditional proportions of fat, carbohydrate, and protein have been lost. In the rebalanced twenty-first-century plate on page 202, we go back to pre-1970s traditional proportions. The amount of fat will stay the same, but the quality will be traditionalized.

Re Carbohydrates: We were eating a lot of sugar and starch even before 1970, as you can see, but the amount and the percentage of both have now almost doubled. Both have become so much more caloric, addictive, and toxic that we've got to scrape them off our plates altogether. Back to more traditional sources and proportions of carbohydrate!

A CLOSER LOOK AT THE FUNDAMENTAL FOODS

THE POWERFUL PROTEINS

Chock-full of amino acids as they are, high-protein foods need to return to a prime place on our plates. About 30 percent of the calories on that plate should come from protein. Most of what we are, from our muscles, bones, skin, and most of our other body parts to our neurotransmitters, are constructed largely of protein. Traditionally, our primary protein sources have been animal-derived. Whether or not you approve of the Homo sapien brain, it is widely acknowledged to have been made possible by the addition of cooked animal protein to the lower-protein fare of our omnivorous primate ancestors.[1] Most of the world's people who now skimp on animal protein do *not* do so by choice—they either cannot afford it or live in regions that have been hunted out of this traditionally prized food. Avoiding animal protein, including red meat, tends to strip us not only of this superfood's amino acids but of its vitamins, minerals, and fatty acids, as well. One example: Red meat is the source of by far the most assimilable forms of the vital iron and zinc in which most of us are now deficient. Adequate protein is linked to reduced cravings, to increased satiety, and to weight loss, just to name a few of the benefits I mentioned in Chapter 3's section on protein (page 70).

Which Kinds of Protein-Containing Foods Are Best for *You*?

Fresh, soaked, organic beans and nuts are lovely, but they are low and incomplete in their protein content, as compared with any animal-derived protein source, such as beef, eggs, turkey, or Greek yogurt. A minimum of four ounces, or thirty-five grams, of meat, poultry, or seafood per meal is what most of our adult female clients have found to be their best dose, at least at first. Any less and they tend to start craving before the next meal. (Males, athletes, and high metabolizers need up to twice as much or more.) To get this much protein, you could eat, per meal, one chicken breast, 2½ cups of garbanzo beans, or two-thirds of a pound of almonds. The bean or nut option would not only be much higher in calories, it would provide you with *in*complete protein, that is, fewer of the nine essential and thirteen other aminos that the human body needs (and too many omega-6 fats). You could combine various types of vegetable-protein sources together, but that would still overload you with extra calories, while shorting you on the amounts of many of the component aminos. Instead, consider combining animal with vegetable sources. I like seeds or nuts with turkey in my whole-meal salads. Beans, combined with animal protein, vegetables, and soaked-whole-corn tortillas have been the staple combination for our southern hemisphere population for millennia. But such carbohydrate-heavy fare may suit neither your tastes, your health, nor your weight loss needs.

Comparing Protein Sources

FOOD SOURCE (LISTED BY PROTEIN CONTENT)	QUANTITY	PROTEIN GRAMS
Meat, Fowl, Fish (without its fat/skin/bone)	4 oz.	35
Cheese	2 oz.	4–26
Cottage Cheese	1 cup	30
Greek Yogurt (full fat)	1 cup	22
Seeds or Nuts	¾ cup	8–19
Eggs, medium	3 whole	21
Beans (pinto, black)	1 cup	5–15
Soy (tofu, tempeh)	4 oz.	25
Milk, Buttermilk, Kefir, Yogurt	1 cup	8–10
Brown Rice, cooked	1 cup	6
Oatmeal, cooked	1 cup	6
Bread	1 slice	2–3
Corn	1 cup	4–10
Vegetables (other than legumes)	1 cup	2
Fruit (apple, banana, orange, etc.)	1	1
*Protein Powder (whey, pea)	varies	20–30

*Do not use protein powders more than once a day, as they are hard on the kidneys, are highly processed, and, other than whey or egg powders, tend to provide poor amino ratios.

How Much Animal or Mixed Protein?

We've found that for women a minimum of four ounces and for men six ounces per meal is almost a universal requirement, three and five ounces too often leaving them feeling hungry, i.e., craving. We recommend four to eight ounces or 35 to 70 grams per meal to our clients, because we've found that it almost always takes this much to reliably provide almost immediate strength, mental clarity, and reduced cravings. Some milder cravers find that this increase in protein alone stops most of their cravings without the amino supplements. The variation in amount depends on sex, activity level, and calorie needs (especially if carbohydrate calories need to drop very low). Remember, the ultimate authority is your response to foods and experimentation is built in after a stabilization and strengthening period.

Complete Animal-Source Proteins (Preferably Pastured and Organic)

MEATS	POULTRY	MILK-DERIVED	SEAFOOD
beef, beef liver	eggs	cow, goat, or sheep cheese	See the list on page 210.
lamb, lamb liver	chicken	cottage cheese	All fish are rich in protein. Wild northern (e.g., Alaskan) fish are safest from mercury. Among farmed fish, standards vary as more regulation is developed. Check the NRDC mercury list, the Monterey Aquarium Seafood Watch list, and other watchdog lists.
mutton (adult sheep)	chicken liver	plain, Greek, full-fat yogurt	
pork	turkey		
ham, bacon (uncured, unsugared)	duck duck eggs		

Include fatty cuts of any of the traditional protein sources above if you're eating organic and/or grass-fed. Residues of pesticides, hormones, antibiotics, and other contaminants accumulate in the fat, so if you cannot buy organic, grass-fed, or wild, choose leaner cuts and add (preferably organic) butter, cream, cheese, extra-virgin olive oil, avocado, or coconut milk sauces. You can also purchase organic chicken or duck fat as well as lard (pork fat).

Traditionally, the *liver* was the most valued part of any animal. We recommend eating sautéed calves' or chicken liver with lots of onions, salt, and pepper weekly. Cutting it into chunks and sautéing it can help the timid. (I make liver hash with leftovers.) The iron content alone makes this organ meat invaluable, but it's also rich in the hard-to-find phospholipids that are so critical for recovery from Techno-Karb glycation, as they are the premier nutrients needed to rebuild any damaged cell walls.

> *Red meat was the primary protein source, and animal protein the primary calorie source, for both native and immigrant Americans until the 1970s.*

In case you're still hesitant about increasing your *egg consumption*, you should know that egg yolks provide another of the few good sources of those invaluable phospholipids required to build, operate, and repair the cell walls of every cell in your body! Even the American Heart Association has relaxed its egg restriction now, and a recent study found that egg consumption lowers blood pressure *and* weight![2] Go back to the ten eggs per week we ate before 1970.[3] It certainly wasn't raising blood pressure or weight or increasing heart disease then!

Have You Avoided Animal Protein Because You Don't Digest It Well?

Do you feel heavy or constipated after eating meat? That's a sign that your digestion is compromised. If you've been avoiding animal protein for a long time, you may have lost some of your capacity to produce the protein-digesting enzyme hydrochloric acid (HCl), or it may have been weak to begin with. Perhaps, like most Americans, you're eating a diet too low in vitamin B_6 and zinc, both required for making your vital HCl. Or perhaps your pancreas is not producing adequate amounts of the enzyme protease, which helps tear high-protein foods into their individual amino constituents. Or you may have been avoiding red meat, which itself stimulates HCl production.

If so, you can take protease as a supplement, alone or in a mix that includes fat- and carbohydrate-digesting enzymes plus some HCl. These combination supplements are called "super enzymes." You should notice a quick difference. You can also test your own HCl levels by taking pure HCl capsules, adding one at a time to each meal (up to four), until you feel a mild burning sensation. If you feel it after one capsule, you don't need any HCl supplementation. If it takes more, you'll benefit from one to four HCl supplements for a while with your meals (see more directions in the Tracking and Testing Tools, page 267).

THE FABULOUS FATS

You can't *see* it on your plate because it melts into the other foods, but traditional fats are as full of nutrients as they are of calories. About 40 percent of our calories (800 for an average woman and 1,000 for an average man), or more, should come from fat. The traditional saturated animal fats, saturated vegetable fats (like coconut oil), and extra-virgin olive oil never did contribute to weight gain or heart disease, so we can and should go back to consuming them in the higher proportion found worldwide in traditional diets. Our own pre-1970s traditional diet consisted of 40 to 45 percent of total daily calories, as I explained in Chapter 2. Multiple studies have shown that people on low-carbohydrate, unrestricted-fat diets lose more weight than those on low-fat diets, even when the calories are equal. Elevated cholesterol and diabetes markers drop lower too![4]

How Much Fat Can You Safely Ingest?

Lots. How do we know? The historical record. For example, arctic people's diets are traditionally 90 percent fat. Consider Julia Child, the 1950s' fit and indefatigable cream queen. Or ask an epileptic. It's been known for many years that epileptics *require* a high-fat diet—a *very* high-fat diet. Their lives depend on 50 to 60 percent of their diet being composed of fat. Dr. Atkins's and other ketogenic diets, whose safety and efficacy are now well researched, contain fat levels up to 80 percent. I offer this rundown as a quick fat-sanity check, since you will need to make fats more of a fuel source to replace the Techno-Karbz you've been consuming. (This is particularly true if you are diabetic, as I explain at the end of Chapter 14.)

Good sources of Omega-3 Fat: Fish, Pastured Meat, and Milk

Acquiring a safe and adequate supply of omega-3 fat is now known to be one of our most important yet increasingly difficult dietary jobs. Fish and other sea- and river foods are tasty and tender sources of the two essential *omega-3* fats. These two fats are called DHA and EPA for short. Here are a few examples of why they are so crucial: The heart doesn't function well without them. Our brain's 60 percent fat content must include critical amounts of DHA, in particular. We now know that we cannot regulate our glucose and insulin levels, maintain normal weight, or repair cellular damage, including glycation, without them. Most aquatic life contains some of them (even algae). *Yet right now, we're consuming almost none of the fish high in these omega-3 fats.* Farmed fish contain some vital omega-3 fat, but much more competing omega-6 fat, unknown in wild fish and unneeded by humans.[5]

We originally acquired our DHA and EPA not just from fish but also from the flesh and milk of land animals, who can convert DHA and EPA from plant forage. Some humans and animals can convert flaxseed, which contains a crude form of omega-3 fat (ALA), into EPA (but never into DHA). We *can* now, once again, derive some DHA and EPA from the fatty meat of land animals, but *only if they're grass fed.*[6, 7] Organic whole-milk products, have recently been found to contain twice as much omega-3 (and much less omega-6—a good thing) as nonorganic (or low-fat) versions.[8] But we need to eat fish as well if we're to experience all the benefits of the omega-3s. On the following page, you'll find a list of fish sources. Most fish fat contains about half DHA and half EPA. All fish on the list are low in mercury as per the Natural Resources Defense Council (NRDC) in 2016, and the few that are farmed are safely farmed (according to the Monterey Aquarium Seafood Watch standards). Please have high or medium omega-3-containing fresh, frozen, or canned fish at least twice a week. (Two pieces of this "fatty" fish per week is the American Heart Association's recommendation.) We recently arranged for one of our staff nutritionists, who averages that much fish per week, plus grassfed meat and organic full-fat milk products, to take two fatty acid blood tests. One was a blood spot home test from Omega Quant and the other was from Health Diagnostics Lab. Her EPA and DHA levels were in the optimal range on both tests. So were her omega-3 to omega-6 ratios.

Having experimented with daily fish consumption myself in the 1990s and become mercury toxic (off the chart) as a result (that was before the NRDC and other groups began to alert us to the dangers of unregulated industrial dumping), I'm reluctant to formally recommend more fish. We must all keep checking for updated fish safety reports.

FISH BY OMEGA-3 CONTENT

HIGH OMEGA-3	MG PER SERVING	MEDIUM OMEGA-3	MG PER SERVING
Salmon: Atlantic, chinook, coho	2.5 mg	Rainbow Trout (farmed)	1.2 mg
Sardines	1.8–2.4 mg	Pink or sockeye salmon	1.2 mg
Herring	1.8–2.4 mg	Arctic char (farmed)	1.2 mg
Caviar/roe (per teaspoon)	1.7 mg	**LOW OMEGA-3**	**MG PER SERVING**
Oysters (farmed)	1.5 mg	Sole	.25 mg
Mackerel, Atlantic and Pacific (but not "king")	1.5 mg	Scallops	.23 mg

See Chapter 12 for fish or algae oil supplement recommendations.

The Fabulous Fats to Add*:

Coconut oil

Organic butter (if you tolerate milk products)

Organic ghee (clarified butter; butter heated to separate the more perishable and allergenic milk "solids"—(the proteins casein and whey and milk sugar)—leaving just the fat, which keeps longer (and does not typically create intolerance)

Organic lard from uncured (sugar-free) bacon/pork fat.

Fresh, leftover fat from your own bacon, chicken, duck, or other meat cooking

For salads and light sautéing: Extra-virgin olive (or macadamia nut or avocado oil, like olive oil, both are high in stable omega-9 fats)

Nuts or seeds, fresh sprouted or dry-roasted (they must be processed one way or the other to remove the digestive blockers) *Note:* Peanut is in the legume (pea/bean) family and a common allergen, besides being highly addictive for many of us. (If in doubt, test per Chapter 15.)

Full-fat milk products, if not addicted or sensitive to them (as per Chapter 15): butter, ghee, cream, yogurt, cheese, milk. *Note:* Pesticides, antibiotics, hormones, and other impurities collect in animals' fatty tissues, so go organic and grass-fed whenever possible.

The Damaging Fats

Partially hydrogenated oils (liquid vegetable oils chemically damaged to harden them, for example, margarine and shortening) are totally banned as of 2018.

Processed vegetables oils: Corn, soy, grapeseed, canola, cottonseed, and so on. These fragile, stripped, and oxidized liquid vegetable oils are also too high in inflammatory omega-6 fats. Even organic, non-GMO status doesn't help here.

Anything deep fat–fried in the above, already damaged vegetable oils: chips, fries, battered foods, doughnuts, pork rinds. Even saturated fats become damaged at this high temperature, so they can't be safely used for repeated frying.

NATURE'S CARBOHYDRATES

The amounts of carbohydrate eaten historically has varied depending on what and how much was locally available, and factors like the season, the weather, and trading or purchasing opportunities. Right now Techno-Karbz comprise 50 percent of the U.S. diet. By subtracting most of the sugar we're eating every year (130 to 160 pounds), and the refined white flours, our total carbohydrate intake can shrink to 20 to 30 percent. We'll do that by raising our fresh produce intake from 8 percent back to over 20 percent of our diet. That produce should be made up primarily of vegetables. Even the lowest-calorie green vegetables contain some carbohydrates along with vitamins, minerals, and fiber. The starchier vegetables, though often frowned on as a class because of their higher carbohydrate content, contain valuable nutrients, fiber, and lots of easily metabolized carbohydrate.

After being poisoned for over forty-five years by overdoses of post-1970s Techno-Karbz, we need to allow our carbohydrate-metabolizing functions to recover whatever degree of carbohydrate tolerance is possible for each one of us. Some people, like the diabetics among us, have become oversensitized to some, or all, of even the most traditional whole-carbohydrate foods. For them, long-term or permanent abstinence from all Techno-Karbz as well as high-carbohydrate foods like fruit, grain, and legumes is often needed. Others of us can tolerate some of these whole high-carbohydrate foods right away as long as the Techno-Karbz are out. To safely find out where each client stands in relation to nature's carbohydrates (and any other foods they're not sure about), we've provided two start-up eating options and a home food-testing process that you'll find out all about in the next two chapters.

Low-Carbohydrate Vegetables

Eat six to twelve cups a day. Eat no less than six cups a day. At first it may seem too difficult and time-consuming. But one salad and two kinds of sautéed, grilled, steamed, or pureed (as a soup) vegetables will do it. You can cook lots of them at a time so they'll be available all day for several days. But don't get stuck on just a few vegetables. Keep rotating them. *Note:* The asterisked veggies contain thyroid inhibitors (goitrogens). Eat these veggies less frequently or not at all (at least for a trial period) and avoid soy, gluten, chlorine, and fluorine as well (all thyroid suppressors) if you have the symptoms of thyroid trouble listed on p. 262.

Low-Carbohydrate Vegetables

Artichokes	Salad Greens—such as lettuces and rapini
Asparagus	Green herbs: parsley, cilantro, thyme, rosemary, etc.
Broccoli	Hearty greens—such as spinach, chard, collards, mustard, kale, arugula
Brussels sprouts	Bok choy
Cabbage	Jicama
Carrots	Kohlrabi
Cassava	Leeks
Cauliflower	Okra
Celery	Onions
Celery Root (Celeriac)	Peppers
Cucumbers	Radishes
Eggplant	Tomatoes
Green Peas	Turnip Greens
	Watercress

Please Go Organic

The nutrient content of organic produce in a multinational study was 60 percent higher than in the conventional equivalents, making them comparable to pre-1970s versions, or better.[9] Organic crops are also getting cheaper all the time as more farms convert. Farmers' markets (or your own garden) make them much fresher, too.

High-Carbohydrate Vegetables

These foods are loaded with nutrients, largely in the skins (this is one of many reasons why organic is better—you can safely *eat the skin*). Take the much-maligned potato. This ancient root originated in the Americas, but it's been incorporated successfully into European and other cuisines for centuries. For example, the Irish were saved from chronic malnutrition by potatoes. They actually grew several inches in height after the spud was introduced in their country. In 2009, the German government issued a report to the nation begging parents to feed their children potatoes again, instead of all the American-style wheat-flour-based Techno-Karbz. Why? Because potatoes are so high in the invaluable mineral potassium, found to be deficient in German children (and in many Americans of all ages). It's true that fried potatoes (and even unfried ones) can be addictive. If that's true for you, cut them out with the help of your aminos. You can always test whether or not they are safe to add back in later. Potatoes aside, we have been surprised at how seldom high-carbohydrate vegetables set off cravings (or retard weight loss).

High Carbohydrate Vegetables

Sweet Potato
Potatoes (white, yellow, purple)
All Winter Squashes (Hubbard, acorn, butternut, kabocha . . .)
Yams (orange, white, purple, red)
Beets
Parsnips
Rutabagas
Cassava Root (yucca or tapioca) (more likely to be allergenic)

Grains

Of course, the most commonly eaten food in America is powdered wheat, used to make countless highly addictive and digestively challenging Techno-Karbz. Wheat and other grains that contain gluten are also harder to digest than high-carbohydrate vegetables or other grains, and they are often more addictive, even in "whole" form. We've had so many clients with gluten intolerance and/or addiction that we always eliminate these grains first and test later by formal reintroduction. Our clients seem to tolerate gluten-free whole grains and nongrains like quinoa and amaranth, but they often become somewhat dependent on them, filling up on these high-carb foods rather than on more nutritious, lower-in-calorie, and better-digested vegetable carbs. Some lose weight nicely just going off of gluten. But others do better off of *all* grains. They provide 150 to 170 calories per cup, cooked, but their effects on weight can vary widely. In this and the next two chapters, you'll find guidelines for preparing, testing, or avoiding grains altogether, whichever works best for you.

Grains and Grain-Like Foods

GLUTEN FREE	GLUTEN CONTAINING
Amaranth	Barley, hulled
Buckwheat	Bulgur
Cornmeal	Farro
Millet	Kamut
Quinoa	Oats
Rice, brown	Rye
Sorghum	Spelt
Sorghum flour	Teff
Teff	Triticale
Wild Rice	Wheat, durum
	Wheat, hard white
	Wheat, red

Quinoa and amaranth are considered pseudocereals (technically not grains). They are both much more like seeds in their protein, fat, and calorie content. Wild rice is not a true grain, like other rice. It is the seed of a different aquatic plant. Buckwheat is a flower. This does not mean that they are necessarily easier to digest. The tolerability of grains depends on you, and on how you prepare them before cooking.

Preparing Grains for Digestibility All grains, beans, and nuts are actually seeds—capable of reproducing. As such, they have a complex nature and contain *digestion inhibitors*, so they require careful preparation before eating. Native North Americans had to process acorns extensively in water before cooking them. Most peoples prepare beans by presoaking them, once or twice, and some soak and sprout seeds and nuts, but we've lost our way when it comes to preparing the "seed" foods called grain. Traditional cultures often prepared grains before cooking them. Fermentation is common in India, where rice (and lentils) are both fermented for at least two days before they are used in staple foods like *idli* and *dosas*. Rice, brown or white, is hard to break down so its calories are the only contents we can easily digest. Yet in some Asian and Latin American countries, *rice* receives a long fermentation to make its nutrients more accessible. In some parts of Africa *corn* and *millet* are fermented for several days to produce a sour porridge called *ogi*; Ethiopians make their bread after fermenting teff for several days; tortilla masa (corn flour) has been presoaked in lime water for millennia to make it more nourishing.

Throughout Europe, oats were soaked overnight, and for as long as several days, in water or soured milk before they were cooked and served as porridge or gruel. (All this makes for grain dishes that are more like mush than the light texture of steamed rice.) The American tradition included sourdough (fermented) breads, pancakes, and biscuits, and whole corn soaked in lime water (hominy) as well as much-kneaded yeast breads. Except for hominy, these preparations are much less practiced in the United States today.

Animals that nourish themselves primarily on grain and other plant matter have as many as four stomachs. Their intestines are longer too, as is their entire digestion transit time. In contrast, humans can digest animal products quickly before they putrefy in the gut, but we're less well adapted to the more recently introduced grains—unless we prepare them through soaking, sprouting, or sour leavening. Then the friendly bacteria do some of our digesting for us.

Buy only organic whole grains and soak them overnight before cooking. If you are gluten *tolerant*, make your own sourdough bread and baked goods or buy organic, stone-ground, sprouted, or sourdough whole-grain bread products.

The best way to negotiate grain, if you're not sure how it affects you and your weight is to avoid all grain for at least a month (gluten grains three months), then reintroduce them, one grain at a time, as per Chapter 15. But if you know that, like our Far Eastern clients, you thrive on a traditional grain-inclusive diet, ignore this!

Note: This section quotes or adapts materials I love from *Nourishing Traditions* page 453 by Sally Fallon, all of whose work (including her 2017 book, *Traditional Fats*) I *highly* recommend to you.

Legumes

Like grains, nuts, and seeds, legumes are nutritious but hard to digest, requiring overnight soaking and long (or pressure) cooking. About a third of any bean is protein; two-thirds are carbohydrate. Legumes seem to be like nongluten grain for our clients: they don't binge on them, but they are sometimes drawn to fill up on them instead of vegetables. Since they are lots higher in calories, this can be a problem. In that case we recommend testing and they sometimes find, as with nongluten grains, some adverse effects such as slowed weight loss or disturbed digestion. (Especially if their blood type is O.) Even when legumes have no adverse effects, the testing period without them prompts many of our clients to get used to eating more veggies instead.

Legumes

Adzuki Beans	Lima Beans
Black Beans	Mung Beans
Black-Eyed Peas	Navy Beans
Dried Peas (split peas)	Pinto Beans
Fava Beans**	Red Beans
Garbanzo Beans (Chickpeas)	Soybeans*
Great Northern Beans	White Beans
Kidney Beans**	White Beans, small
Lentils, dried	

*Minimize soy products (they block iodine in the thyroid, raise levels of estrogens, and are very hard to digest).
**This family of legumes must be very carefully prepared.

What about Fruit?

We've been regaled with studies on the benefits of "fruits and vegetables" for years. But, though both are full of vitamins and minerals, they are not interchangeable. Most vegetables—at least six cups a day of the low-carbohydrate variety—are truly required for craving-free eating. These vegetables contain *much* less of either of the sugars, fructose or glucose, than do fruits. Removing as much of these two sugars as possible allows our blood sugar—and appetite-regulating systems, and the rest of the body as well, so traumatized by decades of fructose overload in particular—to recover. Modern conventional fruit has been bred to be bigger. Ounce for ounce, it is higher in sugars, pesticides, and GMO factors and lower in nutrients and fiber than pre-1970s fruit.[10] In the next chapter, you can choose between some fruit or, at least until testing time, no fruit.

Sugar Contents of Fruits Compared to a Coke

The more of any sugar and the higher the fructose to glucose ratio, the more potentially harmful a sweet food seems to be. In sucrose (table sugar), fructose and glucose contents are bound in equal amounts. Corn syrup, agave syrup, and fruit syrup all contain more free fructose. Whole raw fruits do contain fiber, enzymes, vitamins, and minerals that mitigate the effects of their fructose content. If you can't stop eating a fruit, it's too sweet and having a drug-like effect.

3.5 OZ. OF	FREE FRUCTOSE	FREE GLUCOSE	SUCROSE*
Coca-Cola	7.2	5.8	0
An apple	6.0	2.4	2.1
Grapes	8.1	7.2	0.2
Dried figs	22.9	24.8	0.9
An orange	2.25	2.0	4.3

*Glucose and fructose bound in a 1:1 ratio.

Stevia and Other Non-caloric Sweeteners

All of these products are hundreds of times sweeter than sugar. For example, stevia leaves are 10 to 15 times sweeter, but the extract is 100 to 300 times sweeter.[11] We've almost all become overattached and oversensitized to sweetened foods to one degree or another. Though the aminos make it possible for us to detach I recommend avoiding any sweeteners to avoid the reattachment that can come when they restimulate our brains.

You know from Chapter 2 that the taste, chemical content, and lack of nutrients in zero-calorie sweeteners can trigger some of the same cravings and blood sugar extremes that high-calorie sweeteners can (and imbalance our gut flora). Some of these products are associated with weight gain and diabetes. In spite of the health claims for stevia, it can also perpetuate the sweet fixation. We've found it important that our clients completely desensitize from ultrasweet stimulation, so we encourage them to stay away from anything that's super-sweet. They need a system-wide rest from chemical "sweetness" in *any* form, until they can test their reactions at a future time: "How does it make me feel? Do I crave sweets again since I've been having sweeteners again?"

THE ELEMENTAL FUNDAMENTALS: WATER AND SALT

Water

We (and the earth) are 70 percent water. To maintain that 70 percent is a primal need. We switched to drinking mostly soda by the end of the 1970s and began to consume an average of just 2½ cups of water a day. We're moving away from soda now and drinking a little more water. Let's take that trend all the way!

Dehydration can be a real health hazard. Heat, thirst, activity, altitude, and humidity are important considerations in calculating your water needs. *In general we seem to need to drink ½ to 1 ounce of water a day for every pound of body weight.*[12] A 200-pound person should consume between 100 and 200 ounces—twelve to twenty-four cups—of water a day: 100 ounces if he or she is sedentary and living on a moist, sea-level Hawaiian island, and eats lots of moist fruit and moist raw fish; 200 if he or she is active (sweating) and lives on a mountain eating lots of salty trail mix and jerky. I have a friend who moved to the mountains and felt sick until she learned how much water she *had* to drink daily. Now she's fine.

As for purity, I wish I were sure. Additives, contaminants, political and financial maneuvering, and plastic safety all point to filtration as our best option (since the purity of spring water is often unverifiable). Reverse osmosis (RO) water, installed in our own homes, or purchased, is a reasonable option. But there are some chemicals, notably *chloramine,* often now used in municipal water (like mine—call your water district and ask about yours) that require more filtration. Separate carbon filters are recommended, but the variety of options is daunting.

Salt

There is great debate regarding what the safe and optimal amount of salt is. The AHA urges a 1,500-mg (¼-tsp) cap on daily salt intake.[13] Yet large studies have found that the rates of heart disease among those on such low levels of sodium are much higher than among those on two to three times that amount of salt (½ to ¾ teaspoon).[14] (We used to eat 1 tablespoon [18,000 mg] daily with impunity.) Of course, if you have high blood pressure, start at the lower end and monitor your blood pressure.

We're being inundated with salt now, but, by cutting out most processed foods, you'll automatically reduce your consumption by up to 90 percent. (The seven major sources of excessive salt are commercial yeasted breads, chicken dishes, pizza, pasta, cold cuts, chips, and fries.) Then you'll need to worry about getting enough! By reducing your desire for and consumption of those foods

with amino help, you'll automatically want to increase your intake of the vegetables (and fruits) that are so rich in potassium, which we need in a 4-to-1 ratio to
sodium. Before refrigeration became universal, when salt was our primary preservative, we ate 1 tablespoon of it a day. But our health did not suffer because we
ate enough potassium-rich fresh vegetables (like potatoes) and fruits to balance
the sodium (and we were undoubtedly sweating more, too).[15] Today's commercial diet leaves most of us in the Western world deeply deficient in potassium.
This seems to be even more of a health hazard than too much salt. *Note:* We
recommend Hain's iodized sea salt, to balance out the noniodized salts that are
used now so much commercially. (Iodine is deeply depleted in our soils.)

HOW MUCH AND WHEN TO EAT?

During their Craving Cure process, our clients always say, "I don't feel like I'm
on a diet." That's because they aren't on one. It isn't always easy for them to eat a
pre-1970s diet, not because the food is difficult to prepare or tasteless, but because
it is difficult for them to prepare their *minds* to eat adequate amounts of healthy
food at least three times a day. They've been either overeating, undereating, or
more commonly, both for too long. They've been yo-yoing for so long that they
are disoriented by the concept of three square meals and a few snacks every day.
But they quickly settle into this style of eating when they see how good it makes
them feel.

How Much to Eat?

Human caloric needs vary quite a bit: forest fire–fighters need at least 6,000 calories a day, and we've seen clients with untreated thyroid problems, worsened by
too many diets, gain weight on less than 1,500 calories a day. Each body has its
ideal food and calorie needs. Many of our female clients, who are not big exer-
cises, have needed to eat 2,500 calories a day of traditional foods to achieve a
healthy weight. One woman, who *was* a big exerciser, needed 3,500 calories a day,
but of those calories, she could tolerate *zero* Techno-Karbz without weight gain.
Before 1970, women were eating an *average* of 2,000 calories; men, 2,500. Since
the '70s, we've increased our calorie intake an average of 500 calories a day. We
need to cut out the extra calories from Techno-Karbz, but typical dieters cut
much more than that, leaving themselves with less than the *minimum* number of
calories from healthy foods required to maintain their essential body functions—
including, ironically, metabolic (calorie-burning) functions.

How Many Calories Are Enough?

It depends—on your body. Our clients check their calorie levels before and after starting their new foods, to prevent inadvertently sabotaging their projects by starting to undereat. Usually the Food Log clarifies the issue, but if records are not detailed enough, calorie calculations help. Given the quantity of nutritious food needed for the Craving Cure, we don't like to see any woman go below 2,000 calories a day. She just won't get enough nutrients in the right ratios. *Remember: Eighteen hundred calories a day has been determined by the United Nations Food and Agriculture Organization to be the minimum number of calories required for minimal survival needs.*

For some historical perspective, the world held its breath during the thrilling Berlin airlift, after the USSR shut off road and rail food supplies into the city at the start of the Cold War in 1948, the West was only able to fly 1,800 calories a day per person into the city. "How long can they survive on those starvation rations?" was a very serious concern.[16]

Our goal for needed weight loss to eat as many healthy calories as possible that still allow for steady weight loss up to 4 pounds a month.

Tracking Calories

For tracking calories from specific foods, we suggest sparkpeople.com (or SparkPeople in the app store). While there are plenty of apps and programs available with calorie-count figures, they are not typically as reliable. Like most of the others, SparkPeople gives preposterously low-calorie advice for weight loss, so it's important to just ignore those SparkPeople recommendations when you sign up! For the most accurate calorie calculations, you can use https://ndb.nal.usda.gov/ndb/search at the U.S. Department of Agriculture (USDA). It doesn't calculate an entire meal's calories, but it is the best for single items. The SparkPeople app is fine for rough calculation, to make sure you're basically getting enough food. Please do your first re-calculation by the end of the first month of your Craving Cure, or earlier if you're feeling weak or have started craving for no obvious reason. *Note:* If you'd like to print out a one-page calorie guide for whole foods only, visit cravingcure.com/trackingtools.

Marianne's Calories

Marianne's odyssey illustrates the importance of knowing precisely how much you're eating. Her first diary entry recorded a typical day before this longtime yo-yo dieter had come to see us—100 percent junk food from her morning coffee with CoffeeMate and a jam sandwich to her Coke and pizza lunch to her burger, fries, and 20-ounce Dr Pepper dinner, plus five types of evening chocolate and two ice cream bars before bed. That day totaled 4,003 calories (she kept meticulous records). She had all five Craving Types, so she quickly started all five aminos, lost all her cravings, and chose one of the food plans (which you'll find in the next chapter). The food she was eating tasted fine and she felt good on it. But she relapsed two weeks later. She was, like so many of our clients, at first, so focused on introducing more protein into her diet that she missed the other big (and much less familiar) goal of getting enough overall calories. In all the excitement of losing her cravings after so many years of struggle, she'd assumed she was totally safe. But a tiny, 200-calorie dinner (half a chicken breast) on day seven set her up for her first sugary "snack" in a week. Her unconscious undereating and increased cravings continued and eroded her good intentions until she relapsed completely two weeks later. Had she come in to see us, we would have seen her Food Log and caught it, but she'd thought that the aminos were all she needed and had not yet learned how to analyze her own logs.

Back on the aminos a week later (she'd quit them during her binge) she agreed to increase her calories, and her next log reported no more cravings or slips (and no weight gain on 500 additional whole-food calories!). Her mood and digestion were better, too. We asked her to practice calculating her calories for a few weeks until she got the hang of what "enough" whole-food calories looked and felt like.

When the Scale Helps, and When It Doesn't

Given my clinic's stance on calorie counting, you might be surprised to learn that we *are not* generally pro-scale. We've seen more binges triggered by a disappointing number on the scale than by any other single factor. The result? A much more disappointing number. We prefer to have people watch their clothes instead. But there are exceptions. For example, men may tend to find daily weighing a more productive, helpful reminder.

When might *you* need to use the scale? To keep from fading away. We've learned that calorie counting and weighing yourself can be helpful when it comes to excessive weight loss. It is mandatory with anorexia (but only the clinician or other helper sees the numbers). Weight loss dieting can, totally unintentionally, turn into anorexia. This deadly condition is very hard to correct, though nutrient supplementation (*see The Diet Cure,* Chapters 2 and 10) can help reverse it, reprogramming the brain and body to accept food again. We have had a few clients who lost too much weight on over 2,100 calories and had to fight to get some back. They were not fighting their own minds—they knew they were too thin, but it took a while to work out which foods and quantities would work for them. Meanwhile, they needed the feedback of the scale, along with the calorie app.

How *Often* To Eat?

Eat at least three times a day. Research actually shows that the more often you eat (as long as you're eating non-Techno-Karbz), the slimmer you are. All three meals are crucial, but without that first meal at breakfast, the whole day tends to fall apart. We've seen this thousands of times. As you'll see, snacks can help. The more balanced the better. Our clients eat three to seven times a day, depending on their personal needs.

Breakfast: Our clients find it best to eat breakfast within one hour of awakening, and to eat at least 25 percent of the day's calories (500–700) in the morning. Since we haven't usually eaten for at least eight hours, this first meal of the day literally breaks our fast as it hauls up our blood sugar levels to prevent cravings and generally wakes up our metabolic activity. If you skip breakfast and have some caffeine instead, you'll set off a blood sugar roller coaster that can last all day. You'll crave some quick Techno-Karbz and/or more coffee by late morning, which will throw off your appetite for lunch. Even if you do get in a decent lunch, we've

---

Research on Breakfast

There is so much research on the connection between not eating breakfast and increases in weight gain and diabetes, not to mention the association between no breakfast and fatigue, infertility, heart disease, cognitive defects, and worse grades, that it won't fit into the Notes section![17] Bottom line: Eating breakfast is imperative, and we've found the best amount to be at least 25 percent of the total days' calories.

found that, if breakfast has been missed, the mid-to-late-afternoon cravings usually kick in hard. (Type 2 Cravers are especially vulnerable to this.)

Lunch and Dinner: Let no more than four hours (some people can go five hours) pass between breakfast and lunch, and again no more than six hours between lunch and dinner. Most clients need a snack midafternoon to get them through, at least until they are getting enough food at meals that they no longer need snacks so often.

Snacks: I've looked at snack research as far back as 1964 (when snack foods were mostly healthy!) up to a 2014 study. All showed that weight loss correlated with between-meal snacking. But we've lost the traditional concept of meals and snacks. "Snacking all day" on Techno-Karbz has taken its place. We have to retrieve and restore what I'll call mini meals, real food eaten between full meals to "keep up your strength," as my mother used to say when she dished up the sugar-and-hydrogenated-fat-free peanut butter on whole wheat raisin toast and whole milk after school.

With the help of the between-meal aminos, many of our clients find it easy and comfortable to eat just three meals a day. But other *can't* go for four hours without craving, at least at first. Later they may figure out how much more of which foods they need to take in at meals to keep them satisfied between meals. Our many Type 2s, especially, *have* to have snacks midmorning, midafternoon, at bedtime, or all of the above, long term.

Because it's not always possible to guarantee that all three of your meals will be available at just the right times, always have enough food with you for two snacks. If you find yourself craving, hungry, weak, or stressed *at any time* between meals, have one of those snacks! Taking snacks with you wherever you go probably sounds like a bother, but once you experience this relief from craving and other low-blood-sugar symptoms, you'll see the point. So don't leave home without snacks for at least the first month, until you know for sure how often you'll need them. You'll find snack lists with the recipes on page 358.

With this fundamental food information under your belt, it's time for some food action. The next chapter will help you choose between two culinary options that will define exactly what your own personal plate will look, taste, and feel like— for the first three months, at least.

14

Traditional Cuisines: Choosing What Works Best for You

NOW THAT YOU'VE BEEN REGALED with the facts about the three elemental foods and advised about when and how much of them to eat, I'll help you with implementation. Since there is no single diet that works for everyone, so I'm offering you two! My ultimate goal is to help you factor in your own dietary needs and preferences so that you can develop an anti-craving eating plan that suits, satisfies, and saves you. Our clinic clients begin this food-tailoring process by selecting one of the two jump-start plans. Both are delicious and healthful and both provide adequate calories made up of a balance of the three fundamental foods. But they differ in the types and proportions of the protein-, fat-, and carbohydrate-rich foods they're composed of. Which start-up food plan would be best for you?

I've already urged you to run screaming from newly invented diets and return to the traditional eating habits of your forbears. But there are actually two ancient eating traditions for you to choose from. The first and the most ancient is, of course, the Hunter-Gatherer.

During the time of the omnivorous apes (who were, presumably, our original forbears), we were just gatherers. We ate raw vegetables, fruits, eggs, and very small creatures. Then, two million years ago, we began to also scavenge meat left by carnivorous animals. Over the next million years, we became hunters and cooks. Cooking our meat made it more edible and assimilable. This increase in meat-eating provided the extra proteins, fats, phospholipids, and other nutrients that allowed our brains to double and then triple in size. It's a meat-enabled brain that is allowing you to read this page. The Hunter-Gatherer cuisine included neither dried beans, grains, nor the milk of animals. Now that we can identify the genetic traces of our own ancient ancestry, including the Neanderthal, we can understand that some part of us can still respond to this primitive menu. The popularity of the Paleo diet is a testament to these persisting Hunter instincts.

The second feeding option, the Herder-Planter, developed about 12,000 years ago when we began cultivating plants, herding and milking animals, and doing lots more food preparing. This is the option that most of the planet gradually adopted, until the late twentieth century, when the food industry began to design, produce, and sell us on our current fare.[1]

As both Hunters and Herders, whether we ate wild or domesticated animals and plants, we've been able to count on our strength, health, and genetically appropriate sizes and shapes.

I call the two eating traditions *Hunter* and *Herder* for short. Choosing one of these eating options is not a matter of temperament; whether you think of yourself as a "hunting" or a "herding" sort of person. It certainly has nothing to do with whether or not you're a vegetarian—both traditions include meat. There are several other factors to consider as you decide which plan's contents best suit your tastes, your body, and your life. This chapter will help you take into account your personal trigger foods, food sensitivities, blood type, ethnic diet preferences, and certain health questions.

HUNTER/HERDER BENEFITS AND HOW MY CLINIC CAME TO APPRECIATE THEM

Once you've gone either Hunter or Herder, the positive effects of your new food choices should quickly become obvious. For example, you should experience even fewer cravings than on the aminos alone and more energy, not to mention less weight, bloating, gas, mental fog, wheezing, and constipation. Your Daily Food Log's entries should soon be delightfully different from your original baseline records. After two weeks, you can expect to settle into a consistent eating pattern that will sustain and improve on these benefits.

You may have heard that many common foods can trigger inflammation or water retention and that eliminating these foods can cause an immediate loss of up to 10 pounds. It's true! We've found that jettisoning all toxic Techno-Karbz, even whole *non*gluten-containing grains, and any other "allergy foods" can produce this quick weight drop without any extreme calorie restriction. This weight drop is not only quick, it's also permanent, *as long as you* stay away from whichever foods are causing the *inflammatory reaction*. But how would you know? To find out for sure which food or foods are the cause, you'll need to test—that is, formally reintroduce—each food you'd eliminated. Otherwise you'll take them all back at once, gain back the weight, bloat, and so on, and never know exactly why. In this chapter, we'll embark on the first, food-eliminating phase which clears away potentially harmful foods. In the next phase, described in the next chapter, you'll learn how to experimentally reintroduce some of those foods, one by one, to see how you tolerate them and if you can broaden your food choices at all without retriggering cravings.

Our clinic started out recommending Herder foods, but found that they did not work as well for as many of our clients as the narrower Hunter food plan that we tried about a year later. After we started using the aminos, though, we reintroduced the Herder as an option and found that many of our clients preferred it and did well on it (as their more recent forbears had). Over time, though, our new clients began coming to us in worse and worse shape and more of them seemed to be unable to tolerate even whole grains, fruits, legumes, or milk products as well as they had. And the women weren't losing as much weight as they had. We think that this is because the progressively worse quality of our food has eroded their immune systems and their digestive and metabolic functions. They are just more compromised system-wide now, as are we all. So we began to help them to more carefully choose between these options and to ultimately create their own individualized plans.

COMPARING PLANS: HUNTER-GATHERER OR HERDER-PLANTER?

The following table compares the Hunter and Herder plans, starting with the foods that are recommended for one or both options and ending with the foods that are recommended for neither. In other words, here are the basic yeas (checks) and nays (exes) of craving-free eating:

	HUNTER	HERDER
Animal protein: eggs, meats, poultry, seafood, milk products (if tolerated)	✓	✓
Veggies	✓	✓
Fruit	X	✓
Whole grains (if tolerated)	X	✓
Gluten-containing grains	X	X
Fat: coconut oil, extra-virgin olive oil, avocado oil, macadamia nut oil, organic lard, bacon or chicken fat	✓	✓

Legumes: dried beans, peas, lentils (except soy)	X	✓
Nuts and seeds: dry roasted or sprouted	✓	✓
Vegetable oils (e.g., soy, corn, canola, cottonseed, safflower)	X	X
Hydrogenated oils (even partially)	X	X
Techno-Karbz: sugars, artificial sweeteners, refined (white) flour	X	X
Honey	X	X
Chocolate	X	X
Caffeine	X	X
MSG	X	X
Alcohol	X	X
Any foods causing adverse physical symptoms (see page 248)	X	X

WHAT EXACTLY DO HUNTER-GATHERERS OR HERDER-PLANTERS *NOT* EAT? DETACHING FROM ADDICTIVE AND TOXIC FOODS

I hate talking about food restriction almost as much as I hate talking about weight. You've had too much restriction inflicted on you already. However, as you consider the "ins" and "outs" of each of the Craving Cure's two food plans, remember that you're reading about them for the first time, and have yet to experience the super-powers that your amino supplements will bestow. Until the aminos have wiped out your cravings, it will be nearly impossible for your Techno-Karbz-addled brain to imagine how free of craving you will be and how much easier giving up foods that are chemically engineered to be impossible to give up can be. The aminos make it possible—no, the aminos make it *easy*. Like our clients initially think, you're thinking: "A life without pasta is no life at all!" or "No matter how full I am, I have a separate stomach for dessert" or "I can't get out of bed without caffeine" or "I can't imagine getting through any day without chocolate." But this is the cravings talking. On the aminos, they'll shut up.

Whichever option you start with, you will probably modify to suit your personal needs and tastes over the next twelve weeks, and beyond. You aren't trapped forever in anyone else's rigid concept of what you should eat, including mine! But for now, take that complete extended break from certain foods, like chocolate or gluten-containing foods, that you may have wanted to take for years. Or you may be one of the many who cannot let go of ice cream despite the wheezing, the diarrhea, and the weight gain. But when the aminos come to your rescue, you can finally stop, objectively observe the effects of *any* foods, and make reasoned decisions about whether to continue eating them or not now, and whether to try them again later in a formal food-reintroduction test—or not.

DETOX: WILL THIS ELIMINATION PROCESS BE HARD?

Some diet book authors report awful detox symptoms, and you may have experienced them yourself when trying to follow such programs. In the mid-1980s, our early Hunter clients used to go through at least eight weeks of uncomfortable withdrawal as well. But since we've introduced the aminos, they rarely go through much discomfort at all!

Whether you choose to proceed as a Hunter or a Herder, the craving-busting, mood- and energy-supporting powers of your aminos will make the transition smooth. The therapeutic effects of eliminating foods that really are "bad for you" and eating foods that really are "good for you" will quickly make you feel even better. In case you do have an unusually severe detox reaction for a few days, though, start the process on a weekend or an otherwise undemanding couple of days.

Be sure to drink 7–8 cups of water or chamomile or mint tea a day to assist in the clean-out process. Though taking 2,000–6,000 mg of vitamin C a day can be helpful during any drug withdrawal, our clients rarely seem to feel the need of this extra help. (If you do use vitamin C, cut back if your bowels get loose.) They just don't have much discomfort beyond some manageable fatigue or a headache for a day or two. For *that*, if needed, they can use the OTC anti-inflammatory of their choice briefly.

Our clients swear by our Caffeine Detox Protocol (see the details on page 191 in Chapter 12), which is almost completely infallible when it comes to the dreaded caffeine withdrawal headaches and fatigue.

THE HUNTER-GATHERER OPTION

YES	MINIMUM STARTING SERVINGS	NO
Cooked protein: eggs, meats, poultry, seafood, milk products (if tolerated)	6–8 oz females, 8–10 oz male adults/meal	All Techno-Karbz Fruit
Low-Carb Veggies	4–6 cups /meal	Whole Grains
High-Carb Veggies	½–1 cup/meal	Gluten-containing grains
Fat: coconut oil, extra-virgin olive oil, butter, avocado oil, macadamia nut oil, organic lard, bacon or chicken fat	1 Tb added to each meal	Legumes: dried beans, peas, lentils

Nuts and seeds, sprouted	3 Tb / 3x wk	Vegetable oils (e.g., soy, corn, canola, cottonseed, safflower) Hydrogenated oils (even partially)
<u>Diabetic Hunters:</u> May need to omit all high-carb veggies and increase low-carb to 6 cups/meal		Techno-Karbz: sugars, artificial sweeteners, refined (white) flour Honey, maple syrup, molasses Chocolate Caffeine MSG Alcohol Any foods causing adverse physical symptoms (see page 235)

Adult Female Calories: 2,000–2,500 to start.
Adult Males: Increase all food by a quarter to a third (500–750 calories more).

As a Hunter, right from the start, in addition to stepping away from all Techno-Karbz, you'll also, at least temporarily, forgo some of the Herder-Planter era staples, the higher carbohydrate ones. Grains and legumes are not in the Hunter plan. Neither are fruits. Neither are milk products if you crave them or have any of the symptoms on the food sensitivity list page 235. Later, you should formally reintroduce any or all of these foods, one by one, to see which ones might become "keepers" and which might retrigger cravings or digestive problems, slow down your weight loss, or raise your blood sugar levels too high. The Hunter plan's narrower initial array of foods *does not reduce calories*—your daily total intake will be the same as on a Herder's plan—but it does speed up the food-elimination process and can, as a result, have faster health benefits and faster weight loss.

To make up for the calories you won't be getting from higher carbohydrate foods as a Hunter, you'll eat more whole fats, more protein, and more low-carbohydrate vegetables (plus some high-carb vegetables, especially if you're active). Why cut out fruit, grains, legumes, and milk products if not to lose calories? Fruit goes because of its high fructose content. It was obviously not harmful in our historic past, and even up through the 1960s, when it was not a big part of our diet. But our huge exposure to high-fructose syrups in recent decades has been so destructive that many of us need a break from it, at least temporarily. (Chapter One, page 45 if you've forgotten, explains the glycation problems with "excess free fructose.") Because many fruits have higher fructose than glucose contents, they can be addictive for some people and, more important, can perpetuate the metabolic and genetic damage already well underway under the influence of high-fructose corn, agave, and fruit syrup–sweetened Techno-Karbz.

For its part, *grain*, a relatively recent addition to the human diet and mostly composed of carbohydrate, contains many digestive inhibitors, which can make it hard for some of us to digest. (Especially since we no longer use all the traditional methods of making it more digestible.) *Legumes,* though typically soaked before cooking to remove their digestive inhibitors, are also a relatively modern food. Like grain, they are largely inedible for almost half of us, those with blood type O, the oldest human blood type and the most natural Hunters. As for milk products, they were not part of the human diet till Herder times. We do find that type Os, in particular, can have trouble with them.

MY CLINIC'S EXPERIMENT WITH THE HUNTER OPTION

At my first clinic, we began, in 1983, after much staff debate and expert consultation, to recommend our own version of one of the food plans that seemed to be the most successful of the Overeaters Anonymous's options. It was closer to what we now call a Paleo diet, but with more food. Two of my staff counselors had each lost over 100 pounds on the similar O.A. food plan, and had kept it off for many years. This plan cut out all Techno-Karbz and any other known or potentially addictive "trigger" foods. The plan was both extremely narrow and extremely nutrient-dense. It consisted of:

- 6–8 ounces of animal protein per meal (full fat, skin intact)
- 2–3 T of added oil or butter for cooking, dressing salads, or saucing per meal
- 4–6 cups of cooked or raw, mostly low-carb, vegetables per meal
- No snacks, unless required by the nutritionist or M.D.

It added up to 2,500–3,000 calories per day. No one was hungry. But everyone lost weight. Despite eight to twelve weeks of uncomfortable withdrawal symptoms including negative moods and cravings, our clients eventually raved about their improved mood, energy, digestion, PMS, and encouraging weight loss. For the most part, they enjoyed this food, though some clients complained about having to weigh and measure it and that there was too much of it—an experience they said they'd never had before!

Because of all the protein they were eating, loaded with amino acids, they typically lost most, *but not all,* of their cravings and mood problems. Without the aminos, which we hadn't yet discovered, 70 percent did relapse within two years, though most were able to get back on what they all agreed was this "best ever" food plan, at least for a while. Now, combined with the amino breakthrough, "best ever" can be "Hunter forever."

To give you an idea of the Hunter plan, day to day, here's an example from a Hunter client's Food Log followed by more detail on her experience of becoming a Hunter.

One Day in the Life of Ida the Huntress

"Slept well. I woke up at 8 AM with good energy."

BREAKFAST 9:00 AM

2 cups green beans, steam-sautéed in 2 tablespoons EVOO

3 chicken thighs (skin on), roasted

1 yam, quartered and roasted in with the chicken

2 tablespoons chicken fat over the yam and chicken

"Felt fine all morning."

LUNCH 2:00 PM

4 ounces leftover shredded turkey breast on 3 cups salad greens will

1½ tablespoons of dressing

1½ tablespoons mayo, homemade

1 large artichoke, steamed

"4 PM nice bike ride, 40 min."

DINNER 7:00 PM

2 cups steamed zucchini, pureed to make a soup, topped with fresh herbs

2 duck breasts w/crispy skin (6 ounces), roasted

1 cup sweet potatoes, roasted in pan with duck

3 tablespoons duck fat drizzled over duck and potatoes

"Yummy! Evening energy good"

DAY'S TOTAL CALORIES: 2,358

"Very sleepy by 10:30 PM. The bedtime supplements are really helping this former night owl!"

Ida, a former vegan, was allergic to fish and milk products and leery of red meat. She also had low hydrochloric acid and was waiting to add more red meat until her hydrochloric acid levels improved enough for her to digest it (see HCl test, page 286). (She had a party when she ate her first red meat a month later!) She started with poultry, and did she ever like it! She said that duck breast was the filet mignon of birds. Her "birds" were also simple to prepare and she made enough in a single Crock-Pot batch or soup to supply the protein for two days' worth of meals.

As one of the numerous junk-food vegans who'd come to us, Ida found the unfamiliar high proportion of vegetables and fat, and, of course, animal protein, particularly at breakfast, odd at first, but she got used to it and enjoys it now. The subtle pleasures of vegetables quickly grew on her, and she loved experimenting with a variety of fresh herbs on them. The fat seemed too good to be true. Indeed, she could tell that it was the fat that carried her so easily from meal to meal with very little hunger or blood sugar crashing (and good weight loss!).

THE HERDER-PLANTER OPTION

YES	MINIMUM STARTING SERVINGS	NO
	Women-Men	
Animal protein: eggs, meats, poultry, seafood, milk products (if tolerated)	4–6 oz. (cooked) 35–45 g/meal	All Techno-Karbz Gluten-containing grains
Low-Carbohydrate Veggies	9 cups/day	Vegetable oils (e.g. soy, corn, canola, cottonseed, safflower)
High-Carbohydrate Veggies	1–2 cups	
Fat: coconut oil, extra-virgin olive oil, butter, avocado oil, macadamia nut oil, organic lard, bacon or chicken fat	2–3 Tb. added to each meal	Hydrogenated oils (even partially)
Fruit	2/day	Techno-Karbz: sugars, artificial sweeteners, refined (white) flour
Whole grains (if tolerated)	½–1 cup*	Honey, maple syrup, molasses
Legumes: dried beans, peas, lentils (except soy)	½–1 cup*	Chocolate Caffeine
Nuts and seeds, nut butters (sprouted)	2 Tb. / 3x wk	Alcohol
		Any foods causing adverse physical symptoms (see page 235)

Adult Female Calories: 2,000–2,500 to start.
Adult Males: Increase all food by a quarter to a third (500–750 calories more).
*For the day, 2 cups total beans and/or grains, and/or high carb veggies for females, 3 cups for males.

If you choose this eating option, you'll get to eat eggs, meats, poultry, seafood, plus milk products, if you tolerate them well. (If you have any doubt, stay off milk products till month two and reintroduce as per Chapter 15.) The Hunter's fats, too, are included in this plan: nuts and seeds (preferably sprouted), coconut, extra-virgin olive, avocado or macadamia nut oils; butter or ghee (clarified butter); organic lard, chicken fat, and bacon fat—yes, you read that right: *bacon fat* (so long as the bacon it comes from is free of sugar and chemicals). But you get more: whole grains (*without gluten*), legumes (beans, peas, lentils), fruit, and almost as many bounteous vegetables! (Remember, with your cravings for Techno-Karbz gone, you won't have just eaten two cupcakes, so *you'll be hungry for all of the above.*) As you can see, lots more types of food are available to you as a Herder than are available to Hunters. And on this broader diet, health and weight were excellent for 12,000 years, till the 1970s, for the humans of the world who were no longer hunter-gatherers.

The best way to get a sense of what it's really like to go Herder is to step into one of our Herder clients' footwear.

RICHARD'S HERDER-PLANTER EXPERIENCE

Four months after starting at our virtual clinic for food cravers and overeaters, our client Richard sent us the following e-mail. "I'm the rock star of your program: I'm totally craving-free and eating lots of protein, vegetables, and olive oil, butter, and coconut oil. I'm even going to the farmers' market. I use beans and fruit (which tested well) but no sugars or grains and it's working for me! I'm off of disability and back to my full-time job. And (are you sitting down?) I've lost twenty-five pounds!" (*Note:* Men tend to lose weight faster than women.)

Here's what Richard was up against when we first met him:

At six feet tall and sixty years old, he weighed 300 pounds. A former go-getter, he was so fatigued and unable to focus or produce that he'd spent the previous six months at home, unable to work. For ten years, his diet had consisted mostly of ready-made sweets and starches. He was intelligent and well informed so he knew that this was the wrong food but, because of his craving and his exhaustion, he literally couldn't do any better.

Richard's Craving-Type Questionnaire showed that he had Craving Types 1, 3, 4, and 5—not unusual. On the indicated aminos, he quickly eliminated his insomnia, his fatigue, and his inability to focus, along with much, but not all, of his craving.

Although Richard (who was adopted) had no ethnic clues to guide his food *choices, he began to change his diet the day after he started his aminos. He quit all sweetened food and ate his first breakfast in six years during the first week. By the end of that week, on a scale of 1 to 10, his cravings and overeating had been cut in half, from eights to fours. That was the good news. The bad news was that he was only halfway there. Although he had given starchy foods the highest possible score (10) on his original Trigger-Foods Rating Sheet, he'd tried just cutting out the sugary foods first (he'd scored them as tens, too). Now he understood why his cravings weren't gone completely: he was more addicted to the starchy foods than the sweet ones! But with all his aminos at optimal doses (he'd needed to raise some of them a little), he was ready, willing, and able to take another step. So he jettisoned the bread, the rolls, the pasta, the tortillas, and all whole grains as well. The payoff was remarkable: His craving scores all went to zeros, his chronic constipation disappeared, his weight loss sped up, and his energy spiked. Although he was willing to also cut out legumes and fruit, he didn't need to.*

To make his food prep easier and quicker, especially the vegetables, he bought a fancy blender and a Crock-Pot. He already liked cooking meat on his grill but he learned that vegetables cooked that way were a real pleasure, too. He also went organic, because he discovered that vegetables had so much more flavor if they were organic from local farmers' markets. (He discovered produce was cheaper there, too!)

Richard was working full-time again in two months and stayed craving free on his gradually customized Herder plan. Regular exercise, for the first time in years, also became a frequent and enjoyable part of his life.

FACTORS THAT CAN HELP YOU PICK YOUR PLAN

Now that you have an impression of the two plans, let your own personal trigger foods, food sensitivities, blood type, ancestral diet, and any diabetic condition be your guides to the best eating plan for *you*.

YOUR TRIGGER FOODS

Review your baseline Trigger Foods Rating Sheet (see Tracking and Testing Tools, page 267). This will help you choose which plan will be best for you. What if you have a trigger food that is included in a plan? For example, nuts and seeds are included in both the Hunter and Herder options, but some people can't stop eating them. (I'm one of them.) Or you may find yourself drawing the line at the idea of giving up the Greek yogurt you eat every morning or the cheeses that are part of most of your meals. Yet on the food sensitivity list (coming up) you see several indications that these milk products may be harmful to your health. Just the fact that you want to draw the line so badly ("What else will I eat!? Grrr.") tells you that dairy addiction is a question to consider carefully. *But only consider it after you've started the aminos.* We don't encourage clients to change their diets till they've done their amino trials and begun taking daily supplements. You've had enough racking withdrawals and prolonged feelings of deprivation. I don't want you to see this as just another ordeal.

Whichever option you choose, the foods checked on the Trigger Foods list will comprise your "no" foods (for now, at least). Later, you'll go through it again to decide if you'd like to "trial" some of those nuts or milk products, for example, and see whether they still set-off cravings or other adverse symptoms, or not.

THE FOOD SENSITIVITY FACTOR

Identifying Your Own Food Sensitivities

Food intolerance may express itself through many adverse health symptoms, beyond cravings or weight gain. Here are the symptoms we've found to be the most common and the foods that we've found to most often trigger them. This list will help to steer you toward the initial option, Hunter or Herder, that best fits your sensitivities. Circle the symptoms you have now to compare with once you review it again over time (monthly).

- *Gastrointestinal:* gas, bloat, pain, cramping, diarrhea, constipation (often lifelong). *Most common triggers:* gluten-containing foods and/or lactose-containing milk products, and/or fructose malabsorption.

- *Skin:* rash, acne, psoriasis. *Most common trigger:* gluten.

- *Pain:* head, joints, other. *Most common triggers:* often sugar, sometimes nightshade plants (tomato, peppers, potato, eggplant, and tobacco).

- *Lungs/respiration:* asthma, sneezing, coughing, postnasal drip. *Most common triggers:* milk products or gluten.

- *Fatigue (unrelated to insomnia). Most common triggers:* gluten, sugar
- *PMS: Most common triggers:* sugar, caffeine, gluten.
- *Thyroid: Most common triggers:* soy, gluten, fluoridated/chlorinated water, the Brassica family of vegetables, mercury (e.g., in low-omega-3 fish).
- *Mood:* e.g., depression, anxiety, irritability, inattention, hyperactivity. *Most common triggers:* sugar and/or gluten; many other possible trigger foods include milk, eggs, high-salicylate foods (and food coloring).

Gluten: Not for Hunters or Herders

The most common of the addictions (after sugar), food intolerances, and sensitivity reactions that have plagued our clients have been prompted by gluten-containing foods. That's why they're eliminated in both Hunter and Herder plans. But gluten intolerance is not universal! Only testing will tell, though. And elimination is the first phase of food testing. Many people are now casually (and incompletely) "going gluten free." Most of them don't know why. In fact, weight gain, insulin resistance, and metabolic syndrome are often the result for those who "switch" to the highly processed gluten-free Techno-Karbz substitutes (even if they don't also cheat on wheat).[2]

Anything containing *wheat, rye, spelt,* or *barley* certainly contains gluten, but gluten in some form is in so many prepared foods that I don't have room to list them in this book! Please see the comprehensive list on the Celiac Disease Foundation site at https://celiac.org/live-gluten-free/glutenfreediet/2. The best way to avoid gluten is to do more cooking from scratch—and there are many recipes to encourage that in the Recipe section on page 295.

What about oats? There is ongoing debate about oats, but we find that most people who react to wheat also have problems with oats. A ten-year study found that almost 10 percent of celiacs reacted to oats as well.[3] It tends to be those who eat oats daily who balk at even testing them, yet they're the ones who most need to test! Please remove oats for at least two weeks before reintroducing them separately from wheat, rye, and so on. Be sure to get only *certified gluten-free oats* in any case as, otherwise wheat will almost certainly be present.

Milk Sensitivity

A sensitivity (and/or addiction) to milk products is the second most common negative food reaction we see (after gluten). If you tend to crave or be allergic to milk products, cut out *all* cow-, goat-, and sheep-milk products for at least one month. But do *not* replace milk products with lots of high-omega-6 almond or other nut milk. Mostly use coconut milk (unsweetened) as a substitute. See the Recipe section for nonmilk breakfast ideas.

YOUR BLOOD TYPE IS A GOOD CLUE IN CHOOSING FOODS

Most of the people we've worked with have had either blood type O or blood type A, the two most common types. From them we've learned a lot about these two blood types' genetically programmed affinity for some foods and intolerance of others. It can help vegans, for example, to know that the fact that they have an O blood type means that they have a strong genetic tendency to thrive only on the most ancient diet. O's are the true Hunters, as the O type is the oldest blood type and really does best only on vegetables (including root vegetables), meats, poultry, seafood, as well as some fruits, nuts, and seeds. Type O's, not surprisingly, have the lowest rates of type 2 diabetes. All other blood types have higher rates, with B positives being at the highest risk.[4] (See Recipes and Menus for advice on how to rehab overly restrictive Paleo recipes.) Type O's have usually liked the Paleo-type diets, but like so many Paleos, have cut calories too low and gotten overly attached to coffee, chocolate, and alcohol (the aminos take care of these "attachments"). They all seem to digest and tolerate fruit well, but fruit was only available seasonally and type O Hunters were never deluged by sugar concentrates year-round as we are today. So please take a rest from it and reintroduce it per Chapter 15 in month two.

Blood type A's, we've found, are often drawn to the Herder eating option because they digest beans well, unlike O's, who typically experience lots of gas. (Soybeans and soy products are often hard for *all* types to digest or tolerate.) A's often do not tolerate gluten-containing grains or sometimes milk products well. But they seem to digest nongluten grain pretty well. They thrive on animal protein, as we all tend to do, but may stick with fish and poultry because they feel "heavy" when eating red meat. That is often because blood type A is associated with the low production of hydrochloric acid, which is required for the digestion of dense proteins. If you have type A blood, turn to the Tracking and Testing Tools, page 293, for suggestions on how to assess and, if needed, improve your hydrochloric acid status. People with this blood type have been identified as "natural vegetarians," but we don't agree. They *can* digest more foods than those with the Hunter-Gatherer O blood type can, having evolved later, during the early stages of the development of agriculture. But we didn't *stop* eating animal protein then; we just started *herding* our meat, which we ate along with our newly planted vegetables, beans, and grains. Two naturopathic physicians,

Peter J. and James L. D'Adamo, father and son, have devoted their careers to this subject. What I describe here reflects only those general conclusions of theirs (arrived at independently) that have been confirmed by our clinical observation of the primary blood types O and A. Since we have seen so few of the rare B and AB blood types, I have no actual experience of them to share.

Don't know your own blood type? Get an inexpensive blood test through your doctor or a blood spot test through the Internet. (See Tracking and Testing Tools, page 293.)

YOUR ETHNIC DIET: YET ANOTHER POTENTIALLY HELPFUL CLUE IN FOOD CHOOSING

Should you adopt the Asian diet, heavy on vegetables and rice? Or a diet heavy on corn and beans? Whether of Scandinavian, Italian, Japanese, or Iroquois extraction, our clients almost always respond best to their "native" eating traditions. Their genes actually seem to recognize the ancient foods and correct their appetites and weights accordingly. If you are even close to being pure-blooded, it will be easier for you to determine the foods that might be best for you, right away, with less testing. For example, Asians have adapted to better digest rice.

A Nicaraguan student at a local college spoke up in a class I taught a few years ago. She said that she'd gained a lot of weight when she came to the States, but lost it all when she went home every summer. I asked, "Do you diet when you're at home, or exercise a lot more?" She said, "No and no." I asked how many carbs she ate at home. "Lots of beans and rice, but also meat, poultry, vegetables, and fruit." I asked how often she ate Techno-Karbz when she was at home. "Once a day." And in the United States? "Nothing but sweets and fast food." End of yo-yo weight mystery. Then I asked her if she could eat her "home food" in the United States? "Easily," she said, "I'd just never thought to do it. U.S. food is so glamorous to us at home . . . I didn't know it was so dangerous." She had a ready-made, tried-and-true craving-free eating plan. All she had to do was test to see if she could tolerate any American dulces (sweets) as she could at home. She couldn't.

This is an important point for Herders: If your tradition includes, for example, white rice or sugary sauces as staples, try this long-traditional form of rice and sugar*less* sauces and see how you do. You can trade it in for brown rice if you find yourself craving it. But most of our Asian clients seem fine with it.

Like so many of us in the United States, you may be a genetic mystery mix. But if you don't know your heritage, don't worry. Do a Herder program if you know that your lineage thrived on Asian or Central/South American cuisine. Otherwise, make your best educated guess. If you're a Native American or Native African, do some research. For example, a California client of the Pomo tribe was raised partly on fresh-caught salmon, acorn mush, venison, wild greens, and tule bulbs by his grandmother. Yet he did not have to become a Hunter. He did very well just by avoiding sugar and wheat flour and by going back to fishing. (He was single and both worked and ate at a casino, so this was a blessing.)

TIME TO DECIDE: HUNTER-GATHERER OR HERDER-PLANTER?

This chart sums up the individual factors that can help you pick a plan.

HUNTER	HERDER
If you have blood type O.	If you have, in the recent past, felt well and lost weight on a similar diet (until your cravings drove you back to the Techno-Karbz).
If you've liked Paleo diets.	If you'd like to try an ethnic eating style that includes whole grains and/or beans and/or dairy products that you know worked well for your forbears.
If you have food sensitivities, especially to grains or milk products (see list on page 236).	If you have no or few known food sensitivities (see list page 235).
If you have type 1 or type 2 diabetes.	If you're reluctant to make major dietary changes beyond dumping the Techno-Karbz. At least for now.
If you have non-alcoholic fatty liver disease.	
If you are eager to try cutting out more carbohydrates for weight loss.	
If you have fructose malabsorption, yeast overgrowth, or chronic digestive or other health problems.	

THE *DIABETIC* HUNTER'S THERAPEUTIC OPTIONS

Eliminating Techno-Karbz from your plate, courtesy of the aminos, can stabilize your blood sugar and prevent further glycation, inflammation, *and* weight gain. It can also help prevent further kidney, liver, cardiovascular, circulatory, and pancreatic damage and promote healing. All this in only a few days! In Chapter 7, I told the story of two generations of diabetics whose high blood sugars fell into the normal range within twenty-four hours of starting just the amino acid gluta-mine. Our *prediabetic* clients can do well on either eating plan, but we recom-mend that *all types 1 and 2 diabetics* start as Hunters. Why? Because they have typically become so overreactive to carbohydrates, fructose in particular.

The Hunter plan will shift you as much as possible away from high-carbohydrate foods, not just the Techno-Karbz. Since gluten intolerance is known to be a causative factor in diabetes, gluten certainly must go. Tubers, winter squash, and legumes need to be monitored and sugar-cured meats def-initely won't work at the diabetic table, but feasting will still go on.[5]

If you are not insulin dependent, you may test out legumes and then other higher-carbohydrate whole foods later, as described in the next chapter, moni-toring your reactions with your glucometer and careful Food Log entries. Other-wise, don't bother.

We've found that our Type 1 and progressed Type 2 clients with diabetes can only rarely reintroduce any higher-carbohydrate foods (and much research con-curs).[6] But here is the good news: They can enjoy and thrive on rich, savory sauces made with fats like cheese, nuts, butter, olive oil, coconut cream, and the fat from meat, or poultry, over a marvelous variety of low-carbohydrate vegetables and proteins. Think artichokes with homemade mayonnaise, zucchini pasta with cheese sauce, pork/vegetable-kebabs marinated and cooked with ginger, lime, garlic, and olive oil. I know, you've been told forever to eat low fat (as well as low calorie), but adding traditional, undamaged fats seems to be actually life-saving for diabetics,[7] as it is for anyone with unstable blood sugar. Saturated fats plus adequate protein and low-carb calories equals level blood sugars.

Regarding milk products: Please test them out as soon as possible so that you know whether or not you can use them. I hope you can. The organic, pas-tured, full-fat products are known now to help prevent and ameliorate diabetes.[8] You need such full-fat, high-protein foods to enrich your limited diet, especially for sauces from butter, cheese, cream, milk, and yogurt.

Cooking Tips: Diabetics have long been known to be particularly endangered by any glycated (sweetened or browned) foods. To minimize the latter, try to cook more often with lower heat and increased moisture. Use marinades with meats, poultry, or fish with lemon or vinegar before cooking over more direct heat. Lean toward soups, stews, Crock-Pots, poaching, and steaming.[9] Consult *Dr. Vlassara's A.G.E.Less Diet*, but don't get carried away! Her suggestions are based on the false assumption that no one can give up sugar. (She doesn't yet know about the aminos!) And even so, she has proven that cutting just the *way* diabetics *prepare food at home* by 50 percent stops A.G.E.ing. *Note:* Experts disagree on how to rate all foods' degrees of glycation. One rates butter high, another low, for example.[10] Let's stick with the amount of visible browning for now.

Another Consultant I'd Like to Entrust You to

While our diabetic clients (especially any type 1 diabetic clients or other insulin-dependent diabetics) are getting craving free and clear on which foods they can and cannot tolerate, we refer them to the book *Dr. Bernstein's Diabetes Solution* and to the other resources of Richard Bernstein, M.D. His personal and clinical experience has been so helpful to them.

One of our clients, in her late thirties, had been a type 1 insulin-dependent diabetic since early childhood. Yet she was able to reduce her insulin 75 percent in her first week on the aminos and a Hunter diet.

AN AVERAGE *DIABETIC* HUNTER'S DAY

Meals	3
Protein	30–40% (of calories): 18–24 oz.
Fats	40–60% (of calories): 9 Tb added Fat
Carbohydrates:	10–20%: 18 cups of low-carbohydrate vegetables (or less, if high-carbohydrate veggies are tolerated)
Snacks	0–4, as needed from above food

THE NEXT STEP FOR HUNTERS OR HERDERS

When you've been on your Hunter or Herder plan for at least two months and your Mini Craving-Type Questionnaire and Trigger Food Rating scores have both been close to zeros for at least four weeks, you may be ready to embark on Phase Two of your great food experiment: testing to see if you can broaden the list of foods you're eating by carefully reintroducing certain foods. That's what the next chapter is all about.

15

Personalizing Your Plate: Food-Reintroduction Testing

HOW DO YOU KNOW WHO to trust when it comes to food? You don't. I don't even want you to trust *me*. Do stick with me, though, through this last step of the Craving Cure: discovering which *foods* you can trust. The first phase of this discovery process—the food-elimination phase—was described in the last chapter. This chapter is about phase two: seeing for yourself whether you can bring back any of the questionable foods you eliminated in phase one. This two-part discovery process is what finally relieves our clients of the worrying theories, the guilt, the confusion, and the fears about what they *should* or should *not* be eating. It takes the bias out of the process and provides the evidence so that a rational decision about what foods to keep permanently can be made by the expert—you!

The best way to determine which foods are best or worst for your health, happiness, and weight is to find out how foods actually affect you when you eat them again, one by one, *after* a complete clearing out period.

In the first phase of the testing process, you learned how to eliminate all Techno-Foodz and, at least temporarily, certain questionable *whole* foods. Why and when would you start reintroducing some of those foods you'd removed in phase one? If you've been settled into your new foods for at least one month and the weekly scores on your Mini Craving-Type Questionnaire have been close to zero as well, consider reintroduction testing any *whole* foods that you're not sure about, such as a milk or wheat product.

In my original program, we didn't do *any* food-reintroduction testing because we were afraid of unleashing out-of-control cravings. We just tried to absolutely seal the tomb; identifying and removing all of the general categories of foods that our clients had ever overeaten, permanently. This made for a narrow, rigid, highly nutritious, and allergen-free plan. For some (the Herders) it was too restrictive; for others (the Hunters) it was perfect. But we've found over time that total inflexibility is not helpful to our clients in the long run. Our clients are better off now that they can find out *for themselves* whether to continue avoiding the *whole foods* they had initially eliminated. (The question of whether to trial a Techno-Karb is one I take up later in the section called Playing With Fire.) After we'd introduced the aminos, we saw that, since our clients had been freed from their addictive cravings, they could be safely guided by their own honest and rational reactions to food reintroduction. They could tell whether a particular food, a whole food that had been part of healthful human diets for millennia, was good for *them*—or not—without lapsing back into addictive eating.

Now we even encourage our clients to formally reintroduce foods that they've been "almost positive" were causing them problems so that they can be absolutely sure.

REINTRODUCING THE POSSIBLY PROBLEMATIC FOODS

So, let's identify the specific foods that might be the best (first) or worst (last) candidates for you to reintroduce. Start by reviewing the *whole* foods you'd checked off on your baseline Trigger Foods Rating Sheet. If you've cut out any of them *only for possible sensitivity reasons,* these can be candidates for early reintroduction because they don't trigger cravings, though they might well trigger some other negative symptoms (which could be worse than they'd been when you were eating them regularly and your body had been desensitized somewhat to them). *Note:* If you have many "possibly problematic" foods on your Rating Sheet, you might consider doing lab testing (coming up on page 291).

Look at the Chapter 14 list of foods and the sensitivity symptoms they can evoke again. It helped you decide which foods to eliminate in phase one. Assuming that those adverse symptoms you used to have are now gone, you can use the list to remind yourself what symptoms to look for if you reintroduce foods that are known to cause those symptoms.

An asthmatic client gave up all milk products for two weeks. She immediately stopped wheezing. After three weeks she tested raw, organic, full-fat cow's milk with breakfast and cow's-milk cheese with lunch. The next morning, she woke up wheezing. That was all the information she needed. She did reintroduce goat's- and then sheep's-milk yogurts and cheese later and found them to cause no such problems.

Don't reintroduce a product that contains several foods. Reintroduce pasta, but not stuffed with cheese, for example.

Many problem foods come in families, which makes it easier to test them: cow's-milk products, for example, or cruciferous vegetables, or tree nuts. If all are eliminated and one or two are reintroduced and found to be problematic, usually both home testing and lab testing find that the entire food family is a problem and further reintroductions are unnecessary. But feel free to try each of them if you want to be absolutely sure! One client (a blood type O) had bad reactions to every bean except garbanzo beans.

Any reaction usually emerges between five minutes and seventy-two hours after reintroducing a food. Some foods have *immediate adverse effects*, such as bloating, gas, sneezing, diarrhea, hives, swelling of the throat, sleepiness, or anaphylactic shock. Many people who've experienced these kinds of reactions learn quickly to avoid these foods (if their cravings for them are controllable).

But other foods have *delayed adverse effects* that are much more difficult to identify because they occur up to three days after the instigator has been consumed. By the time you have a reaction, you have also eaten many other foods. But over the years, as we've reviewed the records of thousands of home food tests, our staff has become familiar with the most common delayed effects and which foods cause them. What we've discovered is that the foods that are the most addictive are often the same foods that contribute the most to our clients' chronic health complaints. How did we make this discovery? We helped clients off of their addictive foods and some or all of their adverse health symptoms disappeared. We helped them reintroduce a few possible food culprits later, and the return of adverse reactions was most often prompt and obvious.

Even with all our experience, though, we're often surprised by clients' unpredictable responses. Let your own body be your guide! But these experiments depend on your keeping reliable data and lots of it, so do be *honest* with yourself and document your responses in detail in your Food Log.

Some of our clients have noted that they *felt headachy, queasy, sleepy, fuzzy-headed, bloated, constipated, congested, or achy.* "I won't do that food again. That was a very real experience of toxicity." Other testers *felt nothing* at first but a bit of the old pleasure. They thought, "Maybe I could do that again once in a while, but I'm not sure what I mean by that. I did get some mild cravings over the next few days until I upped my aminos, so that's probably it for me on gluten." Some clients have had *no adverse reactions to a food that used to cause problems.* They monitor their reactions while they proceed to test the next food on their Trigger Food list (at least four days later). If they note the reemergence of cravings or any other adverse effect, they eliminate that food again. (They can always re-test again in three to six months.) If they feel fine after the reintroduction, their ability to tolerate that food is back! The immune system and the structural integrity of the gut may have been strengthened by a nice period free of Techno-Karbz.

Are you resisting reintroduction? Do you fear weight gain? If so, reintroduce slowly and check the scale to be sure. Don't let your diet get more narrow than it needs to be. We've had to force some clients to reintroduce high-carb fruits or vegetables. One doctrinaire Paleo athlete was so grateful to have some fruit back! Others were using caffeine, alcohol, or unsweetened chocolate instead of whole carbs and needed to reverse that (with amino help).

THE THREE-DAY REINTRODUCTION TEST:

First, the three rules of phase two testing:

1. Reintroduce only one "food" or ingredient at a time

After going back to the Trigger Food Rating Sheet and prioritizing the list of foods you're going to try reintroducing. Perhaps wheat gluten will be number one and cow's-milk cheese number two, for example. The effect of each food re-introduction is too specific and important to be casually accomplished by reintroducing a whole a group of foods at once. Do not, for example, do as some compelling diet gurus blithely suggest and just start to eat *all* whole grains (including the gluten-containing ones) after a grain-free period. Even worse are all the "detox" proponents who want you to eliminate many foods (and usually far too many calories) from your diet but give no guidance regarding food reintroduction *at all.* This has created predictable confusion combined with post-starvation super-cravings that make careful, self-monitored reintroductions impossible. The result: Quick and complete loss of benefits (including weight regain, of course), and a lot of unjustified self-blame.

2. Eliminate *100 percent* of the chosen food for four to twelve weeks.

Continuing to eat even small amounts of a food occasionally can perpetuate the irritation so that symptoms remain, confusing the information you would get from reintroducing a food to a truly clean slate. For example, so many people say, "I'm *mostly* gluten-free." This is like being a little pregnant. Speaking of gluten, don't replace it with gluten-free junk food.

3. Keep up with your Daily Food Log.

(It's called "daily" for a reason.) Monitor your physical and mental symptoms and record anything unusual. A change in weight, for example. Food intolerance reactions can be subtle or obvious, quick or slow to emerge. Even if they seem minor, they are likely to increase in severity over time, so do not go into denial. Write everything down honestly. (If you're tempted to ignore the symptoms, your cravings are undoubtedly taking over.)

With these rules in mind, take the reintroduction test one day at a time:

Day 1

Have one serving of the test food at breakfast and one at lunch. Then do not have it again for the rest of the day. Note, in your Food Log, how this goes, especially observing anything unusual.

Note: Some people are very sensitive and can't even tolerate the second serving of the test food on Day 1. Others feel nothing for thirty-six hours after their two Day 1 test meals.

Day 2

Do not eat the food in question at all during Day 2. Observe and record your experience in your Food Log.

Day 3

Continue abstaining from the food throughout Day 3. Again, log your observations in detail.

Day 4: Assess your results

Review your Food Log entries from both before and after any reintroduction. If you noticed any change, especially *any adverse reactions*—from cravings to gas to postnasal drip to weight gain—please avoid that food for another three months, after which you may test it again. If that second test, three months later, is also a bust, wait six months to test again, if you still want to.

REINTRODUCING GLUTEN

You can do a gluten reintroduction any time after you've been totally off it for at least a month. It takes ninety days before the damage to your gut lining and its critical immune system has had a real chance to start healing. The reintroduction of gluten can temporarily disrupt that healing process, but not seriously, and the results will let you know if gluten really is a problem for you or not. After removing *all* gluten-containing foods (including oats) from your diet, preferably for three restorative months, reintroduce a gluten-containing *whole* grain one at a time: wheat, rye, barley, spelt, kamut, or oats. Fatigue and/or digestive distress are by far the most common reintroduction response symptoms, and they usually appear very quickly (often within moments). I reintroduced some fresh whole wheat bread after five years off of gluten, and in five minutes, my dinner companions were asking what was wrong with me; I'd suddenly gone from being the life of the party to almost falling asleep at the table. (One of our clients *did* fall asleep at work on her lunch break!) This foggy state lasted for forty-eight hours.

About 90 percent of our clients have responded badly to the reintroduction of gluten-containing foods. Only about 10 percent of them have been able to eat gluten with no problem. Almost all blood type Os do poorly on gluten (as well as on milk products and legumes).

But, off of these foods, the intestinal permeability (leaky gut) caused by gluten, in particular, has a chance to mend, and the client becomes less reactive. This opens the door to successfully reintroducing other foods. For example, one of our gluten-sensitive clients also seemed to be sensitive to several other foods. She was unable to reintroduce gluten successfully, even after four months, but she *was* able to successfully reintroduce every other food except milk. This is the argument for waiting until month four to start the reintroduction process. Had she tried to reintroduce those foods earlier, before the gluten-caused irritation had healed, she might not have been able to tolerate so many foods.

REINTRODUCING MILK PRODUCTS

Some cow's milk–sensitive people do better eating raw cow's-milk products or goat's- and/or sheeps-milk products (which contain only A2 beta-casein). Clarified butter (ghee), being free of casein, whey, and lactose, works better for many, too. You may be one of them. If you have any doubt, methodical testing is the way to find out.

After removing all cow's-, goat's-, and sheep's-milk products, reintroduce them, one at a time, in whichever order you prefer. About a third of our clients fare poorly when they reintroduce a cow's-milk product. About 10 percent can't even tolerate goat's- or sheep's-milk products. I do encourage you to test raw cow's milk (heating for pasteurization alters milk) as well as the now available and less irritating A2 beta-casein cow's milk before you give up on these products altogether (especially if you can find raw milk from a pure A2 cow).[1,2] Herders did well on A2 milk products for millennia before switching to milk that was all or in part from Holsteins or other breeds that contain the now more common A1-A2 mix.

Lactose intolerance usually expresses itself as loose bowels. Reintroduce lactose-free products first if you suspect this. *Casein intolerance* can set off cravings or bowel, lung, mood, or mental dysfunction. *Whey intolerances* has caused severe bloating.

Should You Use A *Lab Test* for Food Sensitivities?

When our clients seem to be experiencing adverse reactions to many foods, the home testing process can take too long. Or the usual food suspects (gluten and milk) are ruled out and yet the adverse symptoms persist. In these or other cases, we recommend a blood test at Immuno Labs, which analyzes IGG antibodies of up to 250 foods in what seems to be a uniquely effective process. We've found that so many labs have inconsistent results, but because of their lower prices our clients often want to use them. The results can be so meaningless that we've often had to steer them back to Immuno Labs. When our clients go off of the foods identified *there,* they consistently feel better! After three months, they reintroduce the foods identified, one by one, starting with the foods with lower antibody scores. They can usually tolerate many or all of them. They typically find that their discomfort comes back, though, after reintroducing the higher-scoring foods or groups of foods (e.g., all legumes or nuts). It's not infallible, but it's certainly the best we've found so far. Many colleagues concur.

Gluten: We sometimes see high scores on wheat, barley, rye, or spelt, but we rarely request the special add-on anti-gliadin test because we so seldom see scores that reflect our clients' symptoms on elimination and reintroduction. It's been so helpful when it *has* reported a positive antibody reaction on a test because clients take it very seriously and that helps them stay away from hard-to-avoid gluten. A positive reaction really does indicate that they have the most serious form of gluten sensitivity, celiac disease.

Milk and Eggs: The add-on test for casein and whey can be helpful, but the chicken egg add-on often isn't. Duck eggs are a good substitute if chicken eggs fail on reintroduction.

Oxford Clinical Laboratory has a test called the Mediator Release Test. One of our colleagues has been using it for many years and has found that 75 percent of her clients get real benefit when they go off of the foods identified by it. It also includes useful spice- and chemical-sensitivity testing.

- See Tracking and Testing Tools on page 267 for details on Immuno Labs and *a hydrogen breath test* that can help identify *lactose intolerance.*

PLAYING WITH FIRE: SHOULD YOU REINTRODUCE FORMERLY ADDICTIVE FOODS?

You certainly don't have to. However, in the last phase of food reintroduction you may choose to find out what effect foods that have caused you to crave and overeat in the past will have on you now. Perhaps you've been a happy Hunter but you'd like to try brown rice, though you'd binged on white rice in the past.

Techno-Karbz, though, and any other foods you've frequently craved and overeaten, should be saved for the very end, when your brain and body are in the best shape to withstand the shock! At that point re-score your Trigger Foods Rating Sheet again and see if a food that used to call your name has stopped doing so and decide if that food now seems worth a reintroduction. (I try plain, organic, full-fat cow's-milk yogurt annually. No dice. I'm still addicted.)

Since the aminos make it possible to carefully reintroduce foods without being overwhelmed by lust, our clients have shown us that even old Techno-favorites can be hauled back in for phase two testing. If they elicit a craving again, that craving tends to be just strong enough to warn them that they are getting a drug-like effect, which means that this food is not ever going to be for them. Then, because the aminos prevent craving from becoming overwhelming, the door can again be bolted and that food forgotten for good.

But before you do this, ask yourself "why?" And read Chapter 16, Dodging Slips and Shooting Trouble, first. Is there a point to reintroducing foods that ignited a fatal attraction in the past? Most of our clients choose not to do it. They've already failed that test many times!

Here's why we sometimes insist on such experiments, though. We've seen many people who *don't* formally try reintroducing old craving foods but have thoughts that "these might be okay to have in small portions, once in a while." They gradually found themselves eating a bit here and a bit there till they realized that they were hooked again and/or not feeling well. It's better to discover your reactions through the formal challenge (eating two servings in one day instead of in little bits over months).

If you do this, keep in mind that you'll have to monitor your cravings carefully; *even a formal first bite can be like an alcoholic's first drink.* In the next day or two, you may start wanting more. But that's the point of an experiment. If it fails, you adjust your aminos and realize you can't go back to that food at all. If cravings *don't* come back, you may be able to have an occasional bite or serving. (But all need to be *logged* to keep you clear and honest over time.)

If your addictive cravings do come back, you'll have learned that your aminos *cannot* protect you *if you continue to eat that particular, virulently addictive food.*

Caution: I would caution any diabetic against making such an experiment. If you're insulin dependent, the blood sugar spike and crash could actually be life-threatening. I also counsel our bingers and bulimic bingers not to expose themselves to this danger.

IF A THERAPEUTIC DIET IS CALLED FOR

There are many helpful diets targeted to specific health problems. Any of them can be made easier to stick to with the help of the aminos. (Be sure to get enough calories to avoid cravings.) When the Craving Cure fundamentals have not eliminated clients' entrenched health challenges, we suggest that they look for more help from a practitioner who has helped someone they know with a similar problem. Keep in mind that, with a few adjustments, the Hunter plan can be converted into several therapeutic diets: A Hunter with no onions or garlic and no avocado (it is a fruit) becomes a low-FODMAP diet, helpful for certain chronic GI problems. A Hunter without nightshade vegetables (tomato, white potato, eggplant, peppers, and tobacco) can help with gout, arthritis, or herpes. (Herpes also requires avoidance of nuts and seeds.) Without Brassica vegetables or herbs (e.g., broccoli or rosemary) soy, or millet, you could have a more thyroid-supportive diet (though clinical experience of this is sparse). A Hunter who goes ketogenic may improve a wide variety of problems, including yeast overgrowth, diabetes, and cancer. Some clients have had dramatic success in a few days or weeks adapting a Hunter plan. Here is an example:

A Therapeutic Food-Testing Story

One of our Herder clients came back after four years, still craving free, but complaining of months of crippling fatigue, chronic abdominal discomfort, and, though she was basically happy with her looks, ten pounds she couldn't quite lose. Her food's quality had been good, but there were a number of foods she hadn't tested. She'd never felt she needed to, since for the most part she didn't overeat her whole and mostly organic foods. She ate beans, brown rice, or corn tortillas daily. She did tend to overeat cherries, white nectarines, and apricots, but only in season. She'd quit grapes (couldn't ever quit once she'd started), but figured since the other fruits she liked were only available seasonally, they were no big deal. And she had kept twenty pounds off eating this way.

She'd been having herpes "attacks" several days a month or more for years and chronic low thyroid symptoms and test results (but she could not tolerate thyroid supplements or medications). She was also chronically bloated. (Yeasts, bacteria, and other microbes all feed off of the same fructose and glucose and the fiber in the fruits and other whole, but higher-carbohydrate, foods she still ate.) The point is, she'd never tested these foods, so she couldn't know whether or how she'd been affected by them.

With the help of a chronic illness expert we referred her to, she switched to a very narrow Hunter. She dropped all fruit (it helped that her favorites were out of season), onions and garlic (these high-sulfur foods can often cause problems), all Brassica veggies (she didn't like them much anyway), and the nightshades. She also quit brown rice and corn (that was harder) and her beans and peas (hardest of all). The first week, as reported in her log, her stomach pain was much improved and her brain fog was gone (she'd forgotten about that till it disappeared!). Her energy was strong again, too, and she could see, in two weeks, that she'd begun to shed those last persistent pounds. She called a year later, still on her modified Hunter, and said she'd tried reintroducing onions and garlic with no problem, though she found she no longer liked large amounts. She was also able to tolerate very small amounts of fruit (two strawberries or eight blueberries), but a whole pear made her feel sick. Fresh lima and garbanzo beans were fine and so was quinoa, but millet was not. She was feeling so good, and her herpes outbreaks (especially the flu-like symptoms) had so diminished that she felt no urgency to reintroduce more foods.

While you're considering the reintroduction process is a good time to read the next chapter, Dodging Slips and Shooting Trouble. This process can be slippery and there are lots of good (and entertaining) examples in Chapter 16 of how to avoid pitfalls of all kinds.

16

Dodging Slips and Shooting Trouble

MY NUTRITIONISTS HAVE ALWAYS ENJOYED giving out dietary advice. That's because the truly amazing effectiveness of the amino acids makes their advice easy for our clients to follow. In contrast, the nutritionists and dietitians who come to my introductory trainings typically complain about "poor compliance," "poor follow-through," and that their clients disappear after just one or two sessions. *After* the trainings, though, when they've learned about the power of cravings and the *greater* power of the aminos, they contact me to report that their clients, too, have started doing really well.

As successful as we are, though, many of our clients have had some difficulty somewhere along the line. Most of these difficulties have fallen under the category of "slip," a brief return to addictive eating. (Full, permanent relapses back into Techno-Foodz have been very, very rare.) Over the years, we've learned to anticipate the slip problem and have honed some good counterstrategies that I'd like to share with you in this chapter.

We encourage our clients to see their slips as learning opportunities. Slips teach them that, by consulting their Tracking Tools and this chapter's Slip Tips, they can easily correct their course. Some clients, though, run into certain problems that keep them from exercising or eating well. In the second part of this chapter I'll tell you about how we've learned to deal with them.

Take a first pass through the chapter now to get familiar with its backup resources so that you'll know how to use them if the need arises.

THE SLIP TIPS

We are always eager for reports from the front; we enjoy hearing about our clients' nutritional adventures. For example, early on, our clients cut out the foods that are obviously or probably damaging to them. Later, many of them follow Chapter 15's directions and carefully try reintroducing some of those foods back into their diets, one by one. But others have "unplanned exposures" to formerly problematic foods. Sometimes such slips occur *by accident*: "The waiter said there was no wheat in the food I ordered. Suddenly, while I was still eating, I got so tired. But I kept eating because it tasted so good and I assumed it was safe food." Other times it happens on *impulse*: "I just decided to see what would happen. It tasted yummy but I walked away after just a few bites, much to my surprise." Some slips happen *by misfortune*: "My aminos were in my luggage, which was lost when I was on vacation. After a few days *everything* started looking so tempting again and I relapsed badly."

Several clients who'd been longtime bingers actually *planned to slip* and quit taking their aminos so that they could enjoy it more. Those slips don't typically stop for several days. "Oh well," they say to themselves, "I might as well keep going since I've already blown it." Usually this is a very familiar pattern from their many previous dieting attempts, a scenario that just indicates to us that they need higher amino doses. They often do not tell us that they were having any cravings because they have never really believed that they could be totally free of them. They were amazed that we weren't mad at them and more amazed when higher doses of aminos really did stop *all* their cravings.

Returns of cravings and slips aren't usually mysterious at all. The causes are almost always easily traced and corrected. With the Daily Food Log and the weekly Mini Craving-Type Questionnaire for reference, it's easy to assess the cause of the trouble and, with adjusted amino or dietary support, step back into the craving-free zone. The list of slip causes on the following page and the tips that follow are not intended to scare you. On the contrary, they'll help you anticipate a slip and take action to prevent it from actually happening. If you *do* have a slip, this chapter can help you understand why, and to make changes that will prevent future slips.

The Most Common Causes of Slips

1. Forgetting amino doses: "I get so busy" or "I left them at home!"

2. Taking too few aminos: "I ran out" or "I forgot to fill out my weekly Mini Craving-Type Questionnaire this week, so I didn't realize that I needed to raise my dose."

3. Skipping meals or snacks: "I didn't have time." "I woke up too late."

4. Eating too few calories: "I'm afraid I'll gain weight."

5. Eating too little protein: "I'm not used to eating it so often."

6. PMS: "The cravings get so much worse."

7. Thinking you could have "just a little" of a questionable food without formally testing it first: "Just one bite of my son's pizza did me in."

8. Questionable vacations: "There wasn't enough food I could eat."

9. Kitchen remodeling or having no convenient kitchen facilities.

10. Social pressure: "It was a special occasion."

11. Getting on the scale: "I'm not losing fast enough. Why keep trying?"

12. Junk food left all over the house by spouses, children, or roommates.

13. Alcohol, caffeine, or pot set off cravings and poor judgment.

14. Severe and long-term work, family, or relationship stress.

HOW TO PREVENT SLIPS

Remember your aminos. The top threat to your success is *your memory.* Forgetting to have a supply of aminos on hand, to take them along when you go out, or to use them on schedule is actually by far the most common cause of slips. They're usually brief slips because, unless you're on vacation in a remote area, you can go home, take the aminos later, pick yourself right up, and put the cravings and junk foods right down. Make sure to review Chapter 11, page 164, on organization and reminders (e.g., setting alarms on your phone or computer) if forgetting is a regular problem for you.

Remember your meals and snacks. Always keep plenty of good food in the house, including ready-to-eat leftovers and hard-boiled eggs. Take food with you when you leave for long stretches—like for work, school, or travel. Use "alarm" reminders as above if you forget more than once.

Eat enough healthy calories. You've already read (possibly ad nauseum) about one prime slip-promoter: *calorie restriction.* To counter that threat, our clinic has reinstituted monthly calorie counting (for the first three months, anyway) to alert our clients as to how close they might be edging to a slip by, usually inadvertently, *not eating enough.* Be sure to check to see that your calorie intake is not too low using the calorie counter on sparkpeople.com (as advised in Chapter 13, page 201).

Be proactive with PMS. Our menstruating clients often complain of the pre-period blues and PMS cravings. Extra aminos taken during PMS days, plus the support nutrients and freedom from inflammatory foods and beverages (sugar and caffeine are both big PMS drivers), typically wipe out PMS altogether in the first or, at most, the second month. Our clients often report in amazement that they have been surprised by their periods for the first time in years because cravings and all the other usual warning signs have failed to appear. And the periods themselves are typically much more comfortable. If not, we refer them to the suggestions in *The Diet Cure*'s two chapters on hormone rebalancing.

Don't start your cure on vacation. Once you've got the hang of your Craving Cure, vacations can work well, especially well-planned vacations where you can take some of your own food. But at first, it's safer to avoid the disruptions and uncertainty that vacations can inflict on your dietary routines.

Beware kitchen remodeling or not having convenient kitchen facilities, which can undermine your best intentions. It's hard to eat well consistently without being able to stock and prepare your own food. It's been impossible for our clients to succeed until they got access to a working kitchen.

Resist peer pressure. Most of our clients play the "I'm dieting and doing great and I'm not risking it so leave me alone" card and do well. Most of the people in their lives are actually supportive (even envious) and want to find out what kind of diet is working so well for them. If this is a repeated problem, though, get some counseling and/or peer support at Overeaters Anonymous.

Approach the scale with caution. Never use the scale if your weight is all you can think about afterward or you tend to binge after weighing because you never like the numbers. (The exceptions are those who may be afraid to raise calories, have lost too much weight, and/or are having trouble regaining. They *do* need to weigh themselves till they've checked and solved the problem.)

Address chronic stressors. The aminos are amazingly protective, even against big emotional upsets like breakups and deaths that our clients would never have expected to survive without sedative snacks. But occasionally we've seen *chronic* marital or employment stressors or past trauma (PTSD) that cannot be. In these cases, the slips were actually helpful wake-up calls to action. For example, some of our slow weight-losers have only been able to lose weight after leaving a chronically stressful job or separating from a chronically abusive partner. (Here's where counseling and/or support groups like O.A. can really be helpful.)

Be the leader at home. Uncooperative housemates? Most chronic dieters have figured this one out, but it can be very hard, especially if you have to prepare other people's food *as well as* your own. We like it when our parent-clients can say things like, "There will be *no* more junk food in the house. I would be a bad parent [or spouse] if I allowed it *and* I can't take care of myself when it's around. There will always be lots of good meals, leftovers, and snacks here [and there will also always be amino acids here]." But we know that every household has its own dynamic. We support our clients in at least insisting on getting some cooperation in their attempt to care for themselves. Then their success can inspire the rest.

Watch caffeine, alcohol, and cannabis. These substances can get our clients into trouble, even if they aren't addicted to them. Caffeine suppresses our appetite for real food. All three drugs destabilize neurotransmitter and blood sugar levels, which produces cravings. The latter two also distort judgment: "Why not have some dessert?" Your sober self knows why.

Do You Have Addictive Genes?

"What about my anniversary or Christmas with the kids?," you might be asking. "Does this really have to be forever?" It depends on how addicted you are. Each craver has his or her own unique vulnerability to food addiction and relapse. Heredity can play a big part. If there is obvious food, alcohol, or drug addiction in your family, your brain's vulnerability to addiction will typically be much higher than if you come from a family with none of these tendencies. This means that your risk of relapse will be higher and the care you need to take, greater. For example, *you'll probably need to take the aminos longer* than will someone without addiction in the family tree. It's not unusual for our genetically addiction-prone clients to require the aminos for a year or longer. If experiments with addictive foods cause them to slip back into craving, those foods go into the "never again" category and the support of groups like Overeaters Anonymous can be especially beneficial in keeping them there. We're so fortunate to have these nationally accessible support organizations that really understand that overeating is an *addiction* and that there is a physical basis to that addiction, whatever the emotional or spiritual factors may be. Beyond that, meetings vary a lot. Just look for a few people you can relate to. Read the literature and the books and website of Kay Sheppard, author of *Food Addiction.*

We find that some of the food-oriented twelve-step groups (not the original O.A.), such as F.A.A. (Food Addiction Anonymous) and F.A. (Food Addicts in Recovery Anonymous), can be quite restrictive in terms of calories or require carbohydrates like grain or fruit, which may not work for some people. But this varies from group to group. See what suits you.

Note: Avoid any groups that use the "guru" style of sponsorship (where you may never meet or even speak to the sponsor who decides what you should eat).

USING YOUR DAILY FOOD LOG AND CRAVING-TYPE QUESTIONNAIRE FOR SLIP SLEUTHING

Cravings or slips are always trying to tell us something. Your Tracking Tools will help you to listen.

For example, consider a typical case of the Skip that led to the Slip:

Jan suddenly started craving wildly after work. Then she bought her favorite goodie and ate it. Her daily diary reported that nothing upsetting had happened in the prior forty-eight hours, and her weekly Mine Craving-Type Questionnaires revealed that she'd been craving-free for weeks. She began to record what had happened earlier in the day, right before her slip, and discovered that she had gotten very busy and forgotten to eat lunch. She had also forgotten to take her afternoon aminos. Either one of these two boo-boos could have brought on sudden cravings. Case closed. But this was not a crime, it was a lesson. It was no longer a theory—she now knew, in real life, that skipping leads directly to slipping. Back to three squares, plus all her aminos.

Your Tracking Tools will also keep you alert to any *stealth cravings* you might encounter. For example, you might give up all gluten-containing wheat products, but find yourself overeating the refined and sweetened gluten-free substitutes that you'd assumed would be safe. Or maybe when you stopped sweetened foods, you started eating more fruit than it turns out you can tolerate.

MORE COMPLEX TROUBLES: UNABLE TO EXERCISE? MINIMAL WEIGHT LOSS? POOR APPETITE? UNUSUAL CRAVINGS?

Unable to exercise or get no benefit from it? Most of our clients actually start to *crave* exercise once they're on the right food and the right dose of aminos. But some clients can't seem to get going, or have to force themselves to exercise and still see minimal weight loss despite their efforts. They almost always turn out to be suffering from a type of fatigue that the aminos, good food, and the support nutrients can't entirely lift. They need more help, but it may take a while for us to realize it because even these least active clients always gratefully report that they're getting their basic chores done again and that they're not exhausted after work anymore. They're also happy that they've stopped gaining weight, and have quit wanting, and consuming, weight-promoting, health-destroying Techno-Karbz. They have better moods and sleep, too, and they are much healthier because their progression into diabetes and other diet-related health problems has stopped or been reversed. But they're still lacking the energy for exercise and the improved weight loss that exercise often helps make possible.

Our first question is, "Do you have a fatigue problem that's been with you for years?" If so, we ask clients to eliminate gluten and add red meat (if they haven't). Those who have neither responded to the Craving Cure basics nor to these two strategies have tended to have 1) chronic insomnia, 2) adrenal exhaustion, 3) a thyroid problem, or 4) all three.

The amino *sleep-repair* strategies in Chapters 6 and 9 can usually take care of number one. These strategies are also summarized online in my posted article on the three most common types of insomnia at moodcure.com/articles.

If you have *adrenal fatigue,* you often cannot complete a workout, or you become really exhausted afterward. In that case, your adrenal glands are probably producing *subnormal amounts of cortisol,* the energizing hormone best known for helping us to survive stress. You are likely to be a Type 4 Stressed Craver and will benefit from Chapter 9's more extensive information about adrenal exhaustion, as well as the information on this increasingly common problem in both *The Diet Cure* and *The Mood Cure.* Stop any exercise except gentle walking for now and get a four-sample salivary adrenal cortisol testing kit right away. This is the most consistently helpful lab test I've ever come across. Blood testing does not give as sensitive a reading and can only measure levels once in the day. See Tracking and Testing Tools, page 267, for information and directions. If you don't have an adrenal-savvy integrative practitioner to interpret your test results and make suggestions, you can consult one of the nutritionists at cravingcure.com/coach. You can also find a list of health professionals I've trained and certified at juliarosscures.com/practitoner. This problem is typically very responsive to simple nutritional or integrative medical correction. For example, the short-term (up to three-month) use of the herb licorice or natural low-dose cortisol given according to the needs identified by the saliva test results (which will show when your levels are abnormal) can quickly raise subnormal levels of cortisol and bring back your strength and stamina. (Till then just do gentle walks or stretches.)

Thyroid problems are more serious. See the symptom list on page 83. If you're in this group (especially likely if you've been a big dieter) you'll benefit from the thyroid-related suggestions that follow the symptom list.

Possible Causes of Chronic Fatigue

We keep the following list on hand to review with our clients who have struggled to get, or have given up on, exercise. I hope that it will give you some helpful direction.

Insomnia	Chronic infection (herpes, lyme, hepatitis)
Thyroid Dysfunction	Other active illness
Adrenal Exhaustion	Neurotoxins, e.g., mercury
Gluten Intolerance	Mycotoxins, e.g., mold
Testosterone Deficit	Medication side effects
Anemia	Mitochondrial Dysfunction

IS YOUR WEIGHT OR ENERGY TROUBLE
CAUSED BY A SLUGGISH THYROID?

Please read this section if your weight loss is stalled or you're too tired to enjoy exercise—*even if you don't think "a thyroid problem" applies to you.* Thyroid problems frequently go undiagnosed, and yet thyroid medication is often the top prescription drug sold in America. For example, more prescriptions for Synthroid were sold in the U.S. in 2015 than for any other drug.[1] Over 20 million Americans have some forms of thyroid disease.[2] More than 13 million more are undiagnosed.[3] Yet even more have never been tested, or never tested thoroughly. One in eight women encounter thyroid disease in their lifetime.[4] Women are more likely than men to be afflicted, as menstruation, childbirth, menopause, and low-calorie dieting make them more vulnerable.[5] From the time that my clinic opened in 1988, we have seen a steady increase in the number of women coming to us who've turned out to have this problem. (The number of men with the problem has not increased as much.) One of the reasons that low thyroid hormone output reduces energy is that adequate amounts are needed to activate our mitochondria, the ultimate *cellular energy production system* of the body. Thyroid hormone is also required to help activate the genetic program of every cell! But it has even more obvious bearings on our energy and weight, as well. For one thing, thyroid hormones regulate our body temperature as part of their metabolic (calorie burning) function.

The lower the body temperature, the slower the calorie-burning and weight loss can be. Most of our clients who've turned out to be low thyroid have had subnormal body temperatures. Over the past twenty years, so many more of our clients have reported having oral temperatures below the universal human standard of 98.6 degrees that I began interviewing the nurses and medical assistants who take patient temperatures in the general medical department at the local Kaiser Permanente Medical Center. Between 1996 and 2016 the reported average temperatures fell from 98.6 to 97 degrees. They had no explanation for it and I could find no research explaining it. Our clients' temperatures go up when they've improved their thyroid function.

Of the fewer than ten clients we've worked with who have ever actually *gained* some weight, all have been women who've turned out to have lifelong thyroid problems that ran in their families, exacerbated by years of low-cal dieting. They simply could not burn calories normally. Unrecognized or poorly treated thyroid dysfunction is often what keeps our clients from losing *as much* weight, as quickly, as they should. They almost never *gain* any further weight, but, though they have eliminated hundreds of calories worth of Techno-Karbz, these clients drop weight at a very slow pace, even when they force themselves to exercise regularly.

The Most Common Symptoms of Low Thyroid Function

For thirty years, we've been giving clients who don't lose weight readily and continue to be too tired to exercise, a check-off list of the *many* known symptoms of hypothyroidism. Below are the symptoms they have most often checked off. We also ask if parents, grandparents, aunts, uncles, or other family members have had the same symptoms or have been diagnosed with thyroid troubles of any kind:

- Low in energy
- Was a "chubby" child
- Overweight now
- Easily chilled (especially hands and feet)
- Low oral temperature (below 98.6) and low basal temperature (below 97.8 in underarm testing)
- Part of a family that includes people with thyroid problems (who were either formally diagnosed or who share the symptoms on this list)
- Someone who gains weight without overeating; finds it hard to lose excess weight, even on low-calorie diets
- Hard pressed to do even moderate regular exercise
- Very slow to "get started" in the morning
- Low in blood pressure
- Someone whose weight gain began near the start of menses, during or after a pregnancy, or on nearing menopause
- Chronically headachy
- Apt to use chocolate, caffeine, sugar, tobacco, or other stimulating substances to get or keep going

THYROID HELP

If you have many of these low-thyroid symptoms (especially if they run in your family as well), please read the two chapters, based on our clinic's extensive experience with this problem, in my book *The Diet Cure* (2012 edition). It includes a list of many additional, less common symptoms. More importantly, you'll find very specific information there about how to most accurately assess your thyroid function through lab testing and home-temperature-taking (both oral and underarm) and *how to get the professional help you'll need.* Thyroid dysfunction is one problem that we have seldom found a nutritional solution to. Clients often try over-the-counter remedies but they most often end up having to work with a thyroid-intelligent physician and take bio-identical thyroid hormones by prescription. We have often witnessed the successful results: improved ability to exercise, lose weight, and have warm feet.

Note: If you have the symptoms of thyroid dysfunction, do *not* try supplements of iodine or tyrosine until you've had thyroid blood testing done (as per *The Diet Cure*). Either could worsen some types of thyroid dysfunction (Hashimoto's Thyroiditis and Graves Hypothyroidism).

APPETITE LOSS—IS IT ZINC DEFICIENCY?

You could be like a client of ours who was eating enough food, but wasn't enjoying it. "Healthy food doesn't taste good," she complained. She was in danger of undereating and eventually relapsing. What she needed was extra zinc supplementation to improve her appetite. Her Craving Cure multivitamin/mineral was too low in zinc for her special needs.

Zinc is largely responsible for the proper functioning of our taste buds but it is one of the nutrients Americans are most often lacking in. Without enough, you literally can't taste. All you tend to want is food with strong flavor: sweet, spicy, hot, or salty. *Note:* Not surprisingly, anorexics can be profoundly zinc deficient. (Read about them in Chapters 2 and 10 in *The Diet Cure*.)

Zinc Building. The best food-source of zinc has, unfortunately, become very unpopular. It's red meat. If you don't feel you digest red meat easily, *test* your Blood Type (blood Type As are known to be low HCl producers) and your hydrochloric acid levels (HCl is your meat-digesting stomach acid) as outlined in Tracking and Testing Tools, page 267.

One way to determine if zinc deficiency is the problem is to buy and use a *zinc tally,* a bottle of zinc diluted in water. (You can order a sample or a bottle of zinc tally at the cravingcure.com/shop.) Your reaction to its taste indicates whether you're deficient or not (hint: the worse it tastes, the more zinc you have on board and vice versa). If it doesn't taste unpleasant, try one 50 mg zinc supplement daily for two weeks. If your appetite does not improve, take *two* supplements a day for two weeks. Retake the "tally" weekly until it consistently tastes unpleasant, then stop all zinc and re-tally in a month. If the problem persists or comes back when you stop the zinc, you might have an inherited zinc-depletion condition called *pyroluria* and need even more zinc.

Pyroluria has negative effects on mood as well as appetite as other nutrients, notably vitamin B6, are also often deeply deficient. Get the full pyroluria symptom questionnaire and information on testing and treating this condition nutritionally in the book *Depression-Free Naturally* by Joan Matthews-Larson, PhD.

CONTINUED OR INTERMITTENT CRAVINGS FOR SWEETS OR STARCHES: COULD IT BE YEAST (OR PARASITE) OVERGROWTH?

Common indicators of yeast overgrowth: Stubborn cravings for sweet or starchy carbohydrates (whole or processed); brain fog: a history of antibiotic, birth control pill, or cortisone use; bloat after meals that contain significant carbohydrate (yeasts' favorite food). This is a problem that does not usually cause daily cravings, but, even for those on aminos, it can cause "breakthrough cravings" a few times a week, until identified and treated. The Food Log can help you spot whether even whole carbohydrates in meals or snacks trigger bloat and cravings (even off of gluten).

Anti-yeast Remedies: Try a potent (80 billion or more) GI-targeted refrigerated probiotic like Ultra Flora or VSL. Switch to the Hunter eating option, if you aren't on it, or cut out fruit and reduce grains and beans further and replace with increased fat, protein, and low-carb veggies if you are a Herder.

Read *The Diet Cure*'s two chapters on yeast and parasite overgrowth. Reliable lab testing for yeasts and parasites is hard to find. As of 2017, Diagnostic Solutions may be our best bet. After getting no help, as usual, from a large national lab, one of my professional trainees got good results at the small lab at her local university, which did find her parasite with a three-sample test.

Consult an expert practitioner who can help evaluate you for yeast overgrowth (or for internal parasites, which can cause similar cravings and bloat) and give you a potent, individualized antimicrobe protocol.

I hope that the backup I've provided for you in this chapter will help you over any hurdles you may encounter, along with the Tracking and Testing Tools and the Recipes in the Action Resources that follow.

PART V

Vital Resources

TRACKING AND TESTING TOOLS: Timelines, Checklists, Forms, and Testing Guidelines

HERE YOU'LL FIND:

1. Your Twelve-Week Craving Cure Timeline

2. The Craving-Type Questionnaire and Profile

3. The weekly Mini Craving-Type Questionnaire (after once filling out the initial, more elaborate Craving-Type Questionnaire and Profile at the beginning of the book, page 12)

4. The Daily Food Log form and sample

5. The monthly Trigger Foods Rating Sheet

6. The Amino Trialing Record

7. The Supplement Schedule

8. The Lab and Home Testing Guidelines

The above tools are also available online at cravingcure.com/trackingtools.

Your Twelve-Week
Craving Cure Timeline

PRE-CURE SET UP:

- Read *The Craving Cure* in its entirety (except for any of the sections in Parts II and III that don't apply to your Craving Types).
- Fill out the three initial pre-cure Tracking Tools to set your baselines:
  - The Craving-Type Questionnaire and Craving-Type Profile, page 12
  - A three-day Daily Food Log (and calorie calculations, for one day), page 284
  - The Trigger Foods Rating Sheet, page 281

WEEK 1

- Review Part III, the Amino Breakthrough, both the general prep steps in Chapter 11 and the sections on your own Craving Types in Chapter 12.
- Buy your aminos and support nutrients as per Chapter 12.
- *Trial* aminos and record your reactions in the *Trialing Record*.
- Fill out the *Supplement Schedule* to be clear on what, when, and how many supplements to take.
- Review Chapters 13 and 14 to choose your anti-craving food plan. Eliminate all of the specific foods checked off on your Trigger Foods Rating Sheet.
- Study the recipes and meal ideas before going food shopping.
- Start keeping your Daily Food Log as soon as you start your aminos and your anti-craving foods.

WEEK 2

- Fill out your first post-amino *Mini* Craving-Type Questionnaire (and save it to compare its scores to all your past and future scores).
- Log food daily.
- Consult Chapter 12 to adjust your amino doses as needed.
- Reread Chapter 16 any time you have cravings, slips, or other trouble with your Cure.

WEEK 3

- Keep up your Daily Food Log.
- Rescore your Mini Craving-Type Questionnaire to monitor your amino progress and adjust your aminos, if needed, as per Chapter 12.
- Recalculate your calories on a representative day as per Chapter 13, page 201 to make sure you're eating enough.

WEEK 4

- Rescore your Mini Craving-Type Questionnaire
- Rescore your Trigger Food Rating Sheet. Adjust your aminos if any cravings persist. Eliminate any foods you still crave or overeat (however healthy).
- Review the Food Sensitivity Factor list in Chapter 14, page 235. Do you still have some? What foods should you consider eliminating?
- Keep your Daily Food Log as you make these changes to record results.

WEEK 5

- Go to a farmers' market; buy all organic or pasture-raised supplies, if possible. Get fresh herbs and use to flavor your food this week.
- Go all organic all week—or as close to it as you can.
- Keep up your Daily Food Log and your week's Mini Craving-Type Questionnaire. Note any changes during "organic week."

WEEK 6

- Keep up your Daily Food Log and rescore your Mini Craving-Type Questionnaire.

WEEK 7

- Eat no restaurant or prepared food all week. Prepare your own meals. Try new recipes this week from the selections here.
- Keep up your Daily Food Log and rescore your Mini Craving-Type Questionnaire.

WEEK 8

- Decide whether you can quit logging till you start reintroducing foods in weeks 10 to 12. (If your scores are all below 4 and you've had few/no cravings for 4 weeks.)
- If not, go back and analyze your Daily Food Log. Are your meals regular and substantial? Do you need more snacks? Are you taking your aminos? Do you need to raise them? Review Chapter 16 for ideas.
- Recalculate your calories for one typical day. Do you eat enough?

WEEK 9

- Rescore your Trigger Foods Rating Sheet and review the Food Sensitivity Reaction list on page 235 in preparation for possible food reintroduction testing or more eliminations.
- Consider a switch in food plans. Herders and Hunters should switch plans if they're not satisfied with results in weight, health, energy, or craving, or for any other reason.

WEEKS 10–12

- Review Chapter 15, Home Food Testing: Personalizing Your Plate.
- Use your Trigger Foods Rating Sheet to choose and prioritize the foods you'd like to try to reintroduce (or eliminate).

- Reintroduce foods as directed in Chapter 15 at your own pace.

- Keep extra-careful Daily Food Logs during any reintroduction or elimination testing.

- Be prepared to raise your aminos if reintroduced foods trigger cravings. (And remove those foods!)

The Craving-Type Questionnaire

WHAT IS YOUR CRAVING STATUS TODAY?

Directions:

Step 1. To determine your *symptom score,* check off each symptom statement that accurately describes you on a typical day. Each check mark equals a score of one. When you finish a section, add up the number of checks to see if your total symptom score indicates that you have that Craving Type. Then move on to the next section.

Step 2. To determine your *severity rating* on a scale of 0 to 10, rate the *strength* of each symptom statement on the blank line next to any box you've checked off. A rating of 1 is rare and/or quite weak; a 10 is daily and powerful.

Step 3. Enter your symptom score totals on the Profile Graph that follows the questionnaire. This will give you a quick visual perspective: How many Craving Types do you have? How high above the cutoff are your scores?

TYPE 1. THE DEPRESSED CRAVER

Are your cravings caused by a deficiency of serotonin, your brain's inner sunshine?

To determine if you are a Depressed Craver: Check off the box next to each symptom statement that applies to you. Next, rate each *checked* statement on the Severity Scale of 0–10 (0 none, 10 frequent and severe) by placing your number on the blank line next to any checked-off box.

_____ ☐ Your cravings are strongest toward the end of the day—in the afternoon or evening.

_____ ☐ You eat to get to, or get back to, sleep.

_____ ☐ You wake up in the night and head for the fridge.

_____ ☐ You crave more (and perhaps gain more) in fall and winter. Your mood is worse in winter, too.

_____ ☐ You tend to be negative, depressed, or pessimistic.

_____ ☐ You frequently worry or feel anxious.

_____ ☐ You have frequent feelings of low self-esteem, guilt, or shame.

_____ ☐ You are obsessed with certain thoughts or behaviors (e.g., your body, your weight, biting your nails, pulling your eyelashes out).

_____ ☐ You are a perfectionist or a neat freak. You tend to be controlling with others.

_____ ☐ You are subject to irritability or anger.

_____ ☐ You have panic attacks.

_____ ☐ You have phobias: fear of heights, small spaces, crowds, snakes, etc.

_____ ☐ You are hyperactive.

_____ ☐ You often have a nervous stomach (knots, butterflies).

_____ ☐ You are a night owl or have middle of the night insomnia.

_____ ☐ You suffer pain from headaches, TMJ, or fibromyalgia.

_____ ☐ You are using or have used an SSRI antidepressant drug (like Zoloft, Lexapro, or Prozac) with some benefit.

Your symptom total: _____ **(Each check mark equals a score of one.)**

If your symptom score is over 7, especially if most of your severity ratings are over 3, you are a Type 1 Depressed Craver.

TYPE 2. THE CRASHED CRAVER

Are your cravings caused by blood sugar deficits?

To determine if you are a Crashed Craver: Check off the box next to each symptom statement that applies to you. Next, rate each *checked* statement on the Severity Scale of 0–10 (0 none, 10 frequent and severe) by placing your number on the blank line next to any checked-off box.

_____ ☐ Your cravings for sugar or starch are stronger when you have skipped or delayed a meal.

_____ ☐ You tend to skip breakfast and/or other meals.

_____ ☐ Your cravings spike later in the day if you've skipped any earlier meals.

_____ ☐ You suspect you have (or you have been diagnosed with) hypoglycemia.

_____ ☐ You are diabetic or prediabetic. (Your blood sugar levels rise too high, but drop too low at times, as well.)

_____ ☐ You get dizzy, shaky, or headachy if you go too long between meals.

_____ ☐ You find it harder to concentrate when you go too long without healthy meals.

_____ ☐ You can get irritable, or blow up, if you go too long without full meals.

_____ ☐ You feel more stressed the fewer regular meals you eat.

_____ ☐ Hypoglycemia, diabetes, or alcoholism run in your family.

_____ ☐ You are drawn to alcohol on a regular basis.

Your symptom total: _____ **(Each check mark equals a score of one.)**

If your score is over 4, especially if your severity ratings are mostly over 3, you are a Type 2 Crashed Craver.

TYPE 3. THE COMFORT CRAVER

Are your cravings caused by a deficiency of pleasuring endorphin?

To determine if you are a Comfort Craver: Check off the box next to each symptom statement that applies to you. Next, rate each *checked* statement on the Severity Scale of 0–10 (0 none, 10 frequent and severe) by placing your number on the blank line next to any checked-off box.

_____ ☐ You crave—no, love—certain foods. They are treats that give you feelings of pleasure, enjoyment, or reward and taste "sooo goood."

_____ ☐ You think of your comfort foods as your best friends.

_____ ☐ Chocolate is particularly beloved.

_____ ☐ You get extra pleasure if you read, watch TV, or play with the computer, tablet, or phone while you eat.

_____ ☐ You are very sensitive to emotional or physical pain.

_____ ☐ You often feel sad, lonely, or hurt.

_____ ☐ You tear up or cry easily; even at TV commercials.

_____ ☐ You adore animals and need their loving company.

_____ ☐ You get a high from bulimic bingeing or purging or from restricting calories.

_____ ☐ You have a history of chronic physical pain from back or other injuries, or have chronic emotional pain from unresolved trauma or protracted personal ordeals.

_____ ☐ You are a dough lover—bread, cookies, and pasta are at the top of your list. You have trouble eating even whole wheat products moderately.

_____ ☐ Cheese, ice cream, frozen yogurt, butter, and even milk are irresistible.

_____ ☐ Dough and milk *combined* are your top treats: crackers and cheese, pizza, macaroni and cheese or the ultimate, dough and milk with chocolate—chocolate cheesecake, and cookie dough ice cream.

_____ ☐ You may also crave certain other substances or activities that give you similar feelings: painkillers, pot, or alcohol; serious aerobic exercise, porn, or self-harm.

Your symptom total: _____ **(Each check mark equals a score of one.)**

If your symptom score is over 6, especially if most of your severity ratings are over 3, you are a Type 3 Comfort Craver.

TYPE 4. THE STRESSED CRAVER

Do you crave because your brain's levels of calming GABA are too low?

To determine if you are a Stressed Craver: Check off the box next to each symptom statement that applies to you. Next, rate each *checked* statement on the Severity Scale of 0–10 (0 none, 10 frequent and severe) by placing your number on the blank line next to any checked-off box.

_____ ☐ You are overstressed or burnt out.

_____ ☐ You reach for snack food to counteract stress.

_____ ☐ You are unable to relax and loosen up easily.

_____ ☐ You have stiff, tense, or painful muscles.

_____ ☐ Your mind is cluttered and it's hard to focus.

_____ ☐ It's hard to meditate, pray, or be mindful, still, or at peace.

_____ ☐ You feel easily overwhelmed.

_____ ☐ You can feel close to panic.

_____ ☐ You don't get away on regular vacations to relax, rest, and regenerate.

_____ ☐ It is hard to get to sleep (or stay asleep) at times because of the above symptoms.

Your symptom total: _____ **(Each check mark equals a score of one.)**

If your symptom score is over 4, especially if most of severity ratings are over 4, you are a Type 4 Stressed Craver.

TYPE 5. THE FATIGUED CRAVER

Do you crave an energy boost because you're deficient in naturally stimulating catecholamines?

To determine if you are a Fatigued Craver: Check off the box next to each symptom statement that applies to you. Next, rate each *checked* statement on the Severity Scale of 0–10 (0 none, 10 frequent and severe) by placing a number on the blank line next to any checked-off box.

_____ ☐ You gravitate toward the stimulant effect of caffeine, coffees, sodas (including artificially sweetened ones), iced teas, energy drinks, or anything chocolate.

_____ ☐ Your energy is on the low side.

_____ ☐ You frequently feel the need to be more alert and focused.

_____ ☐ You are low in drive and motivation.

_____ ☐ Sweets give you a "pick-me-up."

_____ ☐ You have trouble concentrating, or have attention problems.

_____ ☐ You are easily bored and feel the need for some excitement.

_____ ☐ You have tried, and liked, stimulant drugs like Ritalin, Adderall, diet pills, methamphetamine, cocaine.

Your symptom total: _____(Each check mark equals a score of one.)

If your symptom score is over 4, especially if most of your severity ratings are over 3, you are a Type 5 Fatigued Craver.

THE PROFILE GRAPH

On the blank graph, transfer your total symptom scores for each Craving Type to the corresponding Profile columns. Draw a line across the column where your score falls. See if your scores are above the cutoff score and by how much. Shade in the space below your score. Any score above the cutoff verifies that you have that particular Craving Type. The higher the score above the cutoff line, the more certain it is that you have that particular type of craving and the more severe it usually is, particularly if the severity ratings tend to be over 3.

YOUR PROFILE GRAPH

	TYPE I Depressed Craver	TYPE 2 Crashed Craver	TYPE 3 Comfort Craver	TYPE 4 Stressed Craver	TYPE 5 Fatigued Craver
Max. Possible Score	17	11	15	9	8
	16	10	14		
	15		13	8	7
	14	9	12		
	13	8	11	7	
	12		10		6
	11	7	9	6	
	10	6	8		5
	9	5		5	
	8		7		
Cutoff Score	7	4	6	4	4
	6	3	5		
	5		4	3	3
	4	2	3		
	3	1	2	2	2
	2		1		
	1			1	
					1
Total Symptom Score					

The Mini Craving-Type Questionnaire

Place a number from zero (no symptoms) to ten (severe symptoms) next to each symptom.

TYPE 1 DEPRESSED CRAVER (LOW SEROTONIN)

INITIAL *PRE*-AMINOS DATE: _____

	DATE	DATE	DATE	DATE	DATE
_____ afternoon or evening cravings for foods (or other substances)	___	___	___	___	___
_____ negativity, depression (may be worse in winter)	___	___	___	___	___
_____ worry, anxiety	___	___	___	___	___
_____ low self-esteem	___	___	___	___	___
_____ hyperactivity	___	___	___	___	___
_____ obsessive thoughts or behaviors	___	___	___	___	___
_____ irritability, anger	___	___	___	___	___
_____ panic attacks, phobias (fear of heights, snakes, performing, small spaces)	___	___	___	___	___
_____ migraines, fibromyalgia, or TMJ	___	___	___	___	___
_____ night owl, hard to get to sleep, or have disturbed sleep	___	___	___	___	___

TYPE 2 CRASHED CRAVER (LOW BLOOD SUGAR)

_____ irritable, shaky, stressed, inattentive, or headachy, if too long without a meal	___	___	___	___	___
_____ crave sugar, starch, or alcohol, if too long without full meals	___	___	___	___	___

TYPE 3 COMFORT CRAVER (LOW ENDORPHINS)

_____ crave comfort, pleasure, or numbing from foods (or other substances)	___	___	___	___	___
_____ very sensitive to emotional pain	___	___	___	___	___
_____ cry or tear up easily	___	___	___	___	___
_____ have chronic feelings of sadness or loneliness	___	___	___	___	___
_____ have chronic physical pain	___	___	___	___	___

TYPE 4 STRESSED CRAVER (LOW GABA)

_____ crave foods (or other substances)   ___ ___ ___ ___ ___
for stress relief

_____ stiff, tense, or painful muscles   ___ ___ ___ ___ ___

_____ over-stressed, burned out   ___ ___ ___ ___ ___

_____ unable to relax, loosen up, get to   ___ ___ ___ ___ ___
sleep, be still

_____ often feel overwhelmed   ___ ___ ___ ___ ___

TYPE 5 FATIGUED CRAVER (LOW CATECHOLAMINES)

_____ crave foods or drinks for energy or focus   ___ ___ ___ ___ ___

_____ feel apathetic, bored, flat   ___ ___ ___ ___ ___

_____ lack energy   ___ ___ ___ ___ ___

_____ lack drive   ___ ___ ___ ___ ___

_____ lack focus and concentration   ___ ___ ___ ___ ___

Trigger Foods Rating Sheet

BELOW IS A LIST OF *foods that might be triggering cravings or oth reactions. Score the severity of cravings from 0–10 on its left side. (check off and date when you are eliminate a food. If that food is re later, check off and date. Plan to retake this questionnaire at least r explained in Chapter 11, page 153, and the Craving Cure 12-Week 7 page 268.*

Do not reintroduce an item if you still crave it. Work on eliminating totally first.

Date: _____

CRAVING 0–10	FOODS	ELIMINATE DATE	REINTF
	Grain-based desserts (including gluten-free), e.g., cookies, cake, doughnuts, pie		
	Yeast bread: white or whole wheat flour or gluten-free flour		
	Sweetened quick breads, e.g., muffins, scones		
	Other baked goods, e.g., rolls, croissants, buns		
	Wheat flour tortillas		
	Corn tortillas, e.g., tacos		
	Pasta and pasta dishes: white, whole wheat, or gluten-free		
	Pizza (including gluten-free)		
	Ready-to-eat cold cereals		
	Hot cereal—whole grain		
	Oats, e.g., granola, oatmeal		
	Rice-based dishes, white or brown rice		
	Other forms of gluten: spelt, couscous, rye, barley, or bulgur		
	Nongluten grains		

CRAVING 0–10	FOODS	ELIMINATE DATE	REINTRODUCE DATE
	Ice cream, frozen yogurt, crème brûlée, pudding, custard		
	Cheese		
	Butter		
	Flavored yogurt, low-fat		
	Plain yogurt, full-fat		
	Milk: whole or low-fat		
	Cream		
	BBQ or sweet & sour sauce		
	Peanuts, peanut butter		
	Chips: potato, corn, other		
	Popcorn		
	Candy with chocolate		
	Candy without chocolate		
	Candy with nuts/seeds		
	Gum, sugared or sugarless		
	Nuts or seeds		
	Nut or seed butters		
	Soda, energy/sports drinks (sugar or sugarless)		
	Agave or fruit syrup–sweetened foods or drinks		
	Zero calorie sweeteners		
	Fruit drinks, e.g., Kool-Aid, orange juice, sodas, kombucha		
	Coffee or tea		
	Coffee, lattes, tea, or chai with sugar or artificial sweetener		
	Grain-based alcoholic beverages (beer, liquor)		
	Wine, mixed drinks		
	Potatoes, yams, winter squash, parsnips		
	Fresh fruit		
	Dried fruit		
	Foods sweetened with honey, maple syrup, molasses, etc.		

CRAVING 0–10	FOODS	ELIMINATE DATE	REINTRODUCE DATE
	List any other foods you crave (or have adverse reactions to, however "healthy"):		

Daily Food Log

*Y*OUR GOAL HERE IS TO *give yourself detailed food information. As closely as possible, estimate the quantity of your portions, for example, note ounces, cups, grams, teaspoons, tablespoons, packets, slices, and so on. Give physical as well as emotional symptoms (e.g., bloated, tired, energetic, cheerful, craving a certain food, irritable, jittery). Note any energy shifts through the day and any exercise in the right-hand column. See sample Food Log on page 286.*

Date: _____

Time of Wake-up: _____

Quality of Sleep: _____

TIME	FOODS EATEN	HOW DID YOU FEEL AT OR AFTER EATING? BETWEEN MEALS?
	Breakfast:	
	Morning Snack:	
	Lunch:	

TIME	FOODS EATEN	HOW DID YOU FEEL AT OR AFTER EATING? BETWEEN MEALS?
	Afternoon Snack:	
	Dinner:	
	Evening Snack:	
	Time Asleep:	

SAMPLE DAILY FOOD LOG

Your goal here is to give yourself detailed food information. As closely as possible, estimate the quantity of your portions—for example, note ounces, cups, grams, teaspoons, tablespoons, packets, slices, and so on. Give physical as well as emotional symptoms (e.g., bloated, tired, energetic, cheerful, craving a certain food, irritable, jittery). Note any energy shifts through the day and any exercise in the right-hand column.

SAMPLE LOG

Date: _____

Time of Wake-up: _____

Do *not* fill out this chart as below

TIME	FOODS EATEN	HOW DID YOU FEEL AFTER EATING?
	Breakfast:	okay
	Pancakes	
	Eggs	
	Bacon	
	Juice	
	Coffee	
	Lunch:	tired
	Chicken burrito	
	Diet Coke	

Fill it out with specifics

TIME	FOODS EATEN	HOW DID YOU FEEL AFTER EATING?
7–8 AM	Breakfast:	Energized, bloated
	2 pancakes (4-inch)	
	2 eggs, scrambled	tired by 10 AM, unfocused,
	2 slices of bacon	headache
	6 oz. orange juice	
	1 c. coffee	
	2 tsp. sugar	
	1 Tb.. Half-and-Half	

12 PM	Lunch:	craved a Snickers bar
	1 lg flour tortilla	
	½ c. rice	
	¼ c. jack cheese	
	2 oz. chicken	
	¼ c. tomato salsa	
	Diet Coke (12-oz can)	bloated, still craved sweets

Amino Trialing Record

Date: _____

Below the supplements (and their standard starting dose) make a record of any trial, including the date and 1) the number of mg in your trial dose; 2) what time you trialed; 3) how many minutes later you noticed a response; 4) describe your reaction in as much detail as possible.
 5-HTP example: 25mg (I took half a 50 mg capsule to be cautious) at 5 PM. After 5 minutes, no reaction to 1. Ten minutes later, felt happy 5 minutes after taking the second half.

5-HTP: 50 mg

_____

_____

_____

Tryptophan: 500 mg

_____

_____

_____

GABA: GABA Calm, 125 mg; or Theanine: 100 mg

_____

_____

_____

Tyrosine: 500 mg; or L-Phenylalanine: 500 mg

_____

_____

_____

Glutamine: 500 mg

_____

_____

_____

DLPA: 500 mg

_____

_____

_____

DPA: 500 mg

_____

_____

_____

Melatonin: 1 mg or 3 mg

_____

_____

_____

HCl (Hydrochloric Acid): 1, 2, 3, 4, 5, 6, 7 (circle the number of capsules taken with a meal)

_____

_____

_____

Zinc

_____

_____

_____

Other Supplements Trialed

_____

_____

_____

Supplement Schedule

Date: _____

	BEFORE BREAKFAST	BEFORE LUNCH	MID AFTERNOON	BEFORE DINNER	NIGHT TIME
AMINOS (dose as per Ch. 12)	_____	_____	_____	_____	____
Tryptophan 500 mg	_____	_____	_____	_____	____
5-HTP 50 mg	_____	_____	_____	_____	____
Glutamine 500 mg	_____	_____	_____	_____	____
D-Phenylalanine (DPA) 500 mg	_____	_____	_____	_____	____
DL-Phenylalanine (DLPA) 500 mg	_____	_____	_____	_____	____
Total Amino Solution	_____	_____	_____	_____	____
GABA Calm 125 mg	_____	_____	_____	_____	____
GABA 200–250 mg	_____	_____	_____	_____	____
GABA 500 mg	_____	_____	_____	_____	____
Theanine 100 mg	_____	_____	_____	_____	____
Tyrosine 500 mg	_____	_____	_____	_____	____
L-Phenylalanine 500 mg	_____	_____	_____	_____	____
Melatonin Instant	_____	_____	_____	_____	____
Melatonin 2-Stage	_____	_____	_____	_____	____
_____	_____	_____	_____	_____	____
_____	_____	_____	_____	_____	____
SUPPORT NUTRIENTS					
True Balance	_____	_____	_____	_____	____
Vitamin C, 1,000-mg caps	_____	_____	_____	_____	____
Fish Oil	_____	_____	_____	_____	____
Vitamin D	_____	_____	_____	_____	____
Lecithin	_____	_____	_____	_____	____

	BEFORE BREAKFAST	BEFORE LUNCH	MID AFTERNOON	BEFORE DINNER	NIGHT TIME
OTHER SUPPLEMENTS					
_____	_____	_____	_____	_____	_____
_____	_____	_____	_____	_____	_____
_____	_____	_____	_____	_____	_____
_____	_____	_____	_____	_____	_____
_____	_____	_____	_____	_____	_____
_____	_____	_____	_____	_____	_____
_____	_____	_____	_____	_____	_____

LAB TESTING TOOLS

NEUROTRANSMITTER-LEVEL TESTING

There is only one universally accepted laboratory method of measuring the levels of the four craving-generating neurotransmitters in the brain: that gold standard is cerebrospinal fluid (CSF) testing. When other methods have been tested against it, they compare as follows:

Blood platelet testing is as accurate as CSF, but only for serotonin and the Cats, not for GABA or endorphin, which are not present in blood platelets. Unfortunately, this testing is mostly only available in research facilities. We use Health Diagnostics and Research Lab in New Jersey.

Blood plasma testing does not compare as well but it can give a rough measure. All the large labs use it to measure serotonin levels, mostly to identify carcinoid tumors, which produce pathological amounts of serotonin. (They've actually called us wondering why our clients are getting such *low* serotonin test results!) Unfortunately, plasma levels of GABA and endorphin are typically abnormally high, as their levels alter so quickly in response to the fear of the imminent blood draw, according to New York University's (and Health Diagnostics's) longtime lab director, Tapan Audhya, Ph.D. (in a phone conversation with me in 2014). As a result, we don't recommend these two tests any longer.

Urine testing for neurotransmitters is the *least* reliable method by far, per the above comparison studies by Dr. Audhya and a six-month clinical comparison study that my clinic conducted in 2000. When we first heard about the results of this urine testing, both concluded that this testing gave wildly unpredictable results. We compared testing to the tested clients' scores on our neurotransmitter deficiency symptom questionnaire (the predecessor of the Craving-Type Questionnaire), which they'd filled out just before the urine sample was sent to the lab and before any aminos were given. We found that sometimes test results correlated but that often there was little or no correlation between the test results and the tested clients' symptoms. Of course, we could not use the aminos unless our clients really seemed to need them, so we stopped using the test. Since then, when clients have had this urine test done *before* coming to see us, the aminos recommended to them by the testing lab staff or others, based on results, have sometimes been helpful, but have often made their symptoms much worse. Many health professionals who have had their patients use this testing have called me with the same disappointing experience. (See my article "Urinary Neurotransmitter Testing: Problems and Alternatives" posted on cravingcure.com/exploremore.) So far there has been no research confirming the accuracy of this test, as there has been with the others.

Amino Acid Level Testing: Two clinical authorities on the question of blood versus urine testing for amino levels, Carl Pfeiffer, M.D. (*The Healing Nutrients Within*) and Charles Gant, M.D. (*End Your Addiction Now*), both recommend blood plasma over urine testing. Again, though, plasma levels may change rapidly and so are only a rough measure. Have blood drawn before eating, rather than right afterward.

OTHER TESTING WE FIND VALUABLE

Vitamin D Testing: The essential blood test, 25 OHD, can be ordered from all the big labs. Plan to retest every 3–6 months, if your levels are low, until they get into normal range (which is 35 to 70).

Salivary Adrenal Cortisol Testing: Invaluable if overstress, insomnia, and/or fatigue are serious problems. The salivary cortisol testing lab results we've seen have mostly been helpful. (Genova and Pharmasan have not been as helpful as others.) We've been using Biohealth Diagnostics for almost twenty years with very consistently useful results. It is the only lab that I know of that provides a five-sample kit that allows our sleepless clients to measure their two to four AM wake-up levels as well as their AM, noon, five PM, and ten PM levels. Other labs will supply an extra single vial for this purpose, if you request it. (The normal range is the same as or less than the bedtime range.) Many health practitioners can order this test for you. You can order one yourself through the Canary Club or Direct Access Testing or through cravingcure.com/virtualclinic.

Fatty-Acid Testing: Especially helpful for discovering levels and ratios of omega-6 to omega-3 fats and later to see how your omega-6 flush is progressing. (Retest in six months.) Again, our clients have mostly had this test done at reasonably priced Health Diagnostics and Research New Jersey. It and all the conventional labs do a full-panel blood test of omega-3, omega-6, omega-9, and saturated fats with a doctor's order. An inexpensive blood spot test you can order yourself is available through Omega Quant and elsewhere, but we have just started comparing their results to the full blood-draw testing we're used to, so we're not yet sure of its accuracy.

Food Sensitivity Testing: Immuno Labs is our best suggestion by far. Full food panels and additional casein, whey, and egg fraction testing are what we've done with them and found helpful. *Note:* The gliadin test misses many people with very clear-cut reactions to wheat, although it does pick up wheat pretty often in the full panel. We've not yet found a reliable gluten-sensitivity test. We're waiting to see if the Cyrex Labs test (Cyrex specializes in gluten-sensitivity testing) is better.

Genetic Testing: For folic acid and other important markers. 23 and Me makes it fairly easy to order and to interpret the results.

Blood Type Testing: This is an inexpensive blood test that a physician can order. You can also order a blood spot self-test online for under ten dollars.

THE HOME HYDROCHLORIC ACID TEST:
DO YOU HAVE ENOUGH PROTEIN-DIGESTING HCL?

- Begin by buying HCl (600–700 mg) and taking one capsule in the middle of your next large meal. *If this does not cause any warming or burning sensation*, take two at the next meal; three at the following meal; and four at the meal after that. *Only keep adding on if you experience no warmth at lower doses.*

- Don't take all of the HCl capsules at once. Space them throughout the meals.

- Continue increasing the dose at each meal until you experience a feeling of warmth or burning in your stomach or until you reach four capsules, whichever occurs first. A burning feeling in the stomach means that you have taken too many tablets during that meal.

It tells you that you need to take one *less* tablet for during your next meal.

- Record the number of capsules it took to produce the warm feeling in your Amino Trialing Record.

- Start taking one less capsule with each full meal.

- When you start to feel warmth or burning again, at the lower dose, reduce the number of capsules by one or more again, as needed. It could take days or weeks to reach the point where you no longer need any HCl; over time, your own stomach-acid production will improve and you can stop taking the supplemental HCl completely.

YOUR REACTIONS TO THE HCL TEST

	NOTHING	WARMTH	BURNING
Meal #1: 1 capsule			
Meal #2: 2 capsules			
Meal #3: 3 capsules			
Meal #4: 4 capsules			

Note: HC1 supplementation will sometimes eliminate chronic stomach-burning sensations!

RECIPES AND MENUS:
Two Weeks of Delicious Dishes
for Every Craving Type

TABLE OF CONTENTS

INTRODUCING THE CRAVING-FREE KITCHEN

When you have regained your natural ability to enjoy healthy, nonaddictive food and have chosen either a Hunter or a Herder eating plan, use this chapter to help turn your Craving Cure into a permanent reality. You may have your own easily adapted recipes, you may even have eaten this way before, or you may be feeling quite unsure about where to begin. Regardless of how much time or energy you have, or your cooking expertise, I want to help you quickly start experiencing the pleasures of craving-free eating.

This section of the book starts with a few basic food prep suggestions, followed by a list of meals, recipes, and snacks. Each recipe can be easily adapted to either a Hunter or a Herder plan. Alternatives to grains, legumes, and milk products as well as to other foods (like nuts) that you may be intolerant of, or addicted to, and need to avoid will be provided. Each meal provides healthy, anti-craving proportions of protein, fat, and carbohydrate, and a one-to-four ratio of omega-3 (from fish, flax, pastured meat fat, and organic whole-milk fat) to omega-6 fats (from nuts, seeds, and other sources). The supplemental fish oil in the support nutrients raises this ratio even closer to the ideal one-to-one. The day's recipes are designed to feed three to four people or to give one or two people enough for leftover meals (depending on gender and activity level). They can also be easily cut in half or doubled.

A woman's minimum serving is 2,000 calories a day, and a man's, 2,500, so you'll have to adjust the recipes and add snacks to increase the calories as needed.

For all you rushed and pooped cooks, and you noncooks, my aim is to make your prep work as simple as possible; some techniques will actually allow you to relax while cooking, or avoid most cooking. For example, you'll see the beauty of leftover cuisine: how to prepare enough of a particular entrée for at least two additional and quite different but equally tasty meals. You'll roast and slow cook entire meals (including enough for leftovers) while you read a book, bathe the baby, or call a friend. This leftovers strategy not only helps with feeding you throughout the week, it will also help feed your biome, the trillions of bacteria that populate your digestive tract and can only stay in friendly balance if you feed them particular kinds of foods. Cold potatoes and rice, for example, are biome favorites. They are part of the Salad Bar basics (page 355) that will allow you to vary and expedite this almost-daily feature of your anti-craving cuisine.

MEET THE CREATOR OF THE CRAVING CURE RECIPES

Maia Alpern is a certified health coach, food educator, and talented recipe developer who grew up in the catering business. She is a local legend known for creating health-oriented dishes without sacrificing delicious flavors. She has mastered many cooking styles, from raw and vegan to Paleo, gluten-free, and international. She is passionate about helping people find out if gluten may be the reason for long-standing health issues (as it has been for her). See her website at GlutenfreeFairyGodmother.com.

THE MENUS FOR WEEKS 1 AND 2

WEEK 1 MENUS

Day 1

Breakfast—Oven-Roasted Breakfast
Lunch—Sausage and Bean Salad over Arugula with Parsley Dressing (Q, M)
Dinner—Slow-Cooked Marsala Turkey Thighs with a Sage Butter Cream Sauce and Colorful Brussels Sprouts with Pecans (Q)

Day 2

Breakfast—Nutty Spiced Tea Smoothie (Q)
Lunch—Tuscan Salad with Roasted Chicken and Garlic Rosemary Dressing (Q)
Dinner—Marinated Wild Salmon and Steamed Broccoli, Turnips, and Celery with Lemon Ginger Butter Sauce

Day 3

Breakfast—Ham and Mushroom Bake
Lunch—Salmon Tostada with Cilantro Lime Slaw (L, M, Q)
Dinner—Crispy Duck and Potatoes, Creamy Chard Soup, and Salad

Day 4

Breakfast—Morning Buckwheat Skillet with Baked Eggs
Lunch—Turkey Soup and Salad (L)
Dinner—Beef Short Ribs over Vegetable Noodles and Crimson Salad with Balsamic Dressing

Day 5

Breakfast—Japanese-American Breakfast Soup

Lunch—Pâté-Stuffed Veggies for Liver Haters

Dinner—Slow Cooker Tender Lamb Shanks with a Rosemary, Garlic, Mustard
Rub and Roasted Asparagus and Tomatoes over Spinach

Day 6

Breakfast—Minty Chia Pudding with Prosciutto-Wrapped Shrimp (Q)

Lunch—Almond-Crusted Turkey Schnitzel and Haricots Verts Soup (Q)

Dinner—Shredded Beef Chili (L) and Salad with Avocado Dressing

Day 7

Breakfast—Bacon Egg Foo Young

Lunch—Sliced Steak Salad with Ginger Nut Dressing (L, Q)

Dinner—Lamb and Lemon Sweet Potato Shepherd's Pie (L)

WEEK 2 MENUS

Day 1

Breakfast—Eggamole Salad

Lunch—Nutty Crusted Trout Fillets with Lemon Yogurt Sauce, Asparagus, and
Carrot/Celery Sticks

Dinner—Roast Lamb with Cauliflower Rice, Snap Peas, and Olive Arugula Pesto

Day 2

Breakfast—Leftover Nutty Crusted Trout (Q)

Lunch—Asian Burgers/Meatballs with Peanut Chili Sauce, Miso Vegetable Soup,
and Yam Bakes

Dinner—Chicken Thighs and Peppers Tacos in Romaine, Cauliflower Rice (L),
and a Large Salad with Parsley Dressing

Day 3

Breakfast—Lamb Curry Stew (L) with Spaghetti Squash (M)

Lunch—Baked Scallops with Artichokes and Tomato and Bell Pepper Dip with
Crudités

Dinner—Chicken Thighs and Peppers (L) over Baked Potato with Gazpacho

Day 4

Breakfast—Leftover Baked Scallops with Salad and Dip Dressing

Lunch—Cuban Beef and Potato Bake with Tomato-Basil Soup and Salad

Dinner—Caraway Virginia Ham, Kale, and Kraut Skillet with Steamed Kabocha Squash

Day 5

Breakfast—Ground Turkey Magic Meal with Yam Bakes (L)

Lunch—Wild Salmon in Avocado Half over Large Salad

Dinner—Pulled Slow Cooker Mustard Steak with Celeriac (or Parsnip) Puree and Multicolored Radishes

Day 6

Breakfast—Quiche with Gazpacho (L)

Lunch—Leftover Caraway Virginia Ham, Kale, and Kraut Skillet and Tomato-Basil Soup (Q)

Dinner—Leftover Cuban Beef and Potato Bake (L,Q) and Large Salad with Herbed Tomato Dressing (L)

Day 7

Breakfast—Leftover Pureed Miso Vegetable Soup with Asian Meatballs and Stir-Fried Daikon Rice

Lunch—Leftover Pulled Slow Cooker Mustard Steak over Zucchini Noodles, and Salad

Dinner—Turkey Magic Meal in a Bell Pepper (L)

ORIENTATION TO THE RECIPES

Preparing Your Shopping List

You will need to make a shopping list that is customized to your needs. Are you making these recipes as written or do you want to adjust quantities in half if you are only feeding one and don't want leftovers, or double them for a larger family? Do you need to substitute ingredients due to food sensitivity? Are you a Herder who will need to add extra things like grains and fruit?

Protein Portions

You may be tempted to just buy one or two 4-ounce portions of raw meat thinking you are following the recommendations. If you do this, you will not be eating enough protein or calories.

If you buy a ½ pound (8 ounces) of raw hamburger meat, you'll eat 6 ounces. You'll lose 2 ounces of water and fat during cooking; 25 percent is always lost. If there is a bone in the meat, as in a chicken thigh, we lose another 25 percent.

For a couple: Divide the protein into 4-ounce (when cooked) portions for the average woman and 6-ounce portions for the average man.

For a woman: Divide recipes into 5 equal portions, giving you approximately 4-ounce protein portions. After a few days or a week, evaluate the results. For example, if you divided meals into 5 portions and you were hungry or had cravings, next time divide the recipes into 4 equal 5-ounce portions, then see if that works better for your metabolism and exercise levels. In either case, refrigerate or freeze any extras for quick future back-up meals, soups, or snacks.

For a man: Men will definitely need to add snacks and increase portion sizes in these recipes to meet their greater protein and calorie needs. Divide a recipe into 3 servings (not 4 servings). This will still give you one or two extra meals to freeze or eat as snacks. (Or split a leftover meal in half and use it as 2 snacks.) Or double the recipes if you have the equipment and space and divide it into 6 (not 8) servings.

Men will need to add extra snacks when dividing recipe ingredients in half to create 2 portions to meet their higher nutritional goals. Please note that the *salad meal portions* are very large, so adjust the quantities for each salad to meet your needs or use one large salad for several meals and skip some of the other salad recipes. And if you reduce the amounts and make two different dressings, the salads will taste different even if the ingredients are basically the same.

Write in any *food substitutions or changed quantities* in pencil right on the recipe so you don't get confused when you are cooking. The first time or two, this may take a while but it will become much easier once you know what recipes you like and can create a shopping list and menu plan that can be used over and over again.

Consider your refrigerator and freezer space before you buy your groceries. If you are not used to cooking with a lot of fresh vegetables, you may be surprised how much volume they can take up. If you are only feeding yourself, there are a number of huge "meal" salads that serve four. Reduce the quantities or stretch one salad for four by omitting three other salads so you won't waste food due to spoilage. Luckily, some vegetables do not need to be kept cold before preparing, especially when being used up quickly. Pay attention to how they are being kept at the store and do the same at home. And if you don't have much freezer space, cut the recipes in half if you do not need to consume all the servings of food at that meal and can't store leftovers. Keep this in mind as you create a list for shopping. Do you need one list for a week, or a second list if you will need to shop twice a week to cut down on the quantities of food on hand?

Have your calendar with you as you make your shopping list to be aware of when you won't be eating at home, when you are having guests and need to increase servings, or to make notes on what to eat when. Organize a shopping list divided into sections for meat, produce, fats, and vegetables and a section for high-carbohydrate vegetables and grains. Snack meals also need to be factored in. You may want to add a section for miscellaneous items like spices or containers, too.

This is much easier than it sounds. As you go through each recipe, use a pencil to write in the quantities of each ingredient and increase the quantities each time another recipe used the same ingredient. In other words, if the first recipe uses 1 cup onions and the following recipe uses 1½ cups, change the shopping list quantity from 1 to 2½ cups. Increase it again for any subsequent recipes using onions. And there you have it—a shopping list ready to go.

WEEK ONE RECIPES

Many of the meals are coded as follows: (L)=uses Leftovers, (M)=has items to Make Ahead, (Q)=Quick to make. This will help you to be able to customize or move meals around if necessary. In other words, if you are pressed for time you can substitute a (Q) dish as long as it is of a similar type—like a quick vegetable side dish for a longer-cooking vegetable dish or to choose a different lunch when you did not make something ahead as indicated. And of course, choose (L) dishes when you already have the leftovers ready.

Day 1
Oven-Roasted Breakfast

This is a good meal to make on a weekend when you will be available periodically over an hour. Roast the head of garlic for the lunch salad dressing while you are roasting the potatoes, and prepare the vegetables while the bacon is cooking. I suggest filling the slow cooker with the ingredients for dinner and start cooking it based on when you want to eat dinner.

Serves 4

12 strips of bacon

10 cups fresh spinach leaves

1 large onion, cut in 1-inch chunks

4 cups diced Red Bliss or Yukon Gold potatoes

1 teaspoon salt

Pepper as desired

2 fresh rosemary stems, 3–4 inches long

1 large red bell pepper, cut in large dice

12 eggs (cook 3 per serving as needed just before serving)

¼ cup grated Parmesan cheese (optional; if dairy intolerant)

1. Turn on the oven to 400°F to preheat.

2. Lay the bacon strips on a rack placed on a baking sheet or large roasting pan and put the baking sheet on a rack in the middle of the cold oven when it reaches temperature.

3. Cook for 15–20 minutes. Prep the rest of the meal ingredients while the bacon is cooking. Remove bacon and drain on paper towels.

4. Toss spinach in the hot pan with bacon fat and wilt for 1–2 minutes. Drain on paper towels and divide among four shallow bowls or plates. Pour the remaining bacon fat into a heatproof container and reserve.

5. Put the onion and potatoes in the pan, add 2 tablespoons of the reserved bacon fat, salt and pepper, and toss to evenly coat. Place the rosemary stems on top and cover with foil. Bake in the oven for 20 minutes. Remove the foil and the rosemary and stir the onion and potatoes.

6. Return the pan to the oven, rotating the pan, and stir every 10 to 15 minutes as potatoes get brown and crispy.

7. Carefully crack 3 eggs into a cup or bowl and repeat for each serving so adding the eggs to the roasted vegetables will go quickly. Cut or crumble the cooled bacon into approximately ½-inch pieces.

8. Add the red bell peppers to the pan about 10 minutes before it's done when most of the potatoes but not all are golden and crispy. Continue roasting for another 3 to 4 minutes, remove the pan from the oven, and stir. Salt and pepper to taste.

9. Make 4 big wells in the roasted vegetables (if serving 4) for each serving of eggs using the back of a large serving spoon. Gently pour each cup of eggs into a well and sprinkle each egg serving with a pinch of salt and pepper if desired. (You may also poach, soft boil, scramble, or fry the eggs on the stovetop if you prefer.)

10. Return the pan to the oven and continue to bake 5–8 minutes depending on your desired level of doneness. Remove from the oven. Place each serving of eggs, peppers, and potatoes on top of a portion of spinach. Sprinkle bacon pieces and 1 tablespoon Parmesan cheese on each serving if desired.

Sausage and Bean Salad over Arugula with Parsley Dressing

Serves 4 (If you are a Hunter, make only the amount of salad you need.)

4 Italian pork sausage links (approx. 1 pound)

8 cups arugula, chopped

28 ounces black beans (or a mixture of black and garbanzo beans), cooked or canned, rinsed and drained

2 cups chopped romaine lettuce

2 cups roughly chopped cabbage

2 cups diced celery or fennel

2 cups diced tomatoes

½ cup crumbled feta cheese

¼ cup chopped zucchini

Parsley Dressing (recipe follows)

Sour cream (optional)

4 teaspoons sunflower or pumpkin seeds, as garnish
(omit if sensitive to nuts and seeds)

NOTE: Substitute avocado for feta and sour cream, or diced potatoes for beans.

1. Slice or dice the sausage into small pieces to cook quickly in a skillet over medium-high heat.

2. Combine with the rest of the salad ingredients in a large bowl, except sunflower or pumpkin seeds, or mix just the amount you want to serve, reserving the rest separately for future meals.

3. Mix with the Parsley Dressing as needed, reserving extra dressing.

4. Serve in a large salad bowl or in individual bowls and top with a little sour cream or avocado and garnish with the seeds.

Parsley Dressing

Makes about 1 cup (OK to make the full amount if you like the ingredients and want to have extra dressing to substitute for another dressing recipe or adjust if you need less.)

  1 large bunch parsley, stems removed, chopped (2 cups)
  2 cups peeled and roughly chopped cucumber
  ½ cup olive or other oil
  ⅛ teaspoon salt
  ¼ cup roughly chopped red onions
  1 tablespoon lemon juice
  2 pinches white pepper

Blend together everything in a blender or mini food processor or using an immersion blender. Taste and adjust seasoning if needed.

Slow-Cooked Marsala Turkey Thighs with Sage Butter Cream Sauce

Serves 4 (+2 leftovers)

Marinate the turkey the night before or first thing in the morning. If you prepare the Turkey Soup ingredients before dinner (see page 318) you can quickly add them to the slow cooker after removing the turkey thighs and leave it to cook as you eat dinner. Then a quick and delicious lunch will be ready for later in the week. And why not brew the tea for breakfast tomorrow so it can chill overnight?

  4–5 bone-in, skin-on turkey thighs (about 3⅓ pounds)
  ⅔ cup marsala wine
  ⅔ cup water
  2 onions, thinly sliced
  2 teaspoons minced garlic
  1 teaspoon dried sage
  1 teaspoon dried thyme
  1 teaspoon salt
  ⅛ teaspoon white pepper
  Sage Butter Cream Sauce (page 306)
  Crispy skin garnish (page 305; optional)

1. Combine the ingredients to prepare the marinade, mix well, add the turkey and marinate for at least 15 minutes or overnight.

2. When ready to cook, place the turkey thighs in the slow cooker then pour the marinade around the thighs, including the onions, and cook on high for 4–5 hours or on low for 8 hours.

3. Prepare the ingredients for the Turkey Soup for Day 4 (page 318) to make it very easy to just add them to the slow cooker at serving time

4. About 20 minutes before serving, start preparing the Brussels Sprouts with Pecans but actually cook them while also making the Sage Butter Cream Sauce.

5. About 10 minutes before serving, prepare the Sage Butter Cream Sauce.

6. To serve, place the turkey on a cutting board. Remove the bones, saving them for the soup, and cut turkey into chunks or shred as desired. Plate with side dishes and top the turkey with a tablespoon or two of the sauce and garnish with the crispy skin (if using).

7. Go ahead and add the bones and soup ingredients to the contents of the slow cooker before you sit down to dinner so the Turkey Soup (page 318) will be done tonight and you only have to clean up once, too.

Crispy Skin Garnish (optional)

Turkey skin, removed from the thighs before cooking

Salt

1. About an hour before serving dinner, spread out the skin in a large frying pan on medium-high heat, add 1 cup water, and cover. Turn the skin over every few minutes as you are preparing the sauce and side dish.

2. Once the water is almost gone and a coating of fat is in the frying pan, remove the cover, lower the heat to medium-low, and continue to cook flipping the skin every few minutes.

3. When crisp, golden brown, and fully rendered, place each piece on paper towels and sprinkle with salt. Cut into pieces to use as a garnish for your turkey thighs.

Sage Butter Cream Sauce

Makes about ¾ cup

½ cup ghee or 1 stick unsalted butter

3 tablespoons chopped fresh sage leaves

2–4 tablespoons cream or coconut milk

¼ teaspoon dried sage

Salt and pepper to taste

1. Melt the ghee or butter in a small saucepan over medium-low heat and add the fresh sage leaves when a test leaf begins to sizzle.

2. Cook for a few minutes until butter just begins to brown.

3. Add the cream or coconut milk to lower the temperature and swirl the pan to gently mix the sauce. Add the dried sage and salt and pepper to taste. Be careful not to overheat the sauce once you add the cream—just quickly warm through, stirring or swirling the pan.

4. Remove from heat and serve right away or cool and store in the refrigerator then gently reheat at serving time.

(Consider making extra for adding to potatoes and other vegetables later in the week, as it is so delicious.)

Colorful Brussels Sprouts with Pecans (Q)

Serves 4

1 pound Brussels sprouts

2 tablespoons small-diced red bell peppers

1 tablespoon fat of choice

¼ cup pecans, chopped and lightly toasted

Salt and pepper

4 cups thinly sliced radicchio

1. Shred the sprouts in a food processor.

2. Melt fat of choice over medium-high heat in a skillet large enough to hold all the Brussels sprouts.

3. Add the sprouts and bell peppers and sauté for 3 to 4 minutes. Add pecans and cook for 1 minute.

4. Season with salt and pepper to taste.

5. Remove from heat and toss with the radicchio and serve.

Day 2

Since breakfast is so quick, start cooking the sausage for lunch and make the smoothies while it is cooking. Then prepare the dressing and salad ingredients to make it easy to serve lunch quickly. Depending on your schedule, make the mayonnaise and salt the cabbage for the Cilantro Lime Slaw sometime today so it will be ready to combine for lunch tomorrow. To save time tomorrow morning, take a few moments after dinner to boil some eggs and make either cauliflower rice or regular rice depending on your starchy carb needs.

Nutty Spiced Tea Smoothie (Q)

Serves 2

½ teaspoon ground ginger (or 2–3 tablespoon grated fresh ginger, peeled, grated, and the juice squeezed out)

1 cup double-strength brewed chai tea

¼ cup peanut or almond butter (or other nut butter), or use 2 servings of protein powder if avoiding nuts

1 cup coconut milk plus 1 cup water, or 2 cups almond or whole dairy milk

2 cups fresh ●pinach, or ½ cup frozen

Ice, if desired (use less water)

1. Brew tea or if you are doing it in the morning, use ice cubes when blending.

2. Combine all ingredients in a blender and process until well mixed and frothy. Refrigerate the second serving for another day.

Tuscan Salad with Rotisserie Chicken and Roasted Garlic Rosemary Dressing (Q)

Serves 4

20 cups assorted greens (used 1½ cabbage, 2½ lettuces, 1 spinach per serving)

2 cups chopped radicchio

1 cup parsley, chopped

1 cup cilantro, chopped

2 cups cherry tomatoes

2 cups thinly sliced red onions

2 cups ½-inch-diced bell peppers

1 cup dried garbanzo beans, precooked (or 1 can), or diced potato

2 cups quartered red radishes

Roasted Garlic Rosemary Dressing (page 308)

4 tablespoons toasted sunflower seeds

1¼ pound roasted or rotisserie chicken, diced (include skin) (Divide into 4- or 6-ounce meal portions and 2-ounce snack portions)

1. Toss all the vegetables and beans or potatoes in a large bowl with the dressing. (Only dress the amount you are serving and store extra salad and dressing separately for serving on another day.)

2. Divide among four plates or large bowls and sprinkle on 1 tablespoon of sunflower seeds and add the chicken to each serving.

Roasted Garlic Rosemary Dressing

Makes about 1 cup

1 head of garlic

1 tablespoon fresh rosemary, or 1 teaspoon dried

1½ cups olive or other oil, plus 1 teaspoon to drizzle on garlic

2 cups raw spinach

¼ cup lemon juice

¼ cup champagne vinegar

2 tablespoons sour cream (optional)

2 tablespoons mustard

½ teaspoon anchovy paste (optional)

Salt and pepper to taste

½ cup grated Parmesan cheese (or nondairy version on page 363)

1. Slice the top off the head of garlic leaving a little garlic exposed and the papery skin on. Place on a piece of aluminum foil. Sprinkle the rosemary over the garlic and drizzle with 1 teaspoon of oil and wrap the foil into a little bundle. Bake for 45 minutes to 1 hour.

2. When cool, squeeze out the garlic cloves from the skins and place 2 tablespoons into the blender along with the rest of the ingredients except the olive oil and Parmesan cheese. Add a big pinch of pepper.

3. Blend together to combine and with the blender running, very slowly add the oil a few drops at a time until it begins to come together and emulsify as you continue to add the oil slowly in a thin stream until it is all incorporated.

4. Add the cheese and blend again for a few seconds. Taste for salt and pepper and adjust the seasoning if needed.

5. Dress the salad as needed and reserve the remaining dressing for other salads or to use as a dip for raw vegetables as a snack.

Marinated Wild Salmon and Steamed Broccoli, Turnips, and Celery with Lemon Ginger Butter Sauce

Serves 4 (+4 leftovers)

2¼ pounds center-cut wild salmon fillets with skin on, cut into four 5-oz. similar-sized pieces for this dinner (The size of the rest is less critical as it will be broken into pieces for the tostadas on Day 3. Just make sure that you are careful not to overcook the extra pieces if they are not similar in size to the dinner portions.)

For the marinade:

¼ cup fresh lemon juice with seeds removed (remove the lemon zest before juicing and save for the sauce)

¼ cup olive oil

½ teaspoon ground ginger

Generous pinch of salt

2 teaspoons lemon pepper

¼ teaspoon white pepper

1 tablespoon butter, ghee, or coconut oil, melted

For the sauce:

½ cup reserved marinade

3–4 tablespoons unsalted butter or ghee, or other fat

2 shallots, diced very small

2 tablespoons grated fresh ginger

2 tablespoons sliced scallions

Reserved lemon zest

Large pinch of salt

Small pinch of white pepper to taste

Additional sliced scallions for garnish

1. Preheat oven to 425°F.

2. Combine the ingredients for the marinade.

3. Marinate the salmon for 15 minutes at room temperature, turning once during that time.

4. Pat the salmon dry and place it, skin side up, in a foil lined roasting or broiling pan for easy cleanup. Brush the skin with the melted butter (or melted coconut oil).

5. Put the salmon in the preheated oven and bake for 5–10 minutes depending on the thickness of your salmon and your preference for doneness. (Plan

approximately 8–10 minutes per inch of fish at the thickest part including the broiling time.) Remove smaller pieces from the oven if they are cooking faster than the rest. Preheat the broiler if it is a separate unit when you put the fish in to bake.

6. Meanwhile, pour the reserved marinade into a saucepot and reduce by one-third, cooking it over medium-high heat while the salmon is baking. Once it has been reduced, add the diced shallots, fresh ginger, scallions, lemon zest, salt, and pepper. Just before serving time, add the remaining cold butter, diced, one or two pieces at a time, swirling after each, until combined.

7. Brush the skin again and place under the broiler. Stay close and check often as it only takes 1–2 minutes to crisp the skin. Plate the 4 portions, skin side up, on a serving of sauce so skin will stay crisp. Top with fresh green onions.

8. Refrigerate the rest of the salmon to use for the tostadas. Any extra sauce is delicious drizzled on vegetables.

Steamed Broccoli, Turnips, and Celery (Q)

Serves 4

8 cups broccoli florets

2 cups ½-inch-diced turnips

1 cup ¼-inch slices celery

Salt to taste

Lemon pepper to taste

Lemon Ginger Butter Sauce (see page 309)

1. Place the vegetables in a large steamer basket or colander over a pot with water at a low boil. Cover and steam until tender-crisp. (If not serving immediately, plunge into ice water to set the bright color.)

2. Sprinkle with a little salt and lemon pepper and serve with a drizzle of the Lemon Ginger Butter Sauce.

Day 3

Prepare the cabbage and make the dressing for the slaw in the morning if you didn't prepare it last night. Also, if you prepare the Creamy Kale Soup early in the day it will have time to chill if you want to serve it cold with dinner. Serve it warm if you want to make it right before dinner. Defrost the frozen Turkey Soup from Day 1 to enjoy for lunch tomorrow.

Ham and Mushroom Bake

Serves 4

2 cups sliced carrots or carrot chunks

2 cups ½-inch-diced celeriac

1 cup chopped shallots

3 cloves of garlic, minced

2 tablespoons ghee or butter

2 pounds mushrooms, sliced

4 cups chopped mustard greens

1¼ pounds cooked ham steak, diced

3 tablespoons capers

1¾ cups broth, milk, or cream

1¾ cups grated cheddar cheese (or substitute 2 beaten eggs)

1–2 tablespoons lemon zest

¼ cup walnuts, chopped

2 cups parsley, chopped

1 tablespoon Italian seasoning

1 teaspoon salt

¼ teaspoon pepper

1. Preheat oven to 375°F.

2. Simmer the carrots and celeriac in a large pot of salted water for about 10 minutes. (If carrots are sliced thinner than the celeriac, add them after the celeriac has cooked for about 5 minutes.)

3. While the vegetables are simmering, sauté the shallots and garlic in ghee for 3 minutes over medium heat. Add the mushrooms, Italian seasoning, salt and pepper. Stir and continue cooking for another 6–8 minutes until the mushrooms are cooked.

4. When the carrots and celeriac have cooked for about 7 minutes add the mustard greens to the pot and cook for 5 more minutes.

5. Drain and pour back into the pot.

6. Stir the diced ham into the vegetables.

7. Pour the shallot and mushroom mixture over the ham and vegetables. Add the capers, broth, and half the cheese (or the beaten eggs). Add the seasonings and stir to combine.

8. Lightly grease 9-x-11-inch baking dish with butter and fill with ham and mixture and smooth out in the dish.

9. Top with remaining cheese.

10. Cover with foil and bake for 20 minutes or refrigerate and bake it in the morning for 45 minutes.

11. Remove cover and broil for a few minutes to brown cheese if desired.

12. Remove from oven/broiler and let sit for 5 minutes.

13. Cut into 4 portions.

14. Mix and chop the lemon zest, walnuts, and parsley together and sprinkle over the top before serving.

Salmon Tostada with Cilantro Lime Slaw (L)

Serves 4

I recommend making the mayonnaise the night before; just remember to bring the eggs to room temperature before you want to make it. I would also suggest making the slaw first thing in the morning if you didn't make it the night before. If you can't, you can just add plain shredded cabbage instead, but the slaw makes this so delicious.

> 8 organic corn tortillas (or lettuce leaves if avoiding corn)
> Avocado slices
> 16 ounces leftover salmon (or canned wild salmon, drained)
> Cilantro Lime Slaw (page 313)
> Lime wedges
> Chopped cilantro, tomatoes, and chilies as desired for garnish

1. Crisp tortillas over gas burner or in lightly oiled skillet or place on large lettuce leaves on plates instead of tortillas if desired. (A serving is 2 leaves.)

2. Spread the tortillas with a layer of avocado slices, top with 4 ounces of the salmon and a layer of slaw.

3. Make 2 tostadas per serving and garnish with lime wedges and chopped cilantro.

4. Extra slaw: Serve it on the side. (Hunters: Add an artichoke with mayo.)

Cilantro Lime Slaw (M)

Serves 4

1 cup thinly sliced red cabbage

1 cup thinly sliced napa cabbage (or green cabbage)

Salt and pepper to taste

1 cup shredded carrots

¼ cup thinly sliced red onion

½ cup Cilantro Lime Mayonnaise (recipe follows)

2 Anaheim chiles (or hotter pepper if desired)

½ tomato

2 small or 1 large garlic clove, grated

¼ cup chopped cilantro, for garnish

1. Mix shredded cabbage, carrots, and onion with ½ teaspoon of salt and let it sit in a strainer or colander over a bowl for several hours to allow the liquid to drain off (so that the slaw won't be runny).

2. Mix the cilantro lime mayonnaise with the chiles, tomato, and garlic in a blender or small food processor.

3. After the cabbage has released its liquid, rinse and pat dry.

4. Combine cabbage with the dressing and mix thoroughly. Garnish with cilantro leaves. Refrigerate the extra for an easy side salad for another lunch or dinner.

Note: You can use bagged slaw mix for an even quicker version.

Mayonnaise: Cilantro Lime Variation

Makes about 1½ cups

It is important that the egg is not cold, so taking an egg out of the refrigerator is the first step. And if you don't want to make your own mayonnaise, try Primal Kitchen Avocado Mayo and add the cilantro, lime, and hot sauce. It is made with avocado oil and is available online at Amazon.com, Thrive Market, or at primalkitchen.com.

> 1 large egg, at room temperature*
>
> 1 teaspoon Dijon mustard
>
> ½ teaspoon salt
>
> 2 teaspoons champagne vinegar
>
> 1 teaspoon lime juice
>
> 1 cup olive or avocado oil

(The ingredients up to this point make a basic mayonnaise. Why not make a double batch and save half as is and finish the rest for the Cilantro Lime version if you are feeding a family. If only feeding 1 or 2, split this single batch and make half into Cilantro Lime Mayo for the Salmon Tostadas and save the other half depending on how much mayonnaise you need for the week.)

> ¼ cup fresh cilantro leaves
>
> Zest and juice of 1 lime
>
> Habanero hot sauce (optional)

1. Place the egg and the first group of ingredients, ending with olive oil, in a narrow jar or container.

2. Wait 5 minutes for all the ingredients to separate and settle.

3. Place an immersion blender all the way to the bottom of the container and process for 5–10 seconds then ___very slowly___ begin to move it up and down the cup with slow movements, ___a little at a time___, to slowly incorporate the oil, creating an emulsion.

(If you don't have an immersion blender you can use a food processor or regular blender. Start with just a few drops of oil at a time, then very slowly drizzle the oil into the other ingredients while the food processor or blender is running. Most food processors have tiny holes in the lid just for adding oil at the perfect rate.)

4. After the mayonnaise is created add the cilantro, lime juice, and zest, and briefly blend again until incorporated. Store in the refrigerator up to 1 week to use with salads.

RAW EGG WARNING: Consuming raw and barely cooked eggs may expose you to a small risk of salmonella or other food-borne illness. To reduce this risk use only fresh grade A or AA eggs, refrigerated and stored properly, with clean, intact shells. Avoid contact between the whites and yolks and the shell as you use them.

Crispy Duck and Potatoes with Creamy Chard Soup

Serves 4

8 duck legs (leg and thigh portions)
2 pounds potatoes, diced
Salt and pepper
Steamed greens, for serving

1. Preheat oven to 450°F.
2. Check duck skin for pinfeathers, rinse, and pat dry. Salt and pepper the duck. Roast the duck, skin side down, for 10 to 15 minutes while you cut the potatoes.
3. Remove the duck and place the potatoes and seasonings in the rendered duck fat, and stir. Spread the potatoes in a single layer and place duck on top.
4. Return to the oven for 1 hour, moving the duck to stir the potatoes every 15 minutes.
5. Save any duck fat from the pan and refrigerate to use as desired in other recipes.

Crunchy Option:

6. Remove the duck and place it in a very hot skillet, skin side down and continue to brown the potatoes in the oven. Crisp the duck legs over a medium-high heat for about 8 minutes or until a dark brown.
7. Turn, stirring the potatoes once more, and cook until the second side of the duck is crispy. Serve with the potatoes and steamed greens.

Creamy Chard Soup

Serves 4

Serve this soup warm or cold depending on your schedule today.

> 3 tablespoons butter, ghee, coconut oil, or other fat
>
> 2 large leeks, sliced and carefully washed
>
> 1½ teaspoons salt
>
> 2 bunches fresh chard (or 2 bags of frozen chard, kale, or collards, if you can't find chard), cut the stem into half slices
>
> 4½ cups water or broth
>
> 1 cup half-and-half or full-fat coconut milk
>
> White pepper to taste
>
> 1–2 teaspoons lemon juice to taste
>
> 1 cup fresh or frozen diced red bell peppers
>
> 2 scallions, green part snipped, white part thinly sliced for garnish

1. Melt butter in a soup pot and add the leeks and salt and cook over medium low heat until soft but not brown, stirring occasionally.

2. Add the kale or collards to the pot along with the water or broth and cook for 20 minutes.

3. Puree right in the pot with an immersion blender or transfer the soup to a traditional blender filled only halfway, and blend carefully. (Remove the center plug on the blender lid and cover with a thickly folded towel as you hold the lid so the steam won't build up and cause a painful accident.)

4. Add half-and-half or coconut milk for richness and blend with the soup. Pour it back into the same pot if not using an immersion blender and bring back to a simmer, adjusting the thickness with water or broth to create a nice soup consistency.

5. Add the lemon juice a teaspoon at a time and taste and adjust salt and add white pepper at this time if desired.

6. Add the red peppers and cook for 3–5 minutes.

7. Serve in bowls or chill to serve cold topped with the white part of scallions.

DAY 4

Prepare the Short Ribs in the morning if you didn't prepare the ingredients the night before. After dinner, make the herb paste to rub on the lamb and refrigerate it overnight and if you have no leftovers to use for breakfast, boil eggs for the Egg Salad breakfast tomorrow.

Morning Buckwheat and Baked Eggs

Serves 4

4 tablespoons organic chicken or duck fat, ghee, or unsalted butter, divided

1 large onion, diced

½ pound mushrooms, sliced

1 egg (not for Hunters)

1 cup roasted granulated buckwheat (Hunters: 2 cups each sautéed veggies)

2 cups chicken broth or vegetable broth

½ cup diced red bell pepper (Hunters: 2 cups)

8 chicken or duck eggs

Salt and black pepper

8 slices cooked chicken or turkey or prosciutto

1 cup packed raw spinach (Hunters: 2 cups)

8 tomato slices, for garnish

3 tablespoons chopped fresh parsley

1. Preheat oven to 400°F.

2. Melt 3 tablespoons of the chicken or duck fat in a large skillet or a wide pot that has a cover over medium-high heat and add onion and mushrooms. Stir every few minutes and cook for 10–15 minutes until onion is soft and beginning to brown.

3. Meanwhile, beat one egg in a bowl with a fork and mix in the buckwheat. Stir to coat.

4. When the onion and mushrooms are done, remove them to a plate or bowl and add the buckwheat and flatten it in the pan over high heat for 1 minute. Stir to break up the buckwheat and continue cooking for about 4 minutes, until dry.

5. Add the broth, bell pepper, onion and mushrooms, salt and black pepper, and cover and reduce heat to low and cook for 15 minutes.

6. Prepare the eggs by greasing 8 cups in a muffin pan (or 8 custard cups placed on a sheet pan) with the remaining tablespoon of melted fat.

7. Place a slice of meat in each cup, pressing down to form a little cup. (Test one piece first and if more than ½ inch sticks out above the rim, stack the slices

and cut the slices with a knife, using a large lid or a small plate that will give you the right size to have ¼–½ inch sticking up around each muffin cup.) Place each slice to form a little cup in the muffin tin, and if you do need to trim, chop the extra pieces and divide and place in the bottom of each cup.

8. Carefully break an egg into each cup, making sure not to break the yolk. Sprinkle each with salt and pepper. Bake for 15 minutes.

9. Check the buckwheat and remove from heat if the water or broth has been absorbed. Add the spinach and stir until wilted. Cover and let stand 10 minutes while the eggs are finishing in the oven.

10. About 5 minutes before the eggs finish, fluff buckwheat with a fork and serve a mound on each plate. Using the back of a large serving spoon, make a well in the center of each mound by pressing the buckwheat toward the edges of the plate to make a space. When the eggs are ready (the whites should be cooked but the yolks can still be soft enough to be runny), gently use 2 spoons to lift out each meat and egg cup. Place in buckwheat well. Garnish with sliced tomato sprinkled with parsley and salt.

Turkey Soup and Salad (L)

Serves 3–4

This soup is best made right after making the Slow Cooked Marsala Turkey Thigh recipe and then frozen, or can be almost as delicious with any bones and broth combination you have on hand.

> Contents of the slow cooker after making Marsala Turkey Thighs (page 304)
>
> Water or broth
>
> 2 tablespoons apple cider vinegar
>
> 1–2 bay leaves, depending on their size
>
> 1 teaspoon garlic powder
>
> 1 tablespoon poultry seasoning
>
> Salt and white pepper to taste
>
> 4–5 cups diced fresh vegetables of your choice
>
> 8–12 ounces leftover Marsala Turkey meat
>
> Handful of greens

1. After making Marsala Turkey Thighs, put all the bones, onions, and juices from the slow cooker into a large soup pot with an equal amount of water or

broth of your choice. Add the apple cider vinegar, a bay leaf or two, depending on their size, garlic powder, and poultry seasoning. (Don't add salt or pepper yet as it will get stronger as the soup concentrates as it cooks.)

2. Bring to a boil over high heat and lower the heat to keep it at a gentle simmer. Let it reduce partially covered for least an hour, adding liquid as needed if it reduces past half of the volume.

3. Remove the bones and bay leaf and check for seasonings, adding salt and pepper at this time if needed.

4. Add fresh, diced vegetables to the pot in order of longest to shortest cooking time or cut them to even out the timing. When vegetables are tender, add shredded leftover turkey meat.

5. If making this ahead, cool and freeze in portions. Defrost the night before you need it.

6. When ready to serve, put it in a saucepan over medium heat and add some greens like kale or spinach and cook for a few minutes until the greens are tender and the soup is hot and ready to serve with a large salad.

Beef Short Ribs over Vegetable Noodles

Serves 4 (plus 4 leftovers for chili)

5 pounds beef short ribs (8–10 pieces)

Salt and pepper

1 cup grated onions

1 cup grated carrots

1 cup grated turnip or rutabaga

½ cup grated parsnips

3–4 cloves garlic, whole, peeled

1 teaspoon celery salt

2 tablespoons fresh thyme, or 2 teaspoons dried

2 tablespoons red wine vinegar

1 (14-ounce) can diced tomatoes

1 cup beef broth

2 tablespoons organic grass-fed butter

3 pounds vegetables for noodles (zucchini, winter squash, carrots, or parsnips, cut into thin strips with a spiralizer, mandoline, or a potato peeler and blanched in boiling water)

Red pepper flakes, to taste

1. Sprinkle meat with salt and pepper and brown on all sides adding a small amount of oil of your choice, if needed. Brown in batches rather than crowd the pan, if necessary.

2. Shred the first group of vegetables in food processor and fill the bottom of a slow cooker, adding garlic, seasonings, vinegar, tomatoes, and broth to the vegetables and mix.

3. Lay the ribs on top. Cover and cook 4½–5 hours on high or 8–10 hours on low.

4. Remove ribs to a plate, keep warm, and puree the vegetables with an immersion or regular blender to create a nice sauce, adding butter and adjusting the salt and pepper as needed.

5. Serve ribs with sauce on top of vegetable noodles. Garnish with red pepper flakes for heat, to taste. Serve with Crimson Salad.

Note: Save leftover meat to use for the chili and save the bones and sauce to make a soup or freeze the sauce to serve over something like millet or spaghetti squash.

Crimson Salad with Balsamic Dressing

Serves 4

¼ red onion, thinly sliced

3 red bell peppers, cut in large dice or thin strips

4 large tomatoes, cut into large bite-size pieces

½ large clove garlic, grated

3 tablespoons balsamic vinegar (choose a low-sugar brand)

1 teaspoon orange juice (or a few drops essential orange oil)

1 teaspoon mustard

½ teaspoon fresh thyme leaves

3 tablespoons olive or other oil

1 tablespoon flax oil (optional)

½ teaspoon salt

A few drops of grapefruit essential oil

1. Cut, then rinse the onion under water for 30 seconds to reduce the bite from raw onion. Shake off excess water, pat dry, and add to the peppers and tomatoes in the serving bowl.

2. Mix the remaining ingredients for the dressing, except the essential oils, in a small bowl and whisk together or shake in a jar to combine. Add the

grapefruit oil drop by drop, as essential oils (unlike extracts) are very strong and you can't remove them if you add too much. Mountain Rose is top quality.

3. Gradually add the dressing to the amount of salad you want to serve, toss just before serving and refrigerate any extra salad and dressing separately to serve another day.

Day 5

If you have a rushed morning or a busy day, make rice and boil the eggs the night before. You can also make the pâté and prepare the vegetables to make lunch easy to take with you as you leave in the morning. You can even make the herb paste and marinate the lamb, fill the slow cooker, and keep it in the refrigerator overnight, then start cooking it after breakfast or before lunch so it will be ready for dinner. Yesterday's dinner was very easy and required very little time, so you can shift these tasks without much problem. And remember to soak the beans for the Short Rib Chili for tomorrow's dinner while you sleep.

Americanized Japanese Breakfast Soup (M)

Serves 4 (+4 leftover, steak)

2 cups cooked brown rice

4 hard-boiled eggs, sliced (1 per serving)

2½ pounds London broil steak

1 tablespoon onion powder

1 tablespoon garlic powder

1 teaspoon mustard powder

1 teaspoon salt

½ teaspoon pepper

½ cup macadamia or olive oil

12 cups organic beef broth, chicken broth, or vegetable broth

1 tablespoon organic chickpea miso paste

1 head broccoli

1 bunch watercress

Red pepper flakes to taste

1 cup sliced no-sugar-added dill pickles, or 1 large or 2 small cucumbers, peeled, sliced, and dressed with rice vinegar and sesame oil

1 teaspoon sesame oil

1. Make the rice and hard-boiled eggs if they are not already prepared. (Allow about 45 minutes for this.)

2. Thinly slice the steak across the grain into strips about 2 inches long and ¼ inch thick. (It is easier to slice into thin strips when slightly frozen.) The meat thaws faster if it is spread out instead of in a tall pile.

3. Mix the seasonings together with the oil and rub and toss it on the steak strips until fully coated. Let rest at room temperature for at least 10 minutes.

4. Heat up a grill pan or skillet on top of the stove and quickly sear both sides of the steak in batches. Cook 1–2 minutes per side until medium-rare. Be careful not to overcook. Remove from heat and loosely cover (i.e., with foil) to keep warm.

5. Store 1¼ pounds in the refrigerator to use on Day 7.

6. Peel broccoli stems. Grate by hand or in food processor.

7. Heat the broth of your choice in a pot on the stove, add the grated broccoli, and cook on medium heat for 5 minutes. Make the cucumber quick pickle or place dill pickle into a small dish.

8. When soup is hot but not boiling, add the miso by dissolving the miso paste into half a cup of the broth, then pour into the soup pot and stir. For best health effects, DO NOT LET THE SOUP BOIL ONCE THE MISO IS ADDED.

9. Add the sesame oil. Herders also can add 2 cups cooked rice to the pot and simmer for a few minutes over low heat.

10. Divide the watercress among four 4-cup large bowls, add the broth and rice, and sprinkle with red pepper flakes if desired. Lay the steak slices on top towards one side of the bowl gently and press to submerge in the hot broth. Lay slices of egg on the other side and serve each bowl of soup with a small dish of pickles.

Pâté-Stuffed Veggies for Liver Haters

Serves 4

Note: If you don't need 4 servings now, reduce the vegetables for stuffing to what you need in the next couple of days. I suggest still making the full amount of pâté and using it for snacks by preparing it according to the instructions in the snack section (page 358).

> 20 large mushroom caps, stems removed and chopped (or more raw vegetables to stuff instead)
>
> 8 strips of bacon
>
> 2 large onions, diced
>
> 8 ounces calf's liver
>
> 2 cloves garlic, grated
>
> 1 pound grass-fed ground beef
>
> 2 tablespoons dried rosemary
>
> 2 tablespoons dried thyme
>
> 3 ounces tomato paste
>
> ¼ cup balsamic vinegar
>
> 4 medium red bell peppers, cut in half and seeds removed; can also stuff hollowed-out tomatoes or celery or any other raw vegetables
>
> 8 stalks celery, cut in 3-inch pieces

1. If you are stuffing mushrooms, preheat oven to 400°F. You could also just prepare extra peppers and celery and other raw vegetables like endive leaves, or cucumber slices to eat with the pâté instead.

2. If you are not a fan of liver you might want to soak the liver in milk for an hour to mellow the liver's flavor and discard the milk, though I find that in this recipe it is not that important.

3. Toss the mushroom caps with a little olive oil and place on a baking sheet, cavity side up, and bake for 20–25 minutes until softened.

4. Cook the bacon in a large skillet and drain on paper towels when crisp, leaving the fat in the pan.

5. Add the onions to the bacon fat and cook over medium heat, stirring periodically.

6. Meanwhile remove any veins from the liver and discard the milk (if used).

7. After the onions have cooked for about 5 minutes, add the chopped mushroom stems and garlic.

8. Puree the liver in a food processor until smooth.

9. When the onions are soft and beginning to brown, add the ground beef and stir to brown evenly. Stir in the liver puree when the beef is about halfway browned.

10. Add the herbs and keep stirring until everything is almost cooked.

11. Add the tomato paste and vinegar and cook for another couple of minutes.

12. Pulse the mixture in a food processor, scraping down the sides until it becomes a smooth mixture. Add a little olive oil if the mixture is too crumbly.

13. Stir in the crumbled bacon.

14. Spoon mixture in mounds in the mushroom cavities. Any extra can be stuffed in the red peppers, celery, or any other raw vegetables you want.

Slow Cooker Tender Lamb Shanks with Rosemary, Garlic, and Mustard and Roasted Asparagus and Tomatoes over Spinach

Serves 4 (4 for Day 7)

Make the herb paste and coat the lamb. You can make it in the morning and just cook it right away.

3¼ pounds boneless lamb leg, cut in large cubes

8 small to medium Yukon Gold or Red Bliss potatoes (or use ½ to 1 cup tiny creamer potatoes per serving)

For the herb paste:

1 head garlic, separated into cloves (about 12) and grated

1 teaspoon salt

2 teaspoons freshly grated organic lemon zest

2 tablespoons minced fresh rosemary leaves, or 2 teaspoons dried

⅛ teaspoon white pepper

2 tablespoons olive or other oil

Juice of 1 lemon

2 tablespoons Dijon mustard

1. Put all of the ingredients for the herb paste into a small bowl and mix until it forms a paste and rub the paste all over the meat. Marinate overnight in the refrigerator.

2. In the morning place the meat into the center of a slow cooker, then place the whole potatoes around it and cover. If using a lean cut of lamb or substituting another lean meat like poultry, add a cup of broth or water.

3. Cook on high for 5 hours or on low for 8–10 hours.

4. Place a serving of meat and potatoes topped with some of the juices from the slow cooker and serve with asparagus and carrots and a small green salad.

5. Refrigerate the extra lamb to use for the Shepherd's Pie, Day 7.

Roasted Asparagus and Tomatoes over Spinach

Serves 4

2 pounds fresh asparagus

2–3 tablespoons olive or other oil, divided

½ pound tomatoes, diced

Salt to taste

8 cups fresh spinach

1 lemon, halved

¼ teaspoon lemon pepper

1. Preheat oven to 425°F.

2. Wash asparagus and snap off the end of each stalk. For easy cleanup, you can line a baking sheet with parchment paper.

3. Lay the asparagus on another parchment-lined baking sheet and drizzle 1–2 tablespoons of olive oil over them and toss to coat, then arrange them in one layer.

4. Put the tomatoes in a bowl and sprinkle with a little salt to help release their juices.

5. Bake the asparagus for 10–15 minutes depending on the thickness of the vegetables, rolling them over every 4 or 5 minutes, until tender and beginning to brown. Remove from oven and cut into 1-inch pieces.

6. Put spinach in a large bowl and top with the warm asparagus and diced tomatoes with any juices they released. Squeeze lemon over the top and sprinkle with lemon pepper. Toss and add the remaining olive oil if desired and serve.

Day 6

Make lunch the night before if you will be away all day. You can also take a few minutes to make the tea for breakfast. Once the tea is cool you can add the chia seeds and refrigerate it. After they have soaked at least 30 minutes or if you don't have time for the tea to cool, add the chia if you have time in the morning. Let it soak while you are making the shrimp, then enjoy the pudding after eating them.

Minty Chia Pudding (M)

Serves 4 (Having extra servings in the refrigerator make a good snack.)

5 cups brewed herbal mint tea, double strength, cooled to room temperature

1 cup chia seeds

Fresh mint leaves, chopped for garnish (optional)

1. Combine the tea and chia seeds in a small bowl (or shake in a large jar) and stir several times over the next 20 minutes.

2. Garnish with chopped mint leaves if desired.

Prosciutto-Wrapped Shrimp

Serves 4

2 tablespoons olive or other oil

Juice of ½ lemon

1 tablespoon paprika

1 teaspoon onion powder

½ teaspoon garlic powder

½ teaspoon dried thyme

Pinch of black pepper

1 pound peeled and deveined large raw shrimp (defrosted if frozen)

6–8 ounces prosciutto (or ½ bacon strip for each shrimp)

1. Preheat broiler.

2. Combine oil and spices and toss with shrimp and let rest for a few minutes.

3. Count the shrimp and cut the prosciutto slices in half lengthwise to have one per shrimp. (If using bacon, cut lengthwise diagonally.)

4. Wrap each shrimp with the prosciutto (or bacon) from head end to tail in a spiral fashion and lay ends down on a rack on a lightly oiled baking sheet that will fit in your broiler. (You can secure each with water-soaked toothpicks if desired.)

5. Broil for 3–4 minutes turning once, until shrimp is opaque and prosciutto is crisp.

Almond-Crusted Turkey Schnitzel (Q)

Serves 4

1½ pounds turkey cutlets (turkey or chicken breast or thigh or pork chops will work well too)

¼ teaspoon salt

1¼ cups almond meal

2 tablespoons fresh thyme, or 2 teaspoons dried

¾ cup grated Parmesan cheese (if dairy intolerant leave it out and follow special directions below)

2 egg whites, mixed with 2 tablespoons water (eliminate the water if not using Parmesan cheese)

⅛ teaspoon pepper

2 tablespoons butter, ghee, or other fat

Lemon wedges

1. If you can't find cutlets, you will need to make your own. If using a turkey breast you will need to butterfly it by placing your hand flat on top of the breast, then using a sharp knife to slice parallel to the cutting board, making 2 evenly thick pieces. No need to slice this way if using chicken or boneless pork chops.

2. Pound each piece of meat flat (between parchment, plastic wrap, or food storage bag), using a heavy pan or the heel of our hand if you don't have a meat mallet, until it is ¼ inch thick. Sprinkle both sides of each piece lightly with salt.

3. Mix the almond meal with the thyme and Parmesan cheese (if using the cheese).

4. Beat the egg white and water with a fork or whisk until combined and stir in the pepper. Dip the meat in the egg white, then into the almond/cheese mixture, making sure both sides are well coated. Set aside and repeat until all pieces are coated. (If not using the cheese, mix the egg whites and almond meal together to make a batter and coat the meat.)

5. Melt butter in a large skillet and when the butter is foamy, reduce the heat to medium and place the coated meat into the pan, making sure not to splash yourself. Work in two batches rather than crowd the pan. After 3 minutes,

gently turn and brown the other side. Use a spatula to loosen it if sticking. Cook for 2–3 minutes more. Do not overcook. If working in batches, remove first batch and cover loosely with foil as you cook the second batch, adding more butter to the pan. Serve with lemon wedges.

Haricots Verts Soup (Q)

Serves 4

2 tablespoons bacon fat, or a combination of 1 tablespoon each of 2 different fats

2 pounds haricots verts (very thin green beans), thawed if frozen

3 garlic cloves, grated

½–1 quart chicken broth or vegetable broth

Juice of 4 limes

3 tablespoons lime zest

Salt to taste

1 teaspoon lemon pepper

Splash of champagne vinegar

Pinch of red pepper flakes (optional)

1 tablespoon grated Parmesan cheese (optional)

1. Melt bacon fat or butter or a combination of both over medium heat in a pan or pot large enough to hold all of the green beans.

2. Rinse thawed beans and pat dry.

3. Add the garlic to the pan and stir quickly to prevent burning. As garlic softens over 1 minute or so, add the drained beans and stir to coat with the garlic and fat.

4. Stir every minute over the next 4 minutes, then add broth, lime juice and zest, salt, lemon pepper, and a splash of vinegar and cook until green beans are soft—another 5–10 minutes.

5. Remove from heat and remove half of the liquid and reserve.

6. Using an immersion blender, puree into a soup, adding the reserved liquid as needed to create the consistency you prefer. (You can also puree in small batches in a regular blender, but don't fill the blender and remember to cover the lid with a folded towel to prevent burns/or mess.)

7. Pour back into the pot and rewarm if needed. Serve in bowls and garnish with a little Parmesan cheese if desired.

Shredded Beef Chili (L)

Serves 4

Did you forget to start this by soaking the beans overnight? Use well rinsed canned beans instead.

1 cup dried black, pink, white, or cranberry beans (Hunters can substitute 3 cups of chopped mushrooms and ½ pound of cooked bacon instead.)

1 cup yellow onion

1 cup carrots

1 cup zucchini

1 cup red bell pepper, diced

2 fresh tomatoes, diced

1 14-ounce can crushed, low-salt tomatoes or tomato sauce

1 cup celery (optional)

2 tablespoons chili powder (less if using a super hot one)

½ teaspoon cumin

1 teaspoon salt

¼ teaspoon black pepper

1 Anaheim (or hotter) chili as desired, finely diced

2 cups water

1 pound shredded leftover short rib meat (or brown 1½ pounds ground meat with some chili powder and salt and pepper and add to the vegetables in the beginning if not using leftovers.)

1. The night before, sort beans, remove sticks or rocks if any. Rinse and soak the beans overnight in 2 quarts of water with 1½ tablespoon of salt. (I promise they will not be tough!)

2. In the morning, drain soaked beans, rinse well, and put in a slow cooker.

3. Cut the onions, carrots, celery, and zucchini using a food processor if desired to quickly cut into bite-size pieces.

4. Add the peppers and the fresh and canned tomatoes along with the vegetables and seasonings to the beans in the slow cooker (adding the mushrooms and bacon if not using beans). Add water, stir, and cook on low for 8 hours or 6 hours on high.

5. Half an hour before serving, check if the beans are soft. Add the leftover meat and cook on high without the cover to thicken the chili if there is too much liquid. Stir occasionally until the right consistency is achieved.

6. Garnish with toppings like diced tomatoes, chiles, scallions, shredded cheese, or sour cream (or homemade coconut yogurt, page 362) as desired.

7. Serve with a large green salad.

Day 7

Fry the bacon and prepare the vegetables. (I often keep some chopped cooked bacon in the freezer as it is an easy way to quickly add wonderful flavor to any dish.)

Bacon Egg Foo Young

Serves 4

10 eggs

1 cup bean sprouts, roughly chopped

1 cup thinly sliced onions

½ cup thinly sliced mushrooms

½ cup small-diced red bell pepper

1 cup shredded carrots

(or any combination of fresh or leftover vegetables to equal 4 cups)

1 clove garlic, grated

1 tablespoon grated fresh ginger

½ teaspoon salt

⅛ white pepper

4 strips of bacon, cooked and chopped, fat reserved

1. Preheat the oven to 200°F. Beat the eggs in a large bowl then add the vegetables and seasonings. Mix to combine.

2. Add the bacon pieces to the mixture and stir.

3. Heat a skillet with a little of the reserved bacon fat over medium heat and scoop ½-cup portions of the mixture into the pan for each patty.

4. Cook until each patty begins to brown, turn, and continue to cook the other side for an additional 2–3 minutes.

5. Place the cooked patties, loosely covered with foil, in the oven to keep warm as you continue to cook more patties, adding a thin coating of the reserved bacon fat as needed, until the mixture is totally cooked.

For the sauce:

2 tablespoons reserved bacon fat or other fat

1½ cups sliced scallions (reserve ½ cup for garnish)

3 tablespoons grated fresh ginger

2 cups chicken broth or vegetable broth

2 tablespoons soy sauce (gluten-free if wheat sensitive)

¼ teaspoon sesame oil

1. While cooking the patties, heat the 2 tablespoons of fat in a small saucepan and sauté the scallions and ginger for 1–2 minutes.

2. Add the broth and soy sauce and cook over high heat until reduced by half.

3. Carefully add a few of drops of sesame oil.

4. Blend the scallions, ginger, and broth right in the saucepan with an immersion blender or use a mini food processor or blender, taste, and adjust for seasonings if necessary.

5. Serve 2 patties per plate, with some sauce either underneath or over the top of each one and sprinkle with the reserved green onions to garnish.

Steak Salad with Ginger Nut Dressing (L, M)

Serves 4

4 cups roughly chopped romaine lettuce

4 cups thinly sliced kale

3 cups thinly sliced Napa cabbage

3 cups thinly sliced red cabbage

2 cups thinly sliced celery

4 cups thinly sliced or shredded carrots

2 cups thinly sliced or shredded jicama

2 cups diced cucumber

2 cups diced red or yellow bell pepper

1 cup scallions sliced (on a diagonal)

1 cup chopped fresh cilantro leaves

Ginger Nut Dressing (page 332)

1¼ pounds leftover steak slices (remember to defrost if necessary)

Note: If you don't need to feed 4, dress whatever quantity of salad you need and save the rest for the first few days of next week. Or reduce the ingredient quantities to just what you actually need for this meal.

1. Put all the greens, vegetables, and cilantro in a large bowl. Toss together with the dressing as needed and reserve the extra dressing for other salads. Only dress the salad you are serving and reserve extras for another meal.

2. Top with a serving of the leftover steak strips and serve.

Ginger Nut Dressing

Makes approximately 2 cups

½ cup nut butter (peanut, almond, or cashew, or substitute avocado if sensitive to nuts)

½ cup unseasoned rice vinegar

3 tablespoons fresh lime juice

½ cup oil of choice

1–2 tablespoons soy sauce

1 tablespoon flaxseed oil (optional)

2–3 large cloves garlic, finely grated

1 (2–3-inch) piece fresh ginger, peeled and grated

Stevia to taste (optional)

1–2 teaspoons Sriracha (optional)

1½ teaspoons toasted sesame oil

1. Put all of the ingredients except the ½ cup oil of your choice (or avocado if using) in a blender and process until blended. (I recommend starting with lesser amounts of ingredients where a specific amount is suggested.)

2. Slowly drizzle the oil into the running blender. Taste and add more of any ingredient desired so it will be to your liking.

3. Strain out any remaining pieces of ginger (and then blend in the avocado if using) and store in refrigerator until needed.

Lamb and Lemon Sweet Potato Shepherd's Pie (L)

Serves 4

There are a few steps to this but it is worth it and really doesn't take that long. Prepare the filling while the potatoes are cooking. If you don't have leftover lamb from earlier in the week, you can quickly season and brown ground lamb instead.

For the topping:

2 pounds sweet potatoes, peeled and diced

2 tablespoons butter or coconut oil or other fat

Juice of 1 lemon

2 teaspoons lemon zest

½ teaspoon salt

White pepper to taste

For the filling:

3 tablespoons oil

1 cup chopped onion

2 cloves garlic, minced

2 carrots, peeled and diced small

1 cup sliced mushrooms

1 cup green beans, cut on the diagonal

1 cup chopped kale

(or substitute 5 cups leftover cooked or frozen vegetables for the above)

2 teaspoons tomato paste

½ cup beef broth or chicken broth

2 teaspoons minced fresh rosemary, or about ½ teaspoon dried

1 teaspoon chopped fresh thyme leaves, or ⅓ teaspoon dried

½ cup shelled fresh or frozen peas

1¼ pounds leftover lamb, diced

½ teaspoon salt

½ teaspoon pepper

1. Preheat the oven to 400°F.
2. Cover the sweet potatoes with cold water and bring to a boil over high heat then lower heat to a simmer and cook until tender about 12 minutes depending on the size of your dice.
3. Drain potatoes and return to the saucepan. Mash the potatoes with butter, lemon juice, zest, salt, and pepper until smooth.

4. Make the filling while the potatoes are cooking. Heat the olive oil in a large sauté pan over medium-high heat. Cook the onion, garlic, carrots, mushrooms, green beans, and kale approximately 5 minutes (less for leftover veggies).

5. Add the tomato paste, broth, rosemary, and thyme, and stir to combine. Bring to a boil, reduce the heat to low, cover, and simmer slowly for 10 to 12 minutes or until the sauce is slightly reduced.

6. Add the peas and the leftover lamb to the vegetables and stir. Taste for salt and pepper and adjust if necessary.

7. Place filling into a rectangular baking dish, round casserole dish, or two loaf pans. (Great for freezing one if you don't want to serve the whole thing right away.)

8. Spread the mashed sweet potatoes over the top, sealing around the edge to prevent the filling from spilling over as it bakes.

9. Place on a parchment- or foil-lined sheet tray and bake for 30 minutes or just until the potatoes begin to brown. Cool for 10 minutes before serving.

WEEK TWO RECIPES

Day 1
Eggamole Salad

Serves 4 (Great for snacks)

12 eggs

½ cup guacamole (see page 362)

1 tablespoon plus 1 teaspoon lemon juice

Salt and pepper to taste

1 teaspoon mustard

1 tablespoon olive oil

2 cups shredded or thinly sliced radicchio

4 scallions, thinly sliced

1 tablespoon chopped cilantro

Jicama slices (use instead of bread or crackers)

4–8 cups lettuce (your choice)

1. Hard-boil the eggs in your preferred manner. Cool in very cold water if you haven't prepared them in advance and chilled. Peel off the shells.

2. Dice using an egg slicer by cutting in at least 2 directions or with a fork.

3. Prepare it if you haven't already. Add the guacamole to the eggs and gently mix to combine.

4. Add 1 tablespoon lemon juice and stir again.

5. Taste for salt and pepper.

6. In another bowl, combine the mustard, 1 teaspoon lemon juice, and the olive oil and mix well with a fork. Add the radicchio, scallions, and cilantro, and toss until well coated.

7. Serve ¼ cup per serving. Place appropriately sized mounds on top of the jicama slices and cover with a smaller mound of the radicchio. Alternatively, add the radicchio to a bowl of salad greens and top with a scoop of the eggamole.

Nutty Crusted Trout Fillets with Lemon Yogurt Sauce

Serves 4 (2 for Day 2)

For the Nutty Crust

1 cup lightly toasted hazelnut or almond meal (or replace with an equal amount of potato starch if nut intolerant)

1½ cups potato starch and/or coconut flour

3 tablespoons chopped parsley leaves

1 teaspoon salt

½ teaspoon pepper

1 tablespoon chopped rosemary leaves

½ cup butter or ghee, room temperature

¼ cup Parmesan cheese (optional—do not use nut Parmesan here)

1½ pounds boneless trout fillets

Salt and lemon pepper

1–2 tablespoons grass-fed butter or ghee, room temperature

Lemon Yogurt Sauce (recipe follows)

1. Pulse all the crust ingredients in a food processor until well mixed.

2. Package, label, and refrigerate or freeze and use later to make the crust for the trout.

3. Preheat the oven to 450°F.

4. Check fillets for bones and season each with salt and lemon pepper.

5. Brush a roasting pan with butter. Brush each trout fillet with a generous layer of softened butter and place on the buttered pan.

6. Divide the crust mixture into the same number of pieces as trout. Roll and pat into the shape and size of each fillet and completely cover one side of each fillet. Press firmly with your hand to create a solid coating.

7. Bake for 10–20 minutes or until the fillets are firm and flaky.

8. Carefully lift the trout onto a plate with a large spatula, and drizzle 3 tablespoons of the Lemon Yogurt sauce over the trout and vegetables. *Serve with 2 pounds steamed asparagus and 4 cups carrot/celery sticks (in 4 servings).*

Lemon Yogurt Sauce

Makes about 4 cups

1 cup full-fat Greek yogurt, or homemade coconut yogurt from Week 1 recipes)

¼ cup finely grated cucumber

6 tablespoons chopped fresh mint leaves (optional)

4 teaspoons lemon zest

2 tablespoons lemon juice

Salt and white pepper to taste

Combine the sauce ingredients and serve chilled or at room temperature as a sauce for the trout fillets, and as a dip for the vegetables.

Roast Lamb with Olive Arugula Pesto and "Rice"

Serves 2 (2 for Day 3)

1½ pounds boneless leg of lamb, at room temperature and trimmed of fat

2 tablespoons olive or other oil (to coat before roasting)

Salt and pepper

Olive Arugula Pesto (page 338)

Cauliflower Rice (page 337)

1. Take the lamb out of the refrigerator about 2 hours before you want to eat and let it sit out for about 45 minutes to remove the chill.

2. Preheat the oven to 450°F.

3. Rub the lamb with oil and salt and pepper. Put it in a roasting pan, fat side facing up, and roast for 20 minutes while making the pesto.

4. Set the oven for 350°F and continue roasting for another 20–30 minutes or until the internal temperature reaches 130°F and the meat is golden brown.

5. Take the lamb out of the oven, tent it with foil, and let it rest for about 10 minutes, until the internal temperature reaches 140°F.

6. Slice across the grain into two 6-ounce portions of lamb per serving for dinner and serve with the snap peas, pesto, and "rice."

7. Cut the rest of the lamb into 2 large portions. Do not slice it. Place one package in the freezer and one in the refrigerator. (It may need to be divided into more portions depending on the size of the roast.)

Cauliflower Rice

Serves 4 (2 for Day x)

Both Costco and Trader Joe's sell riced cauliflower at the time of printing.

2 bags of riced cauliflower, or 1 very large or 2 medium heads of cauliflower

2 teaspoons olive or other oil

Salt and lemon pepper

1 bunch scallions, sliced

2 tablespoons capers

1 tablespoon diced preserved lemon (optional)

2 tablespoons kalamata olives, sliced

1. If using whole cauliflower, trim off all the florets from the cauliflower and set the stems aside. Cut any large florets so most of them are about the same size.

2. Put about 2 cups into the food processor. Pulse until the pieces are about the size of rice or use a grater or grating blade. Empty into a bowl and continue with another 2 cups of cauliflower at a time until all the florets are chopped into the size of rice.

3. Heat olive oil in a pot or skillet and add cauliflower and a pinch of salt and lemon pepper when the oil is hot. Stir and cook for 3 minutes, add scallions, and cook another 2–3 minutes until cauliflower is tender.

4. Add the capers, preserved lemon, and sliced olives, stir. Taste the cauliflower. Adjust salt and lemon pepper if needed. Lightly drizzle a little more olive oil for flavor and toss.

Olive Arugula Pesto

Makes about 2 cups

1 cup packed chopped fresh basil leaves

1 cup packed chopped fresh arugula

2 teaspoons black pepper

½ head roasted garlic

¼ 1 cup olive or other oil

¾ cup pitted medium kalamata olives

¼ cup pitted green olives

2 tablespoons walnuts (or omit if nut intolerant)

2 tablespoons capers, drained

1 tablespoon lemon juice, or a drop or two of lemon oil or lemon extract to taste

1. Combine the basil, arugula, and pepper in a food processor and pulse until broken down.

2. Gently squeeze the roasted garlic cloves from the skins into the mixture and, with the food processor running, slowly add the olive oil and blend until it comes together into a smooth paste.

3. Add the olives and walnuts and pulse to chop. Do not overprocess the olives and nuts as you want to create a nice texture. Taste for salt and pepper and adjust if needed. Store in the refrigerator.

Day 2
Breakfast: Leftover Nutty Crusted Trout Meal

Asian Burgers/Meatballs with Peanut Chili Sauce, Miso Vegetable Soup, and Yam Bakes

Serves 2 (makes 2 burgers plus 2 portions meatballs)

8 ounces mushrooms, chopped in a food processor into small pieces

½ onion, small dice

1 tablespoon avocado oil or olive oil

7½ pounds ground pork

½ cup daikon or jicama (chopped in food processor in small pieces)

1 bunch chives

1 egg, beaten

2 tablespoons soy sauce or gluten-free tamari or coconut aminos

1 tablespoon sake (optional) or chicken broth or water

½ teaspoon ground ginger

1 small clove garlic, grated

⅛ teaspoon sesame oil

1 tablespoon potato starch

2 teaspoons Sriracha or garlic chili sauce (optional)

Large portabello mushroom caps, stems removed (to use as bun for burgers), or lettuce leaves to wrap burger

Peanut Chili Sauce (page 340)

1. Preheat oven to 400°F to bake mushroom caps and yam bakes.

2. Sauté the chopped mushrooms and onion in the oil in a pan until softened.

3. Add the cooled mixture to the ground pork with the coconut flour and the rest of the seasonings and gently mix.

4. Divide the meat mixture in half.

5. Form half the meat into 2 burgers, making sure that they are larger than the mushroom caps as they will shrink as they cook.

6. Form the other half into meatballs for variety, using 2 tablespoons of meat for each, to be served Day 7. Freeze until then, raw or cooked.

7. Fry them in a cast-iron skillet or grill pan if you have them or in a lightly greased skillet. Turn once, and cook until browned and cooked through. (Or bake at 400°F until browned and internal temperature is 160°F.)

8. Serve the burgers on the portobello mushroom caps with the Peanut Chili Sauce and crisp lettuce.

9. Freeze leftover meat, cooked or raw, for use on Day 7.

Miso Vegetable Soup

Serves 4 (2 on Day 7)

2 cups bite-size broccoli florets

1 pound bok choy, chopped

2 cups sliced scallions

4 cloves garlic, grated

1 (½-inch) piece fresh ginger, peeled and grated

8 cups organic low-salt chicken broth, reserving ½ cup

¼ cup gluten-free white chickpea miso

¼ teaspoon white pepper

A few drops sesame oil

1. Heat all the ingredients except the meatballs and miso, and bring to a boil. Reduce heat to medium and cook for 10 minutes.

2. Remove 1½ cups of the hot liquid, and in a cup or bowl, stir in the miso until fully dissolved.

3. Place half of the ingredients from the soup pot into a blender. Cover lid with a folded towel and hold down tightly and puree. Add the puree back to the pot, stir, and add more chicken broth or a little water to thin as needed and stir.

4. Add the pepper and the miso dissolved in broth back to the pot, stir to combine, reduce heat to low, and cook for another 3 minutes. Do not boil once miso has been added, to preserve health benefits.

Peanut Chili Sauce

Makes a little over 1 cup

2 tablespoons peanut or almond butter

2 tablespoons soy sauce or tamari, gluten-free

2 tablespoons coconut milk

2 tablespoons lime juice

2 teaspoons hot water, if using nut butter

½ teaspoon cayenne pepper (use more or less to taste)

1. Blend all the ingredients in a mini food processor, or using an immersion blender, until smooth.

2. Place a spoon on each burger. Use the rest to toss over the "rice" later, thinning as needed, and serve with the meatballs.

Chicken Thighs and Pepper Tacos in Romaine, Cauliflower Rice (L), and Salad

Serves 4

2 pounds bone-in chicken thighs

1 pound bell pepper strips, frozen or taken from salad bar veggies

2 onions, sliced

½ cup chicken broth

½ cup diced roasted chile peppers (optional)

1 tablespoon chili powder

1 teaspoon cumin

½ teaspoon onion powder

¼ teaspoon garlic powder

Toppings

Romaine lettuce or Napa cabbage leaves to use as a taco shell

2–3 fresh tomatoes, diced

Sour cream, grated cheese, and/or avocado slices as accompaniments

Chopped cilantro

Hot sauce

1. Mix all the ingredients except the toppings into the slow cooker, bringing the chicken thighs to the top of the vegetables. Cover and cook on high for 4–5 hours or on low for 7–8 hours.

2. When ready to serve, remove chicken from slow cooker and use forks to shred the meat, discarding all the bones. Place meat back in slow cooker and stir to mix.

3. Using a slotted spoon, fill lettuce or cabbage leaves with mixture. Top with desired toppings.

Day 3

Day 3 includes two easy, mostly leftover meals:

Breakfast: Lamb Curry Stew with Steamed Kabocha Squash

Lunch: Leftover Chicken Thighs Over a Baked Potato and Gazpacho (page 353)

Dinner: Fresh Scallops!

Lamb Curry Stew with Spaghetti Squash (L, M)

Serves 2

Prebaking the squash and using canned and frozen organic products will make this a 10–15 minute dish. But if you use fresh produce, cut everything in small pieces and it will be ready almost as quickly, adding the fresh spinach and cubed lamb in the last 5 minutes of cooking.

> 2 tablespoons olive or other oil
>
> 2 onions, chopped
>
> 4–6 fresh tomatoes, diced, or 2 cans whole Muir Glen low-salt tomatoes
>
> 2 pounds cauliflower florets, fresh or frozen
>
> ½ pound peas, fresh or frozen
>
> 1 pound zucchini, fresh or frozen
>
> 4 garlic cloves, grated
>
> 1 (1-inch) piece fresh ginger, peeled and grated
>
> ½ teaspoon ground turmeric
>
> ½ teaspoon garam masala (or substitute 1 teaspoon curry powder for the turmeric and garam masala)
>
> 2 servings of leftover Roast Lamb (page 336), cut into ¾-inch cubes
>
> 1 pound spinach, fresh
>
> ½ cup plain full-fat yogurt or coconut milk
>
> ¼ cup chopped cilantro, for garnish
>
> Spaghetti Squash (recipe follows)

1. Sauté the oil and onions for 5 minutes in a large soup pot, stirring over high heat until starting to brown. Do not let them burn, so reduce heat if you can't watch them closely.

2. Add the rest of the ingredients (except the lamb, spinach, dairy options, and cilantro garnish and spaghetti squash), cover, and stir every few minutes.

3. About 5 minutes before everything is done, remove half of the pot contents and store in the refrigerator for another day. Add the lamb, spinach, and dairy options, and finish cooking for another 5 minutes over medium-low heat.

4. Serve over baked spaghetti squash, garnished with cilantro.

Spaghetti Squash

1 large spaghetti squash or 2 medium
Fat of choice, for brushing

1. Preheat oven to 400°F.

2. Carefully cut the squash in half lengthwise and remove seeds by scraping out with a spoon.

3. Brush with fat of choice and place cut side down on a baking sheet covered with parchment for easier cleanup.

4. Bake 30 to 45 minutes until soft. The cooked flesh will resemble spaghetti noodles as it is removed from the outer skin using a large spoon. Serve under lamb curry stew. For leftovers, add fat and herbs or spices of choice and use as side dish.

Baked Scallops with Artichokes and Tomatoes

Serves 4

For the topping

2 pounds scallops, frozen or fresh

1 bag artichoke hearts, frozen

3 tablespoons ghee or butter, room temperature

4 roasted garlic cloves

4 scallions, trimmed and cut in 1-inch pieces

2 ounces prosciutto, chopped (or bacon, cooked and crumbled)

4 tablespoons fresh parsley

4 tablespoons grated or finely chopped fresh fennel

2 teaspoons lime juice

2 teaspoons lemon juice

1 teaspoon salt

¼ teaspoon white pepper

2 cups cherry tomatoes, cut in half

4 tablespoons dry white wine

4 teaspoons olive or other oil

3 tablespoons Parmesan cheese (or use nut parmesan on page 363)

6 tablespoons crushed Lydia's Kind Italian Herbs Sprouted Crackers (or Mary's Gone Basil & Garlic Crackers for Herders)

Lime wedges, for garnish

1. The day before you want to make this, thaw the scallops and artichoke hearts and topping overnight in the refrigerator.

2. Prepare the topping by putting the ghee, garlic, scallions, prosciutto, parsley, fennel, lime and lemon juice, salt, and pepper in a mini food processor and process to combine. If you don't have one, use a regular one and scrape the sides and redistribute the ingredients several times as you process it. When it is well combined and very finely minced, add the oil slowly the processor running until combined.

3. Preheat the oven to 425°F.

4. Drain the thawed scallops and artichokes toss them with the tomatoes, wine, and olive oil and put in a broiler-safe baking pan large enough so that the scallops are in a single layer. Sprinkle with salt and Parmesan cheese.

5. Bring the prepared butter topping to room temperature. Add the crushed crackers to the butter mixture.

6. Top each scallop with a teaspoonful of the butter and cracker mixture.

7. Bake in the oven for 10–12 minutes, until the topping is golden and sizzling and the scallops are almost done. Turn the oven to broil and cook for 2 minutes until browned. (Move to the broiler if separate from the oven.) Watch carefully so it doesn't burn.

8. Finish with a squeeze of fresh lime and a sprinkling of chopped parsley or fennel fronds and serve in a bowl with crudités and dip on the side.

Red Bell Pepper and Onion Sauce Dip

Makes about 1½ cups

1 cup pureed roasted red bell peppers, or 7-ounce jar roasted bell peppers, drained and chopped

½ cup goat cheese (½ cup frozen and thawed or canned artichoke hearts plus 2 tablespoons extra virgin olive oil and 2 ounces macadamia nuts pureed until smooth if dairy intolerant)

¼ cup sliced scallions

Puree ingredients in a food processor until well combined.

Day 4

Breakfast: Leftover Scallops and Salad with Dip Dressing

Cuban Beef and Potato Bake with Tomato-Basil Soup and Salad

Serves 4 (2 for Day 6)

8 ounces ground beef

4 large potatoes, peeled and grated, or 1 bag frozen hash browns

½ cup chopped scallions

2 tablespoons olive or other oil

½ small serrano chile pepper (or cayenne or red pepper flakes to taste)

4 cloves garlic, finely grated

¼ cup fresh cilantro, chopped

½ cup grated Jack or Pepper Jack cheese or nondairy substitute

8 duck or chicken eggs

¼ cup cream, milk, coconut, or other nut milk

Pinch each of salt and black pepper to taste

1. Preheat the oven to 350°F.

2. Heat the oil in a skillet and sauté the ground beef, potatoes, garlic, chile pepper or pepper flakes, salt, and black pepper stirring until meat is no longer pink, 5–6 minutes. Add cilantro and scallions and stir again and cook until potatoes begin to brown.

3. Let cool and set aside for about 10 minutes.

4. Beat the eggs with a fork or whisk until light yellow then add the cream or milk and mix. Add the ground beef—potato mixture and cheese. Combine and pour into a greased 9-x-9-inch baking dish.

5. Bake for 15–20 minutes until set. Remove from oven and let rest for 10 minutes before turning out of the pan. Cut into 4 servings reserving 2 for another day and serve warm or at room temperature.

Herbed Tomato Dressing

Makes 2 cups + 1 cup to use for Tomato Basil Soup

This can be used as a sauce, dip, or salad dressing.

  1 small red onion

  3–4 ripe medium tomatoes

  1 cup fresh mint

  2 cups fresh parsley

  2 cups fresh cilantro

  2 small serrano chiles

  ½ teaspoon salt

  ¼ cup lemon juice

  ½ cup olive or other oil

  Black pepper and/or lemon pepper

1. Chop the onion and tomatoes.

2. Combine the mint, parsley, cilantro, garlic, chiles, and salt in a food processor and blend.

3. With the machine running, drizzle in the lemon juice and olive oil and process just until fully combined. Taste and adjust seasoning with salt, pepper, and/or lemon pepper if needed.

4. Remove and reserve 1 cup to make into soup below.

5. Thin with a little water if needed for dressing. Refrigerate.

Tomato Basil Soup

Makes 3½ cups (Day 6)

  2 cups organic chicken or vegetable broth

  1 cup Herbed Tomato Dressing (from above)

  3 ounces soaked and drained sun-dried tomatoes or Muir Glen tomato paste

  1–2 cloves garlic, crushed and minced

  2 tablespoons chopped onion

  1 teaspoon garlic powder

  1 teaspoon dried oregano

  Pinch of marjoram

  Salt and black pepper

4–6 leaves fresh basil, stacked, rolled, and sliced into thin strips,
or parsley leaves, for garnish

1. Blend all ingredients except basil or parsley garnish in a blender.

2. Pour into a saucepan and bring to boil.

3. Reduce heat and simmer for 20 to 30 minutes.

4. Save half of the soup and freeze for Day 4.

5. Serve hot or cold garnished with fresh basil leaves or parsley.

Caraway Ham, Kale, and Kraut Skillet with Kabocha Squash

Serves 4

1½ pounds diced Virginia ham (natural without nitrates)

2 tablespoons butter, ghee, or other fat

2 garlic cloves, minced

1 red onion, sliced

1 cup sliced carrots

2 cups shredded kale

2 cups sliced celery

2 cups red or rainbow chard

1 cup raw sauerkraut

1 teaspoon salt

½ teaspoon caraway seed

2–4 tablespoons vinegar of choice

Horseradish, to taste (optional)

Salt and black pepper

Fresh parsley, chopped, as garnish

1. Brown the diced ham in a big skillet or large soup pot with the ghee or
butter.

2. Add and sauté the garlic, onion, carrots, kale, celery, and chard until the
vegetables are cooked to the desired tenderness.

3. Stir in the kraut, seasonings, and vinegar, adding the horseradish if desired.
Season with salt and pepper to taste.

4. Top with chopped parsley. Refrigerate and serve hot or cold as desired with
1 cup of diced, steamed, and buttered squash each.

Day 5

Ground Turkey Magic Meal

Serves 4 (2 for Day 7)

This recipe is easily adapted into many variations by changing the meat, vegetable, and spice combinations used, serving it hot or cold, and works for any meal of the day. You can even roll it up in a coconut wrap or collard or lettuce leaf. What about adding it to a store-bought broth for a quick soup? Have fun and let your creativity fly.

    1 tablespoon olive or other oil
    ¼ teaspoon garlic powder
    ½ teaspoon ground ginger
    ¼ teaspoon onion powder
    1 teaspoon salt
    ½ teaspoon black pepper
    1–1½ pounds ground turkey (not ground turkey breast)
    4 cups green beans, fresh or frozen
    2 cups peas, fresh or frozen
    2 cups tomatoes
    12 cups spinach
    1 bunch scallions, sliced
    ½ teaspoon ground dried sage
    ¼ cup low-sodium chicken broth

1. Sprinkle the spices over the ground turkey and mix gently.

2. Heat oil in a large skillet and crumble turkey into the pan.

3. Sauté the meat over medium-high heat until cooked through, 10–12 minutes, and remove from the pan.

4. Add the vegetables and broth and sauté over high heat, adding more oil if needed. (To cut time in half, cook the vegetables in another large pot or pan at the same time the turkey is cooking and combine when everything is cooked.)

5. Stir every minute or so until almost done. Add the turkey back to finish for the last couple of minutes and serve hot or cold, reserving 2 portions for Day 7.

Wild Salmon in an Avocado Half over Big Salad (Q)

Serves 2–3

6 tablespoons avocado oil or other oil

2 tablespoons champagne vinegar

2 teaspoons grated or minced lime zest

1 teaspoon Dijon mustard

1 teaspoon salt

½ teaspoon lemon pepper

4 tablespoons avocado mayo or homemade mayonnaise

12–14 ounces canned wild salmon, drained (or sardines or mackerel canned in olive oil)

1 avocado, halved

Mixed greens, washed and dried

Lydia's Raw Crackers (Hunters) or Mary's Gone Crackers (Herders) (optional)

1. Whisk the avocado oil, vinegar, lime zest, mustard, salt, and lemon pepper together in a small bowl.

2. Mix mayonnaise with 3 tablespoons of the dressing in a large bowl and save the rest to dress the greens.

3. Add the salmon to the mayonnaise mixture and toss to coat.

4. Scoop about half of the salmon salad onto an avocado half and place over a big green salad or refrigerate until needed.

5. Serve with raw vegetables and some of the dip of the dressing for the salmon, adding gluten-free crackers. Refrigerate the remaining vinaigrette and use for salads as needed.

Pulled Slow Cooker Mustard Steak

Serves 4 (2 for Day 7)

Dry Rub

1 tablespoon dry mustard

1 teaspoon dried oregano

1 teaspoon ground thyme or sage

½ teaspoon onion powder

½ teaspoon garlic powder

½ teaspoon salt

¼ teaspoon lemon pepper to taste

2 tablespoons olive or other oil

1½ pounds London broil or other thick-cut steak (leave the steak in one or two pieces to fit into the slow cooker)

2 cans Muir Glen low-sodium stewed Italian tomatoes and herbs

2 onions, sliced

2 fennel bulbs, sliced

2 tablespoons balsamic vinegar

Juice of 1 lemon

2 tablespoons Parmesan cheese (optional; see page 364 for dairy-free recipe), for garnish

½ cup fresh basil leaves, in thin strips, for garnish

1. Mix the dry rub ingredients, add the oil, and rub over the steak.

2. Wrap and place in the refrigerator.

3. To a container or Ziploc bag, add the vegetables and the rest of the ingredients except the garnishes and place in the refrigerator.

4. When ready to cook, empty the bag of vegetables in the bottom of a a slow cooker, then add the steak.

5. Cover and cook on high for 5 hours or on low for 7–8 hours.

6. Shred the steak with 2 forks and add the meat back into the slow cooker.

7. Garnish with the cheese and basil.

8. Serve with or over Celeriac (or Parsnip) Puree (recipe follows).

Celeriac (or Parsnip) Puree

Serves 4

2 tablespoons bacon fat or other fat

1 tablespoons unsalted butter, ghee, or other fat

2 cups peeled and grated celeriac (or parsnip for Herders)

1 cup peeled and grated turnip

1 medium onion, chopped

1 cup chopped fennel

2 teaspoons dried thyme, or 2 tablespoons fresh

Salt and pepper to taste

¼ cup cream, half-and-half, or milk

1. Wash and peel celeriac using a sharp knife or strong peeler to remove the brown skin. Peel the turnips with a vegetable peeler. Grate both using a food processor or hand grater.

2. Heat bacon fat in a large pot or large skillet over medium-high heat and add the celeriac or parsnip, turnip, and onion and cook for 5 minutes, stirring to prevent burning.

3. Add fennel and thyme and cook until everything is very tender and fully cooked.

4. Put this mixture into a food processor, add butter or other fat, and puree until smooth. Taste for seasonings and add salt and pepper if needed. Adjust thickness of the puree by adding the cream or coconut milk a little at a time and puree again to combine. (Can use broth or water instead of dairy as well if desired.)

5. Save half of the puree to serve later in the week.

Days 6 and 7: Your Leftovers "Weekend"

On these two days, plan to be either too busy to cook or ready to take a rest from cooking. Most of your next six entrées are already made! They are waiting in the refrigerator or freezer. If the latter, let them thaw in the refrigerator the day before, if you have the time.

Day 6

After you whip up a lovely breakfast quiche to enjoy with your leftover Gazpacho, you can relax. All you will have to do is decide which of the following entrées you would like to have for lunch and dinner; whether you'd like to have Caraway Virginia Ham and Vegetable Skillet or Cuban Beef and Potato Bake (both from Day 4). They are both great for either meal.

Bacon and Cheese Quiche with Gazpacho (L)

Serves 4

If you have time, make the quiche filling while dinner is cooking. Bake the quiche during or after dinner.

　8 slices bacon, cooked and chopped

　1 cup sliced mushrooms

　½ red onion, thinly sliced

　1 clove garlic, finely grated

　Large handful of spinach or other greens

　¼ teaspoon salt

　Pinch of white pepper

　2 tablespoons fresh thyme, or 2 teaspoons dried

　2 teaspoons chopped parsley

　6 eggs

　1½ cups half-and-half or full-fat coconut milk

　2 scallions, sliced

　½ cup grated white cheddar cheese

　Pinch of paprika or cayenne

1. Preheat the oven to 375°F.

2. Cook bacon on the stove until crisp and drain.

3. Sauté the mushrooms, red onion, and garlic in the bacon fat until cooked. Add a large handful of spinach or other greens and cook for a minute until wilted. Stir in the salt, pepper, thyme, and parsley.

   If you are making this while making dinner on Day 3, start to cook the Curry Lamb Stew while the vegetables cool slightly.

4. In a large bowl, use a whisk or fork to beat the eggs until light and fluffy. Add the half-and-half or other milk and combine well. Stir in the grated cheese and paprika, then add the bacon and vegetables and stir.

5. Pour into a greased 9-×-9-inch baking dish or pie pan and bake 45 minutes or more until the center of the quiche is firm to the touch.

6. Serve warm or cold.

Gazpacho

Serves 4 (2 for Day 3)

2 cups diced yellow bell peppers (reserve ½ cup)

3 cups peeled (if desired), seeded, and ⅛-inch-diced cucumbers (reserve 1 cup as garnish)

2–3 cups organic low-salt tomato juice

4 medium plum tomatoes, cored, seeded, and cut into ⅛-inch pieces

4 ribs celery, 2 diced to use as garnish

1 small red onion, minced

1 jalapeño, stemmed, seeded, and minced

1 large handful fresh cilantro leaves, minced

½–1 teaspoon table salt

¼ teaspoon ground black pepper

2 tablespoons macadamia nut oil or extra-virgin olive oil

2 tablespoons sherry vinegar

1. Take whatever vegetables you have left from the salad bar and put them into the blender and cut up any more that you need.

2. Reserve all the diced vegetables to add back to the soup after blending.

3. Add all of the rest of the ingredients to the blender, saving half of the tomato juice and all of the water and blend until smooth. Add the saved tomato juice and water as needed to reach the consistency you desire. Stir in the reserved diced vegetables and serve cold.

Day 7

Choose which of three mostly leftover repasts to enjoy when: Steak over Zucchini Noodles, Turkey Magic, raw or baked for 60 minutes at 375° in bell peppers, or the Asian feast below.

Pureed Miso Vegetable Soup with Asian Meatballs (L) and Stir-Fried Daikon Rice

2 servings cooked Asian Meatballs (page 338), defrosted

Leftover Miso Vegetable Soup (page 340)

Additional broth if necessary

1. Puree the defrosted leftover Vegetable Miso Soup if it wasn't fully pureed before freezing.

2. About 15 minutes before you want to eat, combine the soup and meatballs and simmer for 10–15 minutes, adding water or broth if needed. Do not boil. Serve with the Stir-Fried Daikon "Rice" (recipe follows).

Stir-Fried Daikon "Rice"

Serves 4 (or 2 + 2 leftovers)

1 red onion, chopped

1 cup diced celery

1 bok choy, cut crosswise in ¼-inch slices

½ cup carrots, grated in a food processor

3 cups grated daikon radish

1 cup grated parsnip

1 tablespoon oil

1 tablespoon bacon fat or other fat

1 egg, beaten with a few drops of water and sesame oil, optional

½ cup peas, fresh or frozen

5 scallions, thinly sliced

2 teaspoons soy sauce (gluten-free)

Large pinch white pepper

¼ teaspoon sesame oil

1. Heat 1 tablespoon of oil in a large skillet over medium-high heat. Add the red onion and stir for 4 minutes, then add the celery and continue to stir for another 4 minutes. Add bok choy and carrots and stir for 1 minute, then add the cooked "rice" and stir. Cook the daikon and the parsnip before you start the onions or cook it at the same time in another pan. Sauté in a fat of your choice, adding a splash of water after stirring it several times over 6 minutes, stirring a few more times. Cook until softened and set aside until the rest is ready.

2. Stir the "rice" and vegetables and push them to the sides of the pan, leaving an opening in the middle.

3. Add 1 tablespoon of bacon fat in the center and add the egg and let it begin to cook without stirring. Flip it as soon as the egg is set on top, then break it up with a spatula and stir it into the "rice" mixture.

4. Add the peas and scallions and stir again. Add the soy sauce, white pepper and sesame oil and stir for another minute. Taste for seasoning and serve. Save 2 servings for another meal. If feeding 4, add 2 servings of meat (thinly cut beef or chicken) when adding the celery to increase the protein.

Roasted Vegetables

Preheat the oven to 400°F. Roasting times will vary with each vegetable and the size of the pieces.

Yam Bakes: Wash and cut into wedges. Coat wedges with olive oil or melted bacon or duck fat. Toss with salt, pepper, and other seasonings. Herbs should wait until almost done, to avoid burning.

Winter Squash: Carefully cut in half, rub with butter or oil and salt, and place facedown on a sheet tray or baking pan (Spaghetti Squash recipe, page 343).

Roasted Garlic: Pull off the loose outer papery skin of the whole head. Cut a slice off the top end of the whole head. Repeat for more heads and place them on a sheet of foil. Drizzle with olive oil and close up the foil into a packet. For variety, add some fresh rosemary into the packet before closing.

Portobello Mushroom Caps: Wipe the caps clean with a damp paper towel; remove the stems and chop for another purpose. Place the caps stem side down on a baking sheet. Lightly brush with olive oil. Turn over and finish cooking until softened.

Salad and Dressing Bar

Creating an at-home salad bar makes building salads quick and easy as well as having everything ready when it is time to assemble or cook a meal. There are a variety of ways to store the prepared vegetables, from compartmentalized storage containers to plastic or glass individual storage containers or even simple Ziploc bags. Each has pros and cons and your choice will depend on storage space, quantity of ingredients prepared, how often you want to replenish salad ingredients, and how many vegetables are left after preparing your meals. My favorite is to use individual containers, the smaller ones grouped on a tray to make it easy to have a variety of ingredients at your fingertips. And don't forget to have a few dressings on hand to flavor your salads. Remember, it is suggested that you eat 6–8 cups of vegetables minimum per day, so make sure you buy and cut up sufficient quantities. Do a quick calculation after you prepare your shopping list. If storage is limited, you can create a second shopping list to get more fresh fish and vegetables for midweek cooking days. It is very easy to get bags of ready-to-use healthy organic greens these days to add volume to the prepared chopped and sliced salad ingredients in your salad bar.

Here are suggestions to help you choose a variety of ingredients. Cold brown rice, cold yams, or potatoes are great additions for those who can handle the carbohydrates, as the resistant starch helps keep a healthy gut biome fed. It is easy to take a selection of things from your salad bar and completely change the texture so you won't get bored eating so many salads. You can finely chop them and add a dressing to create an almost creamy salad or take other ingredients and blend them with nuts or seeds and herbs and make a dip, soup, or even a cracker to change the texture while still eating an abundance of healthy vegetables. Why not try a couple of things you have never tried before?

LEAFY GREENS
Arugula, Bok Choy, Cabbage, Celery, Chard, Collards, Daikon, Dandelion, Endive, Frisée, Kale, Lettuce, Mustard Greens, Radicchio, Spinach, Watercress

HERBS
Basil, Cilantro, Parsley, Thyme

ROOT VEGETABLES
Beet, Carrot, Celery Root, Fennel, Jicama, Leek, Onion, Radish, Shallot, Turnip

STARCHY VEGETABLES
Bamboo Shoots, Corn, Parsnip, Peas, Potato, Pumpkin, Rutabaga, Squash, Sweet Potato, Water Chestnut

OTHER VEGETABLES
Artichoke, Asparagus, Bean and other Sprouts, Broccoli, Capers, Cauliflower, Hearts of Palm, Kohlrabi, Mushrooms, Peppers, Radicchio, Scallion, Tomato, Zucchini

OTHER INGREDIENTS
Nuts, Seeds, Leftover Potatoes or Rice, Olives, Avocado, Sea Vegetables

Having so many prepared vegetables makes it very easy to make a variety of salads quickly. Why not expand your salads away from the usual greens, tomatoes, and cucumber to something different like the following ideas?

INTERESTING SALAD EXAMPLES FROM THE SALAD BAR

Asparagus Mint Salad

Serves 1–2

1 bunch asparagus spears

3 tablespoons lemon juice

2 tablespoons caper juice

1 tablespoon macadamia nut oil

1 tablespoon finely grated red onion

Fresh chopped mint leaves or parsley

Salt and pepper to taste

1. Lightly steam or roast asparagus until tender-crisp and submerse in ice water immediately to set the bright green color.

2. Combine the rest of the ingredients and marinate for at least 30 minutes.

Fennel Salad

Serves 2 to 4

3 bulbs of fennel, halved or quartered, and *very* thinly sliced

8 ounces mushrooms, thinly sliced

2 cups packed watercress or dandelion greens, chopped

Juice of 2–3 limes

Salt and pepper

¼ cup extra-virgin olive oil

Parmesan cheese (if not dairy tolerant, see page 364)

1. Place all the vegetables in a bowl.

2. Sprinkle with lime, salt, and pepper over and toss.

3. Drizzle olive oil on the vegetables and toss again.

4. Add Parmesan cheese, if desired, and serve.

A Note About Dressings

Running low on dressings? You can use extra sauces, soups, and dips as salad dressings. Think about the base you want to use. Is the sauce too thick as is or is the soup too thin? Does it already have a lot of fat and might benefit from some lemon or vinegar, or vice versa? Or do you want to just add a little broth or even water? Do you want to thicken a soup by adding yogurt, mayonnaise, avocado, or even a pureed vegetable? Do you want to add another flavor like a clove of roasted garlic? Use a blender and play with it, tasting as you go. Is it too bland, salty, sour, sweet, or bitter? If you are not sure if a flavor will be the right thing to add, take a spoonful of the base and add a tiny bit of the new thing and taste again. Is it better or worse? Remember to think about keeping the proportions relative.

And if you don't want to make your own dressings, there are two products made by a company that distributes widely. Bragg has two ready-made salad dressings with extra-virgin olive oil and all-organic ingredients—Vinaigrette and Ginger Sesame. These are handy pantry items not only for salad dressings, but for marinades, too. (If you like creamy salad dressings, add 2 tablespoons of either dressing to a ¼ cup of full-fat Greek yogurt in a jar. Then shake to blend.) Or use the mayonnaise recipe on page 314.

LIST OF DRESSINGS AND THEIR LOCATIONS

DRESSINGS		SAUCES/DIPS THAT CAN BECOME DRESSINGS	
Parsley	PAGE 304	Mayonnaise	PAGE 314
Roasted Garlic Rosemary	PAGE 308	Lemon Yogurt	PAGE 336
Balsamic	PAGE 320	Olive Arugula Pesto	PAGE 338
Ginger Nut	PAGE 332	Peanut Chili	PAGE 340
Herbed Tomato	PAGE 346	Red Bell Pepper and Onion	PAGE 344
		Guacamole	PAGE 362
Avocado	PAGE 358		

Avocado Dressing

Makes approximately 2 cups

2 large avocados, peeled and mashed with 2 tablespoons lemon juice (or blend guacamole (L), page 362, and add oil and vinegar, as below)

½ cup mayonnaise or homemade coconut yogurt

½ teaspoon Worcestershire sauce

⅓ cup chopped onion

¼ cup lemon juice

1 teaspoon salt

Olive oil (optional)

Place all ingredients in a blender or food processor and blend until smooth. Thin with a little olive oil if needed. Use as a dip for vegetables.

HOW TO CONVERT A SAUCE TO A DRESSING

Blend until smooth: approximately 1:1 Red Bell Pepper Onion Dip/Sauce and vegetable broth; 1:1:1 Olive Arugula Pesto, vegetable broth, and lemon juice; 2:1 Peanut Chili Sauce and chicken or beef broth. Lemon Yogurt is okay as is.

Easy Snacks

Olives, nuts (avoid nuts on days that have nuts in the meals), hard-boiled eggs, cheese (if dairy tolerant), raw vegetables and dips, creamy cheese, and vegetables or crackers appropriate for your type. Nut butter and crackers or vegetables, plain full-fat yogurt or Homemade Coconut Yogurt (page 362), or Minty Chia Pudding (page 326). Jerky is easy to carry with you and is available in stores and online. (Consider if you are a Herder or Hunter and choose carefully, looking for healthy, low-sugar brands like Think Jerky—grass-fed, gluten-free, and fruit sweetened; Chef's Cut Chicken Jerky—free range, gluten-free, and 1 gram of sugar for 12 grams of protein; Simply Snackin'—grass-fed, gluten-free, very low sugar; and Country Archer—grass-fed and gluten-free. Fruit can be a good snack for Herders only.)

Leftovers from extra meal portions are the best snacks! Chia seed puddings like Minty Chia Pudding (page 326) are easy and can be flavored in a variety of ways using extracts, nut butters, milks, teas, or other liquids and can be kept in the refrigerator all week to grab when you need a snack, too. Pâté-Stuffed Veggies for Liver Haters (page 323) will make great snacks by being frozen in small portions right after it's been made, using an ice cube tray or placing scoops on a plate or pan and placing in a container once individually frozen. Serve it with raw vegetables or appropriate crackers (Lydia's Kind Foods for Hunters and Mary's Gone for Herders).

Additional Snack Suggestions for Week 2

Extra servings of Quiche or Cuban Beef and Potato Bake can be cut into smaller portions to make quick snacks. They can be refrigerated for a few days or frozen for longer storage and served at room temperature or warmed up. You may need to blot warmed quiche with paper towels to absorb extra moisture that is released. Many other recipes can be used as snacks, too. Just remember that a snack portion is not a full meal portion unless you are a man or very active and need the calories.

Substitutions for Hunters and Herders

There is no diet, menu, or recipe that is right for everyone. Our bio-individuality makes that impossible. So keep your unique traditional foods and tastes and any health conditions in mind as you apply these recipes to your life. To make it easier, we've included the following:

Alternatives to carbohydrates: Are you a Hunter or a Herder? Raise or lower the starchy carbohydrates in these recipes as needed by using the information in Chapter 13. Do you have diabetes? If so, you may need to limit or remove the starchy carbohydrates until you heal enough to better manage your blood sugar. You will need to add more fat and protein as well as to increase your leafy greens and other vegetables to 8–12 cups per day.

Alternatives to dairy products: If you are a Hunter or are dairy intolerant, please make substitutions, even though they may not be specified in every recipe, using the following box. To replace butter many people enjoy using ghee (clarified butter) since the milk solids are removed. Or use coconut oil, extra virgin olive oil, or avocado oil in equal amounts. Coconut milk and nut milks can be substitutes for milk and are easy to make using cashews or almonds, soaked overnight and used with water in a blender then strained through cheesecloth or a cloth paint strainer. And by reducing the amount of water you can create a replacement for cream by using the canned coconut or the tubes. See pages 363 for a recipe for nut cheese to use for sauces and spreads and page 362 for homemade coconut yogurt to substitute for yogurt or sour cream. And when a soup calls for cream you can also puree some of the vegetables with a little fat (from animal fat like lard or chicken fat you have leftover or purchased) to create an added richness and a creamy texture to the soup or top it with the alternative "creams" just described.

DAIRY SUBSTITUTIONS

Butter	Ghee, coconut oil, oil, animal fat
Cow's Milk	Goat's milk, nut milk, coconut milk
Cream	Cashew cream (raw cashew butter thinned with water, or homemade cashew milk using less water), homemade coconut yogurt, cooked vegetables pureed with some fat.
Cow's Milk Yogurt	Goat's milk yogurt, homemade coconut yogurt (commercial brands contain sugar)
Sour Cream	Cashew cream (raw cashew butter thinned with water, homemade cashew milk made with less water), thinned homemade coconut yogurt (add a little vinegar to mimic sour taste)
Cheese	Nut cheese, bean cheese, miso, nutritional yeast

Alternatives to eggs: Many of these recipes include chicken eggs for a number of reasons. They are a quick, easy protein source as well as being very affordable. Luckily, we now realize they got a bum rap for many years and there is no need to fear including them in your diet. That said, some of people are allergic to them and will need to avoid eating them. Unfortunately, they are not as easily replaced as dairy unless you can tolerate duck eggs (many can, Julia has found). If it is a main ingredient, like hard-boiled eggs for breakfast or an egg salad for lunch, choose a protein substitute like a burger patty or a fish or chicken salad instead. You could also select a different meal that is better for your needs. In the case of coating buckwheat with an egg before cooking to keep the grains separate, you can just leave it out without substitution. If it is being used as a binder, mixing flax or chia seeds with water can be used by combining 1 tablespoon ground seeds to and about 3 tablespoons water and letting it gel for about 10 minutes. For something like the Cuban Beef and Potato Bake, adding cheese can help hold something together if you can handle the dairy. However, it may be easier to just select another meal without eggs and replace that meal entirely.

Alternative fats: Here are some questions to help you choose which fat to use: *Is the dish served hot or cold?* Oils will provide a better texture and mouthfeel for cold things like dips and dressings compared to bacon fat or coconut oil that work well in a warm dressing over greens or steamed vegetables. *Is the flavor mild or strong and compatible with the other ingredients in the dish?*

Bacon or duck fat contribute delicious and pronounced flavors or aromas that are desirable in some dishes but may overwhelm more subtle ingredients. A butter sauce will taste different from a sauce made with olive oil, though both can be delicious. The flavor of coconut oil will match well with seasonings in an Asian dish but may seem out of place in an Italian one. Most of the time there is no right or wrong, so think about what you want it to taste like. *Does it provide function like keeping something from sticking to a pan, or adding richness to a sauce, provide volume or flavor in the recipe?* Nut butter, for example, would add richness and flavor but would not the best choice to create a nonstick surface for a sauté. Sesame oil is very strong in flavor and used in very small amounts like a seasoning, versus olive oil, which can provide volume in a dressing. *How will it work with the cooking method?* Avocado is best used uncooked and blended so it would not be a good substitute for butter in a hot sauce, though ghee or coconut oil could work well.

MAKING SUBSTITUTES NEEDED FOR WEEKS 1 AND 2 RECIPES

Dairy Substitutes:

Guacamole

Makes 8 (¼-cup) servings

A nondairy dip or sauce for any vegetable or protein. Good for snacks, dips, to thin with oil and vinegar to make a salad dressing, to garnish dishes, etc.

  4 ripe avocados, pitted and peeled

  1 small red onion, finely chopped

  1 large (or 2 medium) tomatoes

  1 clove roasted garlic

  1 lemon or 2 small limes, juiced

  1 tablespoon chopped fresh cilantro

  Large pinch of ground cumin

  ½ to 1 teaspoon minced jalapeño or serrano pepper (optional)

  Salt and pepper to taste

Place the avocado in a bowl and mash with a fork to create a fairly smooth paste that still has a little texture. Add the rest of the ingredients and stir to combine and taste for seasonings. Serve chilled or at room temperature.

Homemade Coconut (no milk) Yogurt

Serves 4

Make this yogurt a day or two before you need it. Make sure to use coconut milk that is just coconut and water with no stabilizers and that the equipment you use to prepare the yogurt is spotlessly clean by taking all containers and utensils right from the dishwasher or boil them in a pot of water for 5–10 minutes to sterilize. (If your probiotics are old you can test them by adding 1 capsule to ¼ cup of milk or other coconut milk and leave it to ferment in a warm place for 24 hours. If it is still active, the milk will be slightly bubbly and the taste and the smell will have changed.)

  2 cans organic coconut milk, full fat

  1½ teaspoons organic grass-fed gelatin (or 2 tablespoons pectin, white chia seeds, or protein powder; optional for thicker yogurt)

4–5 capsules active probiotics

1 ounce unsweetened, shredded coconut, toasted

1. Spoon the thick part of the coconut milk into a saucepan, pouring the liquid into a bowl or measuring cup.

2. Gently warm the thicker portion only to 120°F and remove from heat.

3. While it is warming, sprinkle the powdered gelatin over the unheated coconut liquid and let it hydrate.

4. When the heated coconut milk has cooled to 115°F, stir in the gelatin and liquid and stir with a clean fork or whisk to create a smooth mixture.

5. Pour into a glass or ceramic container or bowl and from this point on do not use anything metal once the probiotics are added. Carefully open the probiotic capsules and stir with a wooden or plastic spoon. Cover with cheesecloth or a clean kitchen towel so it can breathe but no foreign matter can get in to it.

6. Place in a warm area to ferment, keeping it close to 115°F. You can use an inexpensive yogurt maker, dehydrator, or heating pad on medium heat wrapped around the glass container and nestled inside another close-fitting bowl or larger container and covered. Periodically check the temperature to make sure it is not getting to hot or cold and adjust accordingly. It should take 24–36 hours; taste using a clean spoon until it has the amount of sour tang you like. It will get more sour the longer you leave it and will thicken more after refrigeration. (Add ground chia seeds to thicken if needed.) Top with toasted, shredded coconut.

7. You can take portions of the yogurt and flavor it with herbs and spice combinations and add it to Indian, Greek, or Mexican dishes, too.

Nondairy Spreadable Nut Cheese

This will make a flavorful "cheese" great for snacks, so if you want a plain cheese to add to a recipe, leave out the Italian seasonings, garlic, and tomato. This is a great recipe to play with by changing the seasonings and vegetables to create different flavors or colors of cheese.

1½ cups raw nuts, soaked (cashews, macadamia, Brazil, or pine nuts work best)

1 teaspoon light miso with ¼ cup water

½ teaspoon dried Italian seasoning (or a mixture of dried basil, oregano, and thyme)

    1 clove garlic

    2 tablespoons lemon juice

    1 tomato

1. Blend the ingredients in a blender until as smooth as possible, adding a little water if necessary. Use as little liquid as possible, as you want to end up with a creamy cheese.

2. Put a coffee filter, cheesecloth, or nut-milk bag in a strainer set over a bowl and add the nut cheese mixture. Leave at room temperature for at least 8 hours or overnight so liquid can drain out.

3. Remove resulting cheese from the filter or cheesecloth and place in a container and refrigerate. It will keep for about 1 week.

Nondairy Parmesan

    1 cup raw pine nuts (you can also use raw cashews)

    ¼ cup nutritional yeast flakes

    1 teaspoon garlic powder

    ½ teaspoon dried Italian herbs

    ½ teaspoon sea salt

    Zest of 1 small lemon

1. Pulse nuts until finely chopped; do not overblend.

2. Toast in pan or oven, stirring often. Cool.

3. Add remaining ingredients and mix well. Place in an air-tight container and refrigerate until needed.

GRAIN RECIPES FOR HERDERS

Easy Baked Rice for Herders

Serves 4

    1½ cups brown rice

    2½ cups broth or water

    2 tablespoons fat of choice

    ½ teaspoon salt

1. Preheat oven to 375°F.

2. Rinse and drain rice and put it in an 8-×-8-inch glass baking pan.

3. Heat the remaining ingredients in a pot on the stove until boiling and pour over the rice and stir.

4. Cover the dish with foil and bake for 1 hour. Carefully uncover and fluff with a fork and serve or store as needed.

Quinoa (for Herders)

Serves 4

1 cup quinoa

2 tablespoons fat of choice

2 cups broth or water

½ teaspoon salt

¼ teaspoon pepper

1. Rinse quinoa and drain well.

2. Heat fat in a saucepot over high heat, stirring to toast the quinoa for a few minutes until it smells toasty.

3. Add the liquid and seasonings and heat until boiling. Reduce heat to low, cover, and cook for about 20 minutes.

4. If you still see steam escaping around the cover wait a few more minutes. Remove cover and fluff with a fork, cover again, and leave off of the heat for a few minutes.

5. Serve or store as needed.

6. Optional: Toss the finished warm quinoa with ½ cup of desired dressing, or stir in herbs or seasonings and more fat to add flavor if desired.

Millet (for Herders)

Serves 4

1 cup millet

2 tablespoons butter or avocado oil

3 cups broth or water

½ teaspoon salt

1. Toast the millet by stirring in a dry pan over medium heat for 4–5 minutes until it smells toasted and looks golden brown.

2. Add the butter, liquid of choice, and salt and bring to a boil, cover, reduce heat to low, and cook for 15 minutes.

3. Remove from heat and let stand 10 minutes. Fluff with a fork and spread on a plate to cool quickly.

FOOD PREP 101: SAFETY AND TOOLS

SAFETY

Safe Cooking and Storage Temperatures

Safe refrigerator temperature is 40°F/4.4°C or below

Freezer 0°F/-17.7°C or below

Safe internal cooking temperatures to be reached:

Meats and Fish: 145°F/62.8°C
Ground Meats: 160°F/71.1°C
Poultry: 165°F/73.9°C

Food Handling

Cross Contamination: Raw meat and their juices must be kept away from other foods, especially those consumed without cooking. To prevent food-borne illness place raw meats in leak-proof containers while in the refrigerator so they can't leak on other foods. Good kitchen practices call for using separate cutting boards and knives for raw meats and vegetable and cooked foods during food preparation or washing thoroughly with hot soapy water to prevent cross-contamination. This includes careful hand-washing often with soap and warm water for 20 seconds. (Mentally recite the ABC song.) Use a mixture of 1 tablespoon chlorine bleach to 1 gallon water to sanitize sinks, counters, cutting boards, and other food prep areas if desired.

Thawing and Marinating Foods: Thawing frozen food in the refrigerator is best. For quicker thawing submerge frozen food sealed in a waterproof container in cold water, changing the water 2 or 3 times per hour until thawed. Prepare immediately or refrigerate. Marinating should be done under refrigeration unless it is a very brief period of time.

Leftovers: Store in refrigerator or freezer in containers with maximum surface area within 1–2 hours (less when room temperature is over 90°F/32.2°C). A shallow container will reach safe storage temperatures much quicker than a deep one.

Safe Food Storage Guidelines

Raw fish, poultry, ground meats, and organ meats
Refrigeration: 1–2 days
Freezing: 3 months

Raw steaks, chops, and roasts
Refrigeration: 3–5 days
Freezing: 4–6 months

Processed meats (sausage, bacon, hot dogs, etc.)
Varies so please check the USDA or other food safety websites

Fresh eggs in the shell
Refrigeration: 3–5 weeks
Freezing: Do not freeze

Fresh egg yolks and whites out of the shell
Refrigeration: 2–4 days
Freezing: 1 year

Hard-boiled eggs
Refrigeration: 1 week
Freezing: Do not freeze

Cooked food storage (most foods)
Refrigeration: 3–4 days
Freezing: 3 months

KITCHEN TOOLS

Here is a list of the kitchen equipment that will make it easier for you to prepare these recipes. You may already have many of these things. If not, this craving-free food will allow you to make the permanent food changes that you need. Invest in yourself. The more expensive appliances are nice to have as they will save you a lot of time, but not mandatory. You can spend an hour cutting vegetables by hand, or do it in 15 minutes using a food processor. If budget is an issue, the priority should be buying high-quality food and supplements rather than expensive tools.

THE BASICS

Can opener, manual or electric	Refrigerator thermometer to make sure your refrigerator is cold enough (per safety tips)
Cutting board, 14 × 16-inch wood or bamboo preferred	High-quality knives, minimum 8" chef's knife, 5" utility knife, and 3½" paring knife (Sharp, good knives are actually safer than lightweight, cheap ones.)
Hot pad or oven mitts and towels	Pots and pans (good stainless steel set will last a lifetime. Avoid Teflon coatings): 8-quart stockpot or Dutch oven, 1- 2- and 3-quart saucepans with covers, 8" and 10 or 12" skillet, lids (Heavy bottoms distribute heat evenly and keep food from burning.)
Set of dry measuring cups (¼, ⅓, ½ & 1 cup)	Steamer basket (insert for saucepan)
Measuring spoons (¼, ½ & 1 teaspoon & 1 tablespoon)	2 half sheet pans, approximately 18" × 13" × 1"
Glass liquid measuring cups, 1 cup (2 and 4 cup optional)	8" × 8" or 9"x9" glass or metal baking pan
Nested mixing bowls, set of 3 or more sizes	9" × 5" glass or metal loaf pan
Large colander or mesh strainer	9" glass or metal pie pan
Spatula or turner	9" × 13" × 2" glass or metal roasting pan
Large regular and slotted spoons (Stainless steel and wooden best.)	Muffin pan, best with 9–12 muffin cups
1 cup ladle	Hand grater(s), fine and large holes
Tongs	Timer (1 or more if cooking multiple things at once. Your phone may have one. Or set for earliest time and write down the timing for the other item and reset after the first one is done.)
Vegetable peeler	Storage containers
Wire whisk	Blender
Instant read thermometer if making yogurt and insuring proper cooking of meats	Slow cooker, 5–7-quart oval with removable crock is best—especially handy for whole chickens (3 quart is fine if you are cooking small quantities and don't want a lot of leftovers as slow cookers work best when at least ⅔ full. Note you may have to reduce recipe amounts if using 3-quart size.)

NICE TO HAVE	SUGGESTED EXTRAS WILL SAVE TIME AND EFFORT
Egg slicer	Immersion blender
Silicone rubber scraper	Food processor with chopping blade, large and small slicing blades, and large and small grating blades (Personally, I can't recommend this time-saver enough.)
Salad spinner	Spiralizer (vegetable noodle maker)
Kitchen scale (Nice for packaging portions for later)	Citrus reamer or juicer
Citrus zester (optional if you have a fine Microplane grater)	Inexpensive yogurt maker (if dairy intolerant)

Cooking Terms

Blanch—To partially cook or briefly cook vegetables or fruit in boiling water for 30 seconds to a few minutes then moving the food to ice water immediately to stop the cooking process and set the color. Timing depends on the food and what you are trying to achieve like removing the skin from tomatoes while leaving the flesh raw or to quick cook and set the color of a delicate vegetable to be served later.

Braise—To brown food in small amount of a fat in a pot or skillet to create a caramelized flavor, then add a small amount of liquid and cook slowly on top of the stove or in the oven.

Broil—To cook under the broiler element of a stove or above the coals in a BBQ.

Brown—Creating a caramelized surface on the food by cooking it quickly on top of the stove, under a broiler, or in the oven.

Chop—To create small pieces of food using a knife or food processor.

Dice—To cut food into uniform cubes about ¼ to ½ inch in size.

Drizzle—To slowly add a thin stream of liquid, while moving above another food.

Emulsify—To slowly force liquids to combine that don't normally mix well, such as when making mayonnaise.

Fry—To cook in a small amount of fat in a pan directly over heat.

Garnish—To decorate the food or plate with something, preferably edible, for color or textural contrast to create visual appeal and increase appetite.

Marinate—To soak foods in a flavorful liquid prior to cooking, like oil, vinegar, and herbs or soy sauce, sake and spices.

Mince—To cut into uniform pieces smaller than a dice.

Mix—To combine until the ingredients are evenly incorporated.

Peel—To remove the outer skin of some fruits or vegetables, which can be done with a peeler, knife, spoon, or by hand for something like a banana or tangerine.

Pinch—A very small amount of a powdery ingredient that approximates how much would be picked up between your thumb and finger—about 1/16 teaspoon.

Poach—To cook foods in simmering liquid, often water or broth, with flavoring ingredients.

Preheat—To bring the oven to the required temperature prior to adding the foods.

Puree—To create a uniform, creamy paste of foods, most often using a blender, food processor, or other tools.

Roast—A dry-heat method of cooking food in an oven, rotisserie, or over heat in a pan.

Sauté—To quickly fry in a skillet on top of the stove, turning often, in a small amount of fat until lightly browned.

Sear—To create a brown crust on the surface of food using high heat in the oven or in a pan on top of the stove to develop flavor and seal in juices.

Season to taste—To sample a small amount to see if the flavors are to your liking, usually with regard to salt, pepper, or herbs or any intense ingredient like vinegars, chiles, or horseradish.

Shave—To make wide, very thin slices of food using a vegetable peeler or other tool with a sharp blade.

Shred—To cut food into thin slivers with a knife or grating blade in a food processor. Two forks can often be used to shred very tender meats.

Simmer—To bring and keep a liquid just below the boiling point so that small bubbles break below the surface.

Steam—To cook in a covered container over a small amount of boiling water with the food placed on a rack above the water level.

Stir—To mix until ingredients are well combined.

Toss—To gently bring ingredients together using a lifting motion with fingers or a utensil.

Whip—To cause the food to hold more air so it will increase in volume by beating it by hand or with an electric mixer.

Zest—To remove thin strips of citrus peel using a zester, fine grater, or vegetable peeler, being careful to only remove the colored part, to add essential oils and intensified flavors to food.

Acknowledgments

My lovely agent, Linda Lowenthal, and I had a wonderful time developing the proposal for this book. When it was time to visit publishers, the Flatiron Books team was too dazzling to pass up. My editor there, Whitney Frick, has been a strong hand on the tiller. I needed that, because *The Craving Cure* turned out to be an unexpectedly arduous book to write.

At one point I had to take several months off. When I got back, I needed a lot of help. And I got it! For research, technical, and human support, my original collaborator and friend, Eugenia Dreyfus, was all there for the first three years. When she retired, Krispin Sullivan, CN, my long-time research collaborator, whom I call "the Pearl Diver," once again educated and corrected me, in spite of myself. Nutritionist Barbara Michelson-Harder assisted with research and warmly supported me in so many other ways. Nutritionist Donna Sadler-Kelley was a tireless, meticulous, and gallant support through endless drafts. Later, she was aided by Dawn Kerr of the lightning fingers and mind whose friend, Gail Parmentier, jumped aboard to handle my e-mail and offer wise advice. I thank you all so much.

For the health consults that got me back to the book, I am profoundly grateful to James Reece.

And then there is my staff at the Craving Cure Virtual Clinic: all three of the gifted lead nutritionists there have been with me for many years, thank God:

Kelly Nelson, CNC, also clinic administrator; Karla Maree, CNC, also instructor for the distance training program; and Barbara Clark, CNC, who never stops caring. Our financial and organizational chief, Michele Radcliffe, has been the mainstay behind all of our efforts. Together, they got our new virtual program off and running with very minimal input from me. For that, I apologize and applaud; salute and bow.

My training staff, Pat Loy at the helm, made it possible for me to continue my professional trainings at NNTI—the NeuroNutrient Therapy Institute—until I "got too far along." I'll be so glad to get back into the races with them again. My trainees have been a joy to stay in touch with (as I could). I can't wait to fully reconnect with them and to start new trainings.

In the addiction treatment world, my colleagues and the fellow founders of The Alliance for Addiction Solutions, have been cheering me on as they further pursue our mission to educate those struggling with alcohol, drug, food, and behavioral addictions, their families, and treatment professionals about amino acid and dietary therapies and other effective recovery tools targeting the addicted brain. They've been working away with little help from me, for too long. *Salut, mes braves!* A special thanks to Kenneth Blum, Ph.D., for his pioneering work and for his continuing outpouring of scientific papers on the addictive brain and its response to amino acid precursor therapy. Without you, there would have been no hope.

My friends and family have helped me keep my nose above water (thank you, Fred, in particular) and to faintly recall what life could be like. A.B. Love and thanks to them all, and to The Lighthouse Gospel Singers, who give me weekly joy and remind me that I am *never* alone.

Notes

CHAPTER 1

1. *"Those of us who are still eating several vegetables and fruits . . ."* Ames, B. N. "Micronutrient deficiencies. A major cause of DNA damage." *Annals of the New York Academy of Sciences* 889 (1999):87–106.

2. *". . . and happier."* Stranges, S. Saver, P. C. Samaraweera, F. Taggart, N. Kandala, and S. Stewart-Brown. "Major health-related behaviours and mental well-being in the general population: the Health Survey for England." *BMJl Open* 4:9 (2014). doi: 10.1136/bmjopen-2014-005878.

3. *"Unfortunately, we're now eating less than half of the fresh produce . . ."* USDA Economic Research Service. "Food Availability and consumption." Last modified September 18, 2015. Accessed September 29, 2016. http://www.ers.usda.gov/data-products/ag-and-food-statistics-charting-the-essentials/food-availability-and-consumption.aspx.

4. *". . . when sugar is extracted from the cane and concentrated, . . ."* You can go to the USDA Food Composition Database to find the sucrose levels of sugarcane versus table sugar. https://ndb.nal.usda.gov/ndb/.

5. *"60% of our diet contains none of the nutrients . . ."* Steele, E. M., and L. G. Baraldi, M.L. da Costa L., J. C. Moubarac, D. Mozaffarian, C. A. Monteiro. "Ultra-processed foods and added sugars in the US diet: evidence from a nationally representative cross-sectional study." *BMJ Open* 6:3 (2016). doi:10.1136/bmjopen-2015-009892.

6. *". . . sugar, alone, to be three times more addictive than cocaine."* Lenoir, M., and F. Serre, L. Cantin, S. H. Ahmed. "Intense Sweetness Surpasses Cocaine Reward" *PLoS One* 2(8) (2007). doi:10.1371/journal.pone.0000698.

   Dr. Ahmed, one of the authors of this study, gave us a formula for interpreting the statistics to get a rough numerical comparison between cocaine and sugar

(March 13, 2017). He said that cocaine users become addicted less often than overeaters do. How much less? Since our sources show a range of 20 to 60 percent of eaters becoming addicted to foods and 20 percent of drug addicts becoming addicted, we conclude that food is up to three times more addictive than cocaine. At best, it's *equally* addictive!

7. "*. . . Volkow, Ph.D., has repeatedly made it clear that some foods, like certain drugs . . .*" Volkow, N. D., and R. D. Baler. "NOW vs LATER brain circuits: implications for obesity and addiction." *Trends in Neuroscience* 38(6) (2015):345–52. doi: 10.1016/j.tins.2015.04.002.

8. "*In contrast, there are only about 28 million drug and alcohol addicts. . . .*" "Nationwide Trends." National Institute on Drug Abuse. Published June 2015. Accessed January 8, 2017. https://www.drugabuse.gov/publications/drugfacts/nationwide-trends.

9. "*. . . 190 million people (over 50 percent of the population) . . .*" Szalavitz, M,. "Can food really be addictive? Yes, says national drug expert." TIME.com. Published April 5, 2012. Accessed January 11, 2017. http://healthland.time.com/2012/04/05/yes-food -can-be-addictive-says-the-director-of-the-national-institute-on-drug-abuse/

10. "*That's 20 to 60 percent of the U.S. population.*" Pursey, K. M., P. Stanwell, A. N. Gearhardt, C. E. Collins, and T. L. Burrows. "The prevalence of food addiction as assessed by the Yale Food Addiction Scale: a systematic review." *Nutrients.* 6(10) (2014): 4552–4590. doi: 10.3390/nu6104552.

11. "*. . . considered several times more addictive than crack.*" Pursey, K. M., and P. Stanwell, A. N. Gearhardt, C. E. Collins, T. L. Burrows. "The prevalence of food addiction as assessed by the Yale Food Addiction Scale: a systematic review." *Nutrients.* 6(10) (2014): 4552–90. doi: 10.3390/nu6104552.

12. *Re Yale food addiction study*: Schutte, E., N. Avena, and A. Gearhardt. "Which foods may be addictive? The roles of processing, fat content and glycemic load." *PLoS One* 10(2) (2015):e0117959. doi: 10.1371/journal.pone.0117959.

13. "*portion sizes doubled in fast food and chain restaurant outlets:.*" Nestle, Marion. "Today's 'Eat More' Environment: The Role of the Food Industry." in *A Place at the Table: The Crisis of 49 Million Hungry Americans and How to Solve It,* ed. P. Pringle. (New York: PublicAffairs, 2013), chapter 7.

14. Overeaters Anonymous. "*Are you a compulsive eater?*" Accessed September 16, 2016. https://oa.org/newcomers/how-do-i-start/are-you-a-compulsive-overeater/.

15. "*Most cold cereals' started out at 20% sugar.*" Harris, J. L., M. B. Schwartz, K. D. Brownell, V. Sarda, M .E. Weinberg, S. Speers, J. Thompson, A. Ustjanauskas, A. Cheyne, E. Bukofzer, L. Dorfman, and H. Byrnes-Enoch. "Cereal FACTS: Evaluating the nutrition quality and marketing of children's cereals." Rudd Center for Food Policy and Obesity (2009).

16. "*. . . Kellogg's Honey Smacks, for example, were 60% sugar . . .*" Harris, J. X. L., and M. B. Schwartz, K. D. Brownell, V. Sarda, M. E. Weinberg, S. Speers, J. Thompson, A. Ustjanauskas, A. Cheyne, E. Bukofzer, L. Dorfman, and H. Byrnes-Enoch. "Cereal FACTS: Evaluating the nutrition quality and marketing of children's cereals." Rudd Center for Food Policy and Obesity (2009).

17. "*. . . and Lieber's Cocoa Frosted Flakes were 88% sugar.*" Undurraga, D., and O. Naidenko, R. Sharp, N. Bruzelius. "Children's cereals: Sugar by the pound." Environmental Working Group (2014). http://static.ewg.org/reports/2014/cereals/pdf/2014-EWG-Cereals-Report.pdf?_ga=1.165904830.1843646902.1488645704.

18. "*Chillingly, children's cereals typically contain much more sugar than do 'adult' cereals.*" Pestano, P., M.S., E. Yeshua, J.D, J. Houlihan, M.S.C.E. "Sugar in Children's

Cereal." Environmental Working Group. Published December 12, 2011. Accessed January 8, 2017. http://www.ewg.org/research/sugar_in_childrens_cereals.

19. *"Our rate of diabetes . . . In 2016, it was 50 percent."* CDC. *Long-term Trends in Diabetes.* April 2016. http://www.cdc.gov/diabetes/data.

20. *". . . pre-diabetics, most becoming full-fledged diabetics in six to ten years . . ."* Harding, Anne. *"Stopping prediabetes in its tracks."* MSNBC. Published October 30, 2013. Accessed January 11, 2017. http://www.nbcnews.com/id/3341560/ns/health-diabetes /t/stopping-prediabetes-its-tracks/#.WHbplJI5Q6Y

21. *"Five percent of children . . ."* CDC. "Prevalence of Overweight and Obesity among Children and Adolescents: United States, 1963–1965 Through 2011–2012." Last modified September 19, 2014. Accessed February 26, 2016. http://www.cdc.gov/nchs/data /hestat/obesity_child_11_12/obesity_child_11_12.htm.

22. *". . . 20 percent of teens . . ."* Tucker, Miriam E., "Nearly one in five American teens has prediabetes or diabetes." *Medscape.* Published July 19, 2016. Accessed January 8, 2017. http://www.medscape.com/viewarticle/866326.

23. *". . . high rates of often-fatal forms of heart, kidney, and liver disease."* Fougère, B., and E. Boulanger, F. Nourhashémi, S. Guyonnet, and M. Cesari. "Chronic inflammation: Accelerator of biological aging." *The Journals of Gerontology. Series A Biological Sciences and Medical Sciences* p.ii (2016): glw240. doi: 10.1093/gerona/glw240.

24. *"Almost all cancers."* Scappaticcio, L., et al. "Insights into the relationships between diabetes, prediabetes, and cancer." *Endocrine* 56(2)(2016): 231–239. doi: 10.1007/ s12020.016-1216-y.

25. *". . . Alzheimer's disease is now being called diabetes III."* Kroner, Z. "The relationship between Alzheimer's disease and diabetes: Type 3 diabetes?" *Alternative Medicine Review* 14(4) (2009): 373–379.

26. *". . . several studies have found sugar to be the specific factor that correlates world-wide with diabetes incidence."* Basu, S., P. Yoffe, N. Hills, and R. H. Lustig. "The relationship of sugar to population-level diabetes prevalence: an econometric analysis of repeated cross-sectional data." *PLOS ONE.* 8(2) 2013: e57873. doi:10.1371/journal.pone .0057874.

27. *". . . excess fructose glycation is ten times more damaging."* McPherson, J. D., B. H. Shilton, and D. J. Walton. "Role of fructose in glycation and cross-linking of proteins." *Biochemistry* 27(6) (1988):1901–7. doi: 10.1021/bi00406a016.

28. *"[glycation as a] primary cause of diabetes."* Aeberli, I., et al. "Moderate amounts of fructose consumption impair insulin sensitivity in healthy young men. A randomized controlled trial." *Diabetes Care* 36(1)(2013):150–156. https://doi.org/10.2337/dc12-0540.

29. *". . . glycation is a major contributor to heart disease and stroke . . ."* Kizer, J. R., D. Benkeser, A. M. Arnold, J. H. Ix, K. J. Mukamal, L. Djousse, R. P. Tracy, D. S. Siscovick, B. M. Psaty, and S. J. Zieman. "Advanced glycation/glycoxidation endproduct carboxymethyllysine and incidence of coronary heart disease and stroke in older adults." *Atherosclerosis* 235(1)(2014):116–21. doi: 10.1016/j.atherosclerosis.2014.04.013.

30. *"[glycation is a contributor] to our increasing number of diet-related cancers"* Turner, D. P. "The role of advanced glycation end-products in cancer disparity." *Advances in Cancer Research* 133(2017):1–22. doi: 10.1016/bs.acr.2016.08.001.

31. *". . . cutting glycated food consumption by 50 percent resulted in a decrease in AGES . . ."* Vlassara, H. *Dr. Vlassara's A.G.E.Less Diet.* New York: Square One Publishers, 2017, p. 39.

32. *"Triglycerides are an essential storage fuels . . . When amounts are excessive, they can certainly raise your risk of heart disease."* Siri-Tarino P. W., Q. Sun, F. B. Hu, and and R. M. Krauss. "Meta-analysis of prospective cohort studies evaluating the association

of saturated fat with cardiovascular disease." *American Journal of Clinical Nutrition* 91(3) (2010):535–46. doi: 10.3945/ajcn.2009.27725.

33. "*. . . paid scientists from Harvard and elsewhere to blame saturated fat, instead of sugar . . .*" Kearns, C., L. A. Schmidt, and S. A. Glantz. "Sugar Industry and coronary heart disease research: A historical analysis of internal industry documents." *JAMA Internal Medicine* 176(11)(2016): 1680–1685. doi:10.1001/jamainternmed.2016.5394.

34. "*Heart damage starting in infancy*" Vos, M. B., J. L. Kaar, J. A. Welsh, L. V. Van Horn, D. I. Feig, C. A. M. Anderson, M. J. Patel, J. C. Munos, N. F. Krebs, S. A. Xanthakos, and R. K. Johnson. "Added sugars and cardiovascular disease risk in children." *American Heart Association Scientific Statement* (2016). doi: 10.1161/CIR, 00439. http://circ.ahajournals.org.

35. "*Drinking two high-fructose corn syrup-sweetened sodas a day for eight weeks . . .*" Stanhope, K. L., and A. A. Bremer, V. Medici, K. Nakajima, Y. Ito, T. Nakano, G. Chen, T. H. Fong, V. Lee, R. I. Menorca, N. L. Keim, P. J. Havel. "Consumption of fructose and high-fructose corn syrup increase postprandial triglycerides, LDL-cholesterol, and apolipoprotein-B in young men and women." *Journal Clinical Endocrinology Metabolism* 96(10)(2011): E1596–E1605. doi: 10.1210/jc.2011-1251.

36. "*Drinking two high-fructose corn syrup-sweetened sodas a day for eight weeks . . .*" Aeberli, I., and M. Hochuli, P. A. Gerber, L. Sze, S. B. Murer, L. Tappy, G. A. Spinas and K. Berneis. "Moderate amounts of fructose consumption impair insulin sensitivity in healthy young men. A randomized controlled trial." *Diabetes Care* 36(1)(2013): 150–156. https://doi.org/10.2337/dc12-0540.

Lustig, Robert, M.D., and Michael Goran, Ph.D. "Viewpoints: Don't believe industry-paid 'experts' on soda and diabetes." *The Sacramento Bee*. Published July 23, 2014. Accessed March 7, 2016. http://www.sacbee.com/opinion/op-ed/article2604563 .html

37. "*drug and alcohol addicts die because of their addictions every year.*" National Institute on Drug Abuse. "Overdose Death Rates." Published January 2017. Accessed January 8, 2017. https://www.drugabuse.gov/related-topics/trends-statistics/overdose-death-rates "Alcohol Poisoning Deaths." Published January 2015. Accessed January 11, 2017. https:// www.cdc.gov/vitalsigns/alcohol-poisoning-deaths/index.html.

38. "*almost 5 million smokers are killed by their tobacco use every year.*" "Tobacco" World Health Organization Fact Sheet. Published June 2016. Accessed January 12, 2017. http://www.who.int/mediacentre/factsheets/fs339/en/.

39. "*. . . contributes to 35 million deaths worldwide annually.*" Lustig, Robert H., M.D., L. A. Schmidt, and C. D. Brindis. "Public health: The toxic truth about sugar." *Nature* 482 (2012): 27–29. doi:10.1038/482027a.

CHAPTER 2

1. "*What resulted was a crystalline concentrate eight hundred percent sweeter.*" USDA Food Composition Database lists the sucrose levels of sugarcane versus table sugar. https://ndb.nal.usda.gov/ndb/.

2. "*The list of sucrose's early pharmaceutical uses . . .*" Mintz, S. W. *Sweetness and Power: The Place of Sugar in Modern History.* New York: Viking Adult, 1985, p. 96–99.

3. "*The French used a popular expression for centuries to . . .*" Macinnis, P., *Bittersweet: The Story of Sugar.* Australia: Allen & Unwin, 2003, chapter 1, p. 18.

4. "*In England, in as late as the 1880s, it was . . .*" Bentley, R., and H. T. *Medicinal Plants: Being Descriptions with the Original Figures of the Principal Plants Employed in Medicine and an Account of the Characters, Properties, and Uses of Their Parts and Products.* London: Churchill, 1880.

5. *"In the 1900s, sucrose began to be extracted in the US from . . ."* Beghin, J. C., and H. H. Jensen. "US sweetener consumption trends and dietary guidelines." Iowa Ad Review Online 11(1) (2005). Accessed September 29, 2016. http://www.card.iastate.edu/iowa _ag_review/winter_05/article5.aspx.

6. *"By the 1970s, the average American was consuming a hundred and . . ."* Allshouse, J. E., and J. J. Putnam. "Food consumption, prices and expenditures, 1970–97." *USDA Economic Research Service Statistical Bulletin* (1999). Last updated May 27, 2012. Accessed September 29, 2016. http://www.ers.usda.gov/publications/sb-statistical-bulletin/sb965.aspx.

7. *"That was partly because the sucrose industry began fighting to protect . . ."* Kearns, C., L. A. Schmidt, and S. A. Glantz. "Sugar industry and coronary heart disease research: A historical analysis of internal industry documents." *JAMA Internal Medicine* (2016). doi:10.1001/jamainternmed.2016.5394.

8. *"Between 1970 and 1999, our sweets intake overall went from . . ."* Wells, H. F., and J. C. Busby. "USDA dietary assessment of major trends in U.S. food consumption, 1970–2005." USDA Economic Research Service. ix. (2008). www.ers.usda.gov/media/210681 /eib33_1_.pdf.

9. *"The HFCS in foods and beverages can contain anywhere from 42 percent to 90 percent fructose."* Walker, R. W., K. A. Dumke, and M. I. Goran. "Fructose content in popular beverages made with and without high-fructose corn syrup." *Nutrition* 30(7–8) (2014): 928–35. 10.1016/j.nut.2014.04.003.

10. *"Between 1970 and 1999, our sweets intake overall went from 120 pounds. . . ."* Wells, H. F., and J. C. Busby. "USDA dietary assessment of major trends in U.S. food consumption, 1970–2005." *USDA Economic Research Service. Economic Bulletin Number 33* (2008). www.ers.usda.gov/media/210681/eib33_1_.pdf.

11. *"Perhaps the most important are the hormones ghrelin, leptin, and insulin:"* Lustig, R. H., M.D. *Fat Chance: Beating the Odds Against Sugar, Processed Food, Obesity, and Disease* New York: Hudson Street Press, 2012, pp. 127–128.

12. *"Close to 60 percent of the sugar in these drinks is fructose and only 40 percent is glucose.* Walker, R. W., K. A. Dumke, and M. I. Goran. "Fructose content in popular beverages made with and without high-fructose corn syrup." *Nutrition* 30(7–8) (2014): 928–35. 10.1016/j.nut.2014.04.003.

13. *"90 percent of the highly concentrated syrup from the agave cactus . . ."* Willems, J. L., and N. H. Low. "Major carbohydrate, polyol, and oligosaccharide profiles of agave syrup. application of this data to authenticity analysis." *Journal of Agriculture & Food Chemistry.* 60(35) (2012): 8745–54. doi: 10.1021/jf3027342.

14. *"Additional studies have found that apple juice alone contains 67 percent . . ."* Walker, R. W., and K. A. Dumke, M. I. Goran. "Fructose content in popular beverages made with and without high-fructose corn syrup." *Nutrition.* 30(7–8)(2014): 928–935. http://dx.doi.org/10.1016/j.nut.2014.04.003.

15. *"[Fructose] is also responsible for our increased rates of often fatal fatty liver disease . . ."* Bhatt, H. B., and R. J. Smith. "Fatty liver disease in diabetes mellitus." *Hepatobiliary Surgery and Nutrition* 4(2)(2015): 101–108. doi: 10.3978/j.issn.2304-3881.2015.01.03.

16. *"[Fructose] is also one major cause of the degradation of the microbiome, . . ."* Payne, A. N., and C. Chassard, C. Lacroix. "Gut microbial adaptation to dietary consumption of fructose, artificial sweeteners and sugar alcohols: implications for host-microbe interactions contributing to obesity." *Obesity Review* 13(9)(2012): 799–809. doi: 10.1111/j.1467-789X.2012.01009.x.

17. *"As much as 30% of the population is affected."* Ebert, K. and H. Witt. "Fructose malabsorption." *Molecular and Cellular Pediatrics* 3(2016): 10. doi: 10.1186/s40348-016-0035-9.

18. *"No matter which type or brand, these are almost all bizarre chemicals . . ."* Mercola, J., and K. D. Pearsall, N.M.D. *Sweet Deception* Nashville, TN: Thomas Nelson, Inc., 2006.

19. *"Artificially sweetened sodas contain as much synthetic caffeine. . . ."* Gardener, H., T. Rundek, M. Markert, C. B. Wright, M. S. V. Elkind, and R. L. Sacco. "Diet soft drink consumption is associated with an increased risk of vascular events in the Northern Manhattan study." *Journal of General Internal Medicine* 27(9)(2012): 1120–1126. doi: 10.1007/s11606-011-1968-2.

20. *"Unfortunately, through their effects on your taste buds, your gut bacteria . . ."* Pepino, M. Y. 2015. "Metabolic effects of non-nutritive sweeteners." *Physiology & Behaviour* 152(Part B) (2015): 450–455. Accessed October 2, 2016. doi:10.1016/j.physbeh.2015.06.024.

21. *"The French study that found sugar to be more addictive . . ."* Lenoir, M., F. Serre, L. Cantin, and S. H. Ahmed. "Intense sweetness surpasses cocaine reward" *PLoS One* 2(8) (2007). doi:10.1371/journal.pone.0000698.

22. *"One study showed a 7 percent increase in BMI for diet sugar users . . ."* Fowler, W., S. Fowler, and H. Hazuda. "Diet soda intake is associated with long-term increases in waist circumference in a biethnic cohort of older adults: The San Antonio longitudinal study of aging," *Journal of the American Geriatrics Society*, 63(4) (2015): 708–715. Accessed October 2, 2016. doi: 10.1111/jgs. 13376.

23. *"A disrupted microbiome is known to promote weight gain and diabetes . . ."* Suez, J., T. Korem, D Zeevi, G Zilberman-Schapira, C. A. Thaiss, O. Maza, D. Israeli, N. Zmora, S. Gilad, A. Weinberger, Y. Kuperman, A. Harmelin, I. Kolodkin-Gal, H. Shapiro, Z. Halpern, E. Segal, and E. Elinav. "Artificial sweeteners induce glucose intolerance by altering the gut microbiota." *Nature* 514 (2014): 181–186. Accessed October 2, 2016. doi:10.1038/nature13793.

24. *". . . vegetarian Egyptians died grossly overweight . . ."* Cockburn, T. A. *Mummies Disease & Ancient Cultures.* England: Cambridge University Press, 2008 (2d., paperback) I was directed to this fascinating work by the authors of a favorite book of mine from the late '90s, *Protein Power*, by M. R. Eades, and M. D. Eades. (New York: Bantam, 1997).

25. *". . . we are eating thirty-five pounds more wheat flour products a year . . ."* Kasarda, D. D. "Can an increase in celiac disease be attributed to an increase in the gluten content of wheat as a consequence of wheat breeding?" *Journal of Agriculture & Food Chemistry* 61(6) (2013): 1155–9. doi: 10.1021/jf305122s.

26. *". . . mixing a gliadin concentrate called 'vital gluten' into most baked goods . . ."* Kasarda, D. D. "Can an increase in celiac disease be attributed to an increase in the gluten content of wheat as a consequence of wheat breeding?" *Journal of Agriculture & Food Chemistry* 61(6) (2013): 1155–9. doi: 10.1021/jf305122s.

27. *"incidence of Celiac Disease and gluten sensitivity has increased . . ."* Lewis, R., Ph.D., "Pediatric celiac disease diagnoses triples in 20 years." *Medscape Medical News.* Last updated January 23, 2015. Accessed October 3, 2016. http://www.medscape.com /viewarticle/838622.

28. *". . . documented concerns about gluten-free foods."* Reilly, Norelle R., M.D. "The gluten-free diet: Recognizing fact, fiction and fad." *The Journal of Pediatrics* 175 (2016): 206–10. doi: 10.1016/j.jpeds.2016.04.014.

29. *"This may be better tolerated and less addictive milk."* Bell, S., G. T. Grochoski, and A. J. Clarke. "Health implications of milk containing beta-casein with the A2 genetic variant." *Critical Reviews in Food Science and Nutrition* 46(1) (2006): 93–100.

30. *"Fat is simply not as chemically addictive as sugar or starch."* Snoek, H. M., L. Huntjens, L. J. van Gemert, C. de Graaf, and H. Weenen. "Sensory-specific satiety in obese and normal-weight women." *American Journal of Clinical Nutrition* 80(4) (2004): 823–831.

31. *". . . salt has moderate effects on endorphin and dopamine."* Gold, M. S., and D. M. Blumenthal. "Neurobiology of food addiction." *Current Opinion in Clinical Nutrition and Metabolic Care* 13 (2010): 359–365. doi: 10.1097/MCO.0b013e32833ad4d4.

32. *". . . they must be balanced in a ratio of 1 to 4 with the potassium and magnesium . . ."* Morell, S. F. "Why salt is essential to health and happiness." The Weston A. Price Foundation. Published July 4, 2011. Accessed January 5, 2017. http://www.westonaprice.org /health-topics/abcs-of-nutrition/the-salt-of-the-earth/.

33. *". . . coffee also has pleasure-promoting properties . . ."* Arnold M. A., D. B. Carr, D. M. Togasaki, M. C. Pian, and J. B. Martin. "Caffeine stimulates beta-endorphin release in blood but not in cerebrospinal fluid. *Life Sciences* 31(10) (1982): 1017–24.

34. *"THC contents have increased from .5 percent to levels as high as 90 percent in "dabs," 'wax,' and other super-concentrated and toxic preparations."* Gillet, S., LCSW, CRNC. *True Bud.* New York: BIRD, 2016.

35. *"We have found that this plant can impact any or all of the brain's five Craving Types, amplifying the naturally mellowing effects of brain neurotransmitters like serotonin, endorphin, and GABA for some, but also able to trigger energizing (or even psychotic) symptoms in others."* Study from *True Bud* by Scott Gillet.

36. *"The new potencies are having many disturbing consequences such as a doubling of ER visits with psychotic symptoms."* Volkow, N. D., R. D. Baler, W. M. Compton, and S. R. Weiss. "Adverse health effects of marijuana use." *New England Journal of Medicine.* 370(23)(2014): 2219–27. doi: 10.1056/NEJMra1402309.

CHAPTER 3

1. *". . . 70 percent of us are overweight . . ."* Fryar, C. D., M.D. Carroll, and C. L. Ogden. "Prevalence of Overweight, Obesity, and Extreme Obesity Among Adults: United States, Trends 1960–1962 Through 2009–2010." CDC. Accessed December 14, 2016. https://www.cdc.gov/nchs/data/hestat/obesity_adult_09_10/obesity_adult_09_10 .htm.

2. *". . . half of us are on the diabetic spectrum."* Babey, Susan H., J. Wolstein, A. L. Diamant, and H. Goldstein. "Pre-diabetes in California: Nearly half of California adults on path to diabetes." *Health Policy Brief,* UCLA Center for Health Policy Research. March 2016.

3. *". . . free of industrially processed food, overweight and diet-related diseases . . . are virtually unknown."* Price, Weston A. *Nutrition and Physical Degeneration.* La Mesa, CA: Price-Pottenger Nutrition Foundation, 2009.

4. Fallon, S., and M. G. Enig. *Nourishing Traditions: The Cookbook that Challenges Politically Correct Nutrition and Diet Dictocrats.* Washington, DC: New Trends Publishing, 2001. p. 6. I have used the term "traditional" throughout this book. In fact, this principle is the foundation of my clinic's approach to dietary safety and sanity. The resource on traditional nutrition that has been the most helpful has always been the Weston A. Price Foundation (WAPF). WAPF, named for the scientist who studied traditional peoples and their diets directly before, and as they were, increasingly subjected to modern foods. His invaluable firsthand observations and photos and the continuing research and dietary activism it has led to, are disseminated throughout this worldwide organization. (http://www.westonaprice.org/)

5. *"Whole milk consumption, . . . quickly dropped by 66 percent . . ."* Allshouse, Jane E. and Judith J. Putnam. "Food Consumption, prices and expenditures, 1970–97." USDA Economic Research Service, 1999, p. 19.

6. *". . . reduced American meat consumption for years."* Teicholz, N."How Americans Got Red Meat Wrong." *The Atlantic,* June 2, 2014. Accessed September 29, 2016.

http://www.theatlantic.com/health/archive/2014/06/how-americans-used-to-eat
/371895/.

7. *"... studies that condemned hydrogenated fat specifically vindicated saturated fat."*
Teicholz, N. *The Big Fat Surprise: Why Butter, Meat and Cheese Belong in a Healthy
Diet*. New York: Simon & Schuster, 2014, p. 119.

8. *"saturated fat was not associated with increased risk of heart disease."* Siri-Tarino P. W.,
Q. Sun, F. B. Hu, and R. M. Krauss. "Meta-analysis of prospective cohort studies evaluating the association of saturated fat with cardiovascular disease." *American Journal
of Clinical Nutrition* 91(3) (2010): 535–46. doi: 10.3945/ajcn.2009.27725.

9. *"Another exhaustive review, published in 2015, confirmed this yet again."* de Souza R. J.,
A. Mente, A., Maroleanu, A., Cozma, V. Ha, T. Kishibe, E. Uleryk,, P. Budylowski, H.,
Schünemann, J., Beyene, and S. S. Anand. "Intake of saturated and trans unsaturated
fatty acids and risk of all cause mortality, cardiovascular disease, and type 2 diabetes:
systematic review and meta-analysis of observational studies." *BMJ* 351 (2015): h3978.
doi: http://dx.doi.org/10.1136/bmj.h3978.

10. *Re ban on hydrogenated fats by 2018*: "Final determination regarding partially hydrogenated oils." US Department of Health and Human Services, Food and Drug Administration. June 17, 2015. http://federalregister.gov/a/2015-14883.

11. *"Saturated fat had been made a decoy to protect the sugar industry..."* Kearns, D. E., L. A.
Schmidt, and S. A. Glantz. "Sugar Industry and Coronary Heart Disease Research: A Historical Analysis of Internal Industry Documents." *JAMA Internal Medicine.* 176(11) (2016):
1680–85. doi:10.1001/jamainternmed.2016.5394.

12. *"Sugar was known then to raise our levels of* heart damaging *cholesterol as well as
triglycerides"* Kearns, Cristin E., DDS, et al. "Sugar Industry and Coronary Heart
Disease Research: A Historical Analysis of Internal Industry Documents." *JAMA
Internal Medicine.* 176(11) (2016): 1680–85. doi: 10.001/jamainternmed.2016.5394.

13. *"These facts had been documented as early as 1962, but discredited by the sugar industry's paid Harvard scientist and others."* Kearns, D. E., L. A. Schmidt, and S. A. Glantz.
"Sugar Industry and Coronary Heart Disease Research: A Historical Analysis of
Internal Industry Documents." *JAMA Internal Medicine.* Published online September 12, 2016. Accessed October 5, 2016.

14. *"Now the sugar-heart connection is again being laid open by studies that clearly link
sugar consumption with death by cardiovascular disease."* Siri-Tarino P. W., Q. Sun, F. B.
Hu, R and M. Krauss. "Meta-analysis of prospective cohort studies evaluating the association of saturated fat with cardiovascular disease." *American Journal of Clinical
Nutrition* 91(3) (2010):535–46. doi: 10.3945/ajcn.2009.27725.

Yang, Q., Z. Zhang, E. W. Gregg, W.D. Flanders, R. Merritt, F. B. Hu. "Added sugar
intake and cardiovascular diseases mortality among US adults." *JAMA Internal Medicine.* 174(4)(2014): 516–24. doi: 10.1001/jamainternmed.2013.13563.

15. *"Saturated fat consumption was not associated with high cholesterol, nor with heart
disease."* Castelli, W. P. "Concerning the possibility of a nut..." *Archives of Internal
Medicine* 152(7) (1992):1371–2.

16. *"... drop in their cholesterol, the subjects experienced an 11 percent increase...."* Mann,
G. V., F. Pearson, T. Gordon, T. R. Dawber, L. Lyell, and D. Shurtleff. "Diet and cardiovascular disease in the Framingham study." *American Journal of Clinical Nutrition*
11(3) (1962): 200–225.

17. *Re 2006 US Women's Health Initiative*: Teicholz, N. *"The Big Fat Surprise: Why
Butter, Meat and Cheese Belong in a Healthy Diet."* New York: Simon & Schuster,
2014, p. 3.

18. *"lowering intake of saturated fats can drop heart protective HDL levels by one-third."* Knopp, R.H. "Sex differences in lipoprotein metabolism and dietary response: basis in hormonal differences and implications for cardiovascular disease." *Current Atherosclerosis Reports.* 7(6) (2005): 472–9.

19. *Re Israeli high vegetable oil diet associated with high rates of heart disease*: Teicholz, N. "The Big Fat Surprise: Why Butter, Meat and Cheese Belong in a Healthy Diet." New York: Simon & Schuster, 2014. p. 82

20. *". . . milk fats are specifically protective against Type 2 diabetes . . ."* Mozaffarian, D., H. Cao, I. B. King, R. N. Lemaitre, X. Song, D. S. Siscovick, and G. S. Hotamisligil. "Trans-palmitoleic acid, metabolic risk factors, and new-onset diabetes in U.S. adults: a cohort study." *Annals of Internal Medicine* 153(12) (2010): 790–9. doi: 10.7326/0003-4819-153-12-201012210-00005.

21. *". . . milk fats are specifically protective against . . . heart disease."* Soedamah-Muthu, S. S., E. L. Ding, W. K. Al-Delaimy, F. B. Hu, M. F. Engberink, W. C. Willett, and J. M. Geleijnse. "Milk and dairy consumption and incidence of cardiovascular diseases and all-cause mortality: dose-response meta-analysis of prospective cohort studies." *American Journal Clinical Nutrition* 93(1) (2011): 158–71. doi: 10.3945/ajcn.2010.29866.

22. *"The Finns proved . . . saturated fat was the preferred fuel of the heart and protective against stroke."* Pietinen, P., A. Ascherio, P. Korhonen, A. M. Hartman, W. C. Willett, D. Albanes, and J. Virtamo. "Intake of fatty acids and the risk of coronary heart disease in a cohort of Finnish men. The alpha-tocopherol, beta-carotene cancer prevention study." *American Journal of Epidemiology* 145(10) (1997): 876–87.

23. *". . . eggs are specifically protective against stroke."* Alexander, D.D., P.E. Miller, A.J. Vargas, D. L. Weed, and S. S. Cohen. "Meta-analysis of egg consumption and risk of coronary heart disease and stroke." *Journal of the American College of Nutrition* 35(8) (2016):704–716. Doi: 10.1080/07315724.2016.1152928.

24. *". . . saturated fats like butter assist vitamin A absorption in this life-preserving function, ..."* Sani, B. P., R. D. Allen, C. M. Moorer, and B. W. McGee. "Interference of retinoic acid binding to its binding protein by omega-6 fatty acid." *Biochemistry and Biophysical Research Communication* 147(1) (1987): 25–30.

25. *"Butter is also rich in its namesake, butyrate, the fastest burning of all fats, used extensively in the brain and is well known to protect us from colon cancer."* Stilling, R.M., M. van de Wouw, G. Clarke, C. Stanton, T. G. Dinan, and J. F. Cryan. "The neuropharmacology of butyrate: The bread and butter of the micro-gut-brain axis?" *Neurochemistry International* 99 (2016): 110–132. doi: 10.1016/j.neuint.2016.06.011.

26. *"the earlier that patients start to have lower cholesterol concentrations, the greater the risk of death"* McGee, D., D Reed, G. Stemmerman, G. Rhoads, K. Yano, and M. Feinleib. "The relationship of dietary fat and cholesterol to mortality in 10 years: the Honolulu Heart Program." *International Journal of Epidemeology* 14(1) (1985): 97–105.

27. *". . . low cholesterol causes hemorrhagic stroke and cholesterol protects against cancer."* Knekt, P., A. Reunanen, A. Aromaa, M. Heliovaara, T. Hakulinen, and M. Hakama. "Serum cholesterol and risk of cancer in a cohort of 39,000 men and women." *Journal of Clinical Epidemiiology* 41(6) (1988): 519–30.

28. *"Many studies agree that low cholesterol is firmly associated with autism . . ."* Moses, L., N. Katz, and A. Weizman. "Metabolic profiles in adults with autism spectrum disorder and intellectual disabilities." *European Psychiatry* 29(7) (2014): 397–401. doi: 10.1016/j.eurpsy.2013.05.005.

29. *"cholesterol is essential for the production of our natural anti-depressant, serotonin."* Scanlon, S. M., D. C. Williams, and P. Schloss. "Membrane cholesterol modulates serotonin transporter activity." *Biochemistry* 40(35) (2001):10507–13.

30. *"We initially reduced the amount of fat we ate . . ."* Teicholz, N. *The Big Fat Surprise: Why Butter, Meat and Cheese Belong in a Healthy Diet.* New York: Simon & Schuster, 2014, p. 4.

31. *". . . our fat intake, in 2011, was 850 calories a day, somewhat higher . . ."* Cohen, E., M. Cragg, J. deFonseka, A. Hite, M. Rosenberg, and B. Zhou. "Statistical review of US macronutrient consumption data 1965–2011: Americans have been following dietary guidelines coincident with rise in obesity." *Nutrition* 31(5) (2015): 727–732. doi: http://dx.doi.org/10.1016/j.nut.2015.02.007.

32. *"Natural omega-9 oils—the only stable liquid oils—are concentrated in olives, avocados, and macadamia nuts, but they also compose up to one-third of animal fat (including bacon fat) . . ."* Enig, M., and S. Fallon. *Eat Fat, Lose Fat: The Healthy Alternative to Trans Fats.* New York, Penguin 2005.

33. *"Farmed fish have less omega-3 and much more omega-6 fat."* Sprague, M., J. R. Dick, and D. R. Tocher. "Impact of sustainable feeds on omega-3 long-chain fatty acid levels in farmed Atlantic salmon, 2006–2015." *Scientific Reports* 6(2016). doi:10.1038/srep21892.

    Strobel, C., G. Jahreis, and K. Kuhnt. "Survey of n-3 and n-6 polyunsaturated fatty acids in fish and fish products." *Lipids in Health and Disease* 11(2012):144. doi: 10.1186/1476-511X-11-144.

34. *"we are now among the lowest consumers of omega-3 fats in the world . . ."* Starka, K. D., M. E. Van Elswykb, M. R. Higgins, C. A. Weatherfordd, and N. Salem. "Global survey of the omega-3 fatty acids, docosahexaenoic acid and eicosapentaenoic acid in the blood stream of healthy adults." *Progress in Lipid Research* 63(2016):132–152. doi: 10.1016/j.plipres.2016.05.001.

35. *"Because of this, the ratio of omega-3 to omega-6 fat we consume is no longer 1 to 1, it is now closer to 20 to 1."* Simopoulos, A. P. "An Increase in the omega-6/omega-3 Fatty Acid Ratio Increases the Risk for Obesity." *Nutrients* 8(3) (2016):128. doi: 10.3390/nu8030128.

36. *". . . caused our total omega-6 fat intake to be higher by a third than it was before 1970"* Ramsden, C. E., D. Zamora, S. Majchrzak-Hong, K. R. Faurot, S. K. Broste, R. P. Frantz, J. M. Davis, A. Ringel, C. M. Suchindran, and J. R. Hibbeln."Re-evaluation of the traditional diet-heart hypothesis: analysis of recovered data from Minnesota Coronary Experiment (1968–73)." *BMJ* 353 (2016):i1246. doi:10.1136/bmj.i1246.

37. *"Teicholz' review of animal studies is alarming."* Teicholz, N. *The Big Fat Surprise: Why Butter, Meat and Cheese Belong in a Healthy Diet.* New York: Simon & Schuster, 2014, p. 231–35.

38. *". . . for every unit of cholesterol reduced by a high vegetable oil diet, the risk of death rose 22%."* Ramsden, C. E., D. Zamora, S. Majchrzak-Hong, K. R. Faurot, S. K. Broste, R. P. Frantz, J. M. Davis, A. Ringel, C. M. Suchindran, and J. R. Hibbeln."Re-evaluation of the traditional diet-heart hypothesis: analysis of recovered data from Minnesota Coronary Experiment (1968–73)." *BMJ* 353 (2016):i1246. doi:10.1136/bmj.i1246.

39. *Re oil oxidizing and being processed to deodorize it:* Gavin, Arnold M. "Edible oil deodorization." *Journal of the American Oil Chemists' Society* 55(11) (1978):783–791. doi:10.1007/BF02682649.

40. *". . . the more omega-6 fat we consume, . . . , the more metabolically impaired and overweight we become."* Simopoulos, A. P. "An increase in the omega-6/omega-3 fatty acid ratio increases the risk for obesity." *Nutrients* 8(3) (2016):128. doi: 10.3390/nu8030128.

41. *". . . lean subjects have tended to have higher omega-6 fat levels and lower omega-3 levels than obese subjects."* Pickens, C. A., L. M. Sordillo, S. S. Comstock, W. S. Harris, K. Hortos, B. Kovan, and J. I. Fenton. "Plasma phospholipids, non-esterified plasma polyunsaturated fatty acids and oxylipids are associated with BMI." *Prostaglandins, Leukotrienes and Essential Fatty Acids.* 95 (2015):31–40. doi: 10.1016/j.plefa.2014.12.001.

42. *". . . adding in just a small amount of omega-3 fat . . . can reverse the adverse effects of a formerly 100 percent omega-6 diet."* Alvheim, A. R., M. K. Malde, D. Osei-Hyiaman, Y. H. Lin, R. J. Pawlosky, L. Madsen, K. Kristiansen, L. Frøyland, and J. R. Hibbeln. "Dietary linoleic acid elevates endogenous 2-AG and anandamide and induces obesity." *Obesity* (Sliver Spring) 20(10(2012): 1984–94. doi: 10.1038/oby.2012.38.

43. *". . . fish oil diet (even though carbohydrates were still high) cured 100 percent . . ."* Maciejewska, D., P Ossowski, A. Drozd, K. Ryterska, D. Jamioł-Milc, M. Banaszczak, M. Kaczorowska, A. Sabinicz, J. Raszeja-Wyszomirska, and E. Stachowska. "Metabolites of arachidonic acid and linoleic acid in early stages of nonalcoholic fatty liver disease—A pilot study." *Prostaglandins and Other Lipid Mediators* 121(Pt B) (2015): 184–9. doi: 10.1016/j.prostaglandins.2015.09.003.

 Vernon, G., and A. Baranova, and Z. M. Younossi. "The Epidemiology and Natural History of Non-alcoholic Fatty Liver Disease and Non-alcoholic Steatohepatitis in Adults." *Alimentary Pharmacology and Therapeutics* 34(3) (2011): 274–85. doi: 10.1111/j.1365-2036.2011.04724.x.

44. *"This can be done by providing more omega-3 fats to reform the fat-protein content of the phospholipids . . ."* Skórkowska-Telichowska, K., J. Kosińska, M. Chwojnicka, D. Tuchendler, M. Tabin, R. Tuchendler, Ł. Bobak, T. Trziszka, and A. Szuba. "Positive effects of egg-derived phospholipids in patients with metabolic syndrome." *Advances in Medical Science* 61(1) (2016): 169–74. doi: 10.1016/j.advms.2015.12.003.

45. *"So we were downing even more Techno-Karbz as half of our food was eaten 'out' by then."* Todd, Jessica E., L. Mancino, and Bling-Hwan Lin. "The impact of food away from home on adult diet quality." *USDA Economic Research Report* Number 90, February 2010.

46. *". . . 60 percent of our diet is 'pure' Techno-Food with no helpful nutrient content . . ."* Steele, E. M., and L. Galastri Baraldi, M. L.da Costa Louzada, J.-C. Moubarac, D. Mozaffarian, and C. A. Monteiro, "Ultra-processed foods and added sugars in the US diet: evidence from a nationally representative cross-sectional study." *BMJ* Open 6(3) (2016). doi: 10.1136/bmjopen-2015-009892.

47. *". . . sugar intake went up to 120 pounds a year in the 1960s."* Hollander, Gail M. "Renaturalizing sugar: narratives of place, production and consumption." *Social and Cultural Geography* 4(1) (2003): 59–74. doi: 10.1080/1464936032000049315.

48. *"By 2000 we were consuming about 155 pounds of sugar per year, most of it high-fructose corn syrup."* Ibid., p. 47.

49. *"Our consumption of white flour went way up too—by 35 pounds per year."* Kasarda, D. D. "Can an increase in celiac disease be attributed to an increase in the gluten content of wheat as a consequence of wheat breeding?" *Journal of Agriculture & Food Chemistry* 61(6) (2013): 1155–9. doi: 10.1021/jf305122s.

50. *". . . we're eating over 500 calories more per day than we were eating before 1970."* USDA Economic Research Division. "Food Availability (Per Capita) Data System: Summary Findings." Last updated, August 3, 2016. Accessed September 29, 2016. http://www.ers .usda.gov/data-products/food-availability-(per-capita)-data-system/summary-findings .aspx.

51. *"Now they make up just 8 percent, mostly as processed tomatoes and potatoes."* USDA Economic Research Division. "Food availability (per capita) data system: Summary

findings." Last updated, August 3, 2016. Accessed September 29, 2016. http://www.ers
.usda.gov/data-products/food-availability-(per-capita)-data-system/summary-findings
.aspx.

52. *"Of 15,000 overweight Dutch women ..."* Salmerón, J., and J. E. Manson, M. J. Stampfer, G. A. Colditz, A. L. Wing, and W. C. Willett. "Dietary fiber, glycemic load, and risk of non-insulin-dependent diabetes mellitus in women." *JAMA* 277(6) (1997): 472–7.

Shai, Iris, et al."Weight Loss with a Low-Carbohydrate, Mediterranean, or Low-Fat Diet." *The New England Journal of Medicine* 359(3) (2008): 229–41.

53. *"A similar study found 50% greater incidence of diabetes ..."* Beulens, J. W., L. M. de Bruijne, R. P. Stolk, P. H. Peeters, M. L. Bots, D. E. Grobbee, and Y. T. van der Schouw. "High dietary glycemic load and glycemic index increase risk of cardiovascular disease among middle-aged women: a population-based follow-up study." *Journal of the American College of Cardiology* 50(1) (2007): 14–21. doi:10.1016/j.jacc.2007.02.068.

54. *"We used to eat about 10 per week. "* Cha, A.E. "Eggs are okay again." *Washington Post.* Published January 7, 2016. Accessed January 11, 2017. https://www.washingtonpost .com/news/to-your-health/wp/2016/01/07/cholesterol-new-u-s-dietary-guidelines -remove-warnings-making-eggs-okay-again/?utm_term=.5e6367cbcda8.

55. *"... the satiety power of protein, which is known to be greater. ..."* Dhillon, J., B. A. Craig, H. J. Leidy, A. F. Amankwaah, K. O. Anguah, A. Jacobs, B. L. Jones, J. B. Jones, C. L. Keeler, C.E.M. Keller, M. A. McCrory, R. L. Rivera, M. Slebodnik, and R. D. Mattes. "The effects of increased protein intake on fullness: A meta-analysis and its limitations." *Journal of the Academy of Nutrition and Dietetics* 116(6) (2016): 968–983. doi:10.1016/j.jand.2016.01.003.

56. *"When amino supplies are limited by a high-carbohydrate, low animal-protein diet, athletes often lose ..."* Loosli, A. l. and J. S. Ruud. "Meatless diets in female athletes: a red flag." *The Physician and Sportsmedicine* 26(11) (1998): 45–8. doi:10.3810/psm.1998 .11.1194.

57. *"Buddhist communities worldwide are split in half between those who eat eggs and milk products and those who eat meat as well."* Liusuwan, N. "What stereotypes surround Buddhism?" *The Huffington Post.* Published April 29, 2016. Accessed January 11, 2017. http://www.huffingtonpost.com/nicholas-liusuwan/what-stereotypes-surround_b _9783566.html.

58. *"A similar "lacto-ovo" diet is followed by 40% of those in India,. ..."* *The Hindu,* August 14, 2006. Accessed October 6, 2016. http://www.thehindu.com/todays-paper/the -food-habits-of-a-nation/article3089973.ece.

59. *"Children in India have twice the incidence ..."* Alvarez-Uria, G., P. K. Naik, M. Midde, P. S. Yalla, and R. Pakam. "Prevalence and severity of anaemia stratified by age and gender in rural India." *Anemia* (2014). doi:10.1155/2014/176182.

60. *"Low iron and B$_{12}$ are serious and common among Western vegans and ..."* Pawlak, R., S. J. Parrott, S. Raj, D. Cullum-Dugan, and D. Lucus. "How prevalent is vitamin B(12) deficiency among vegetarians?" *Nutrition Reviews* 71(1) (2013): 110–117. doi: 10.1111/ nure.12001.

61. *"Children show mental as well as physical detriment."* Michalak, J., Xiao C., Zhang, and F. Jacobi. "Vegetarian diet and mental disorders: Results from a representative community survey." *International Journal of Behavioral Nutrition and Physical Activity* 9(2012):67. doi: 10.1186/1479-5868-9-67.

CHAPTER 4

1. *". . . over 70 percent of US adults and 30% of children have become overweight . . ."* Fryar, C. D., M.D. Carroll, and C. L. Ogden. "Prevalence of overweight, obesity, and extreme obesity among adults: United States, Trends 1960–1962 through 2009–2010." Centers for Disease Control and Prevention. https://www.cdc.gov/nchs/data/hestat/obesity _adult_09_10/obesity_adult_09_10.htm. Accessed December 14, 2016.

2. *". . . more than half of them are obese."* "Overweight in Children." American Heart Association. http://www.heart.org/HEARTORG/HealthyLiving/HealthyKids/Childhood Obesity/Overweight-in-Children_UCM_304054_Article.jsp#.WFKZQpI5Q6Y. Updated July 5, 2016. Accessed December 14, 2016.

3. *". . . diets fail the majority of dieters . . ."* Wing, R. R., and J. O. Hill. "Successful weight loss maintenance." *Annual Review of Nutrition* 21 (2001): 323–41. doi: 10.1146/annurev.nutr.21.1.323.

4. *"Frequent dieters, for example, are 12 times more likely to become bingers than nondieters."* Field, A. E., S. B. Austin, C. B. Taylor, S. Malspeis, B. Rosner, H. R. Rockett, M. W. Gillman, and G. A. Colditz. "Relation between dieting and weight change among preadolescents and adolescents." *Pediatrics* 112(4) (203): 900–6.

5. *Re eating disorders caused by dieting*: Ross, J. *The Diet Cure*. Penguin, New York, 2012, chapters 2 and 10.

6. *". . . fast food and chain restaurant portion sizes doubled at that time . . ."* Nestle, M. "Today's 'eat more' environment: The role of the food industry." in *A Place at the Table: The Crisis of 49 Million Hungry Americans and How to Solve It*, ed. P. Pringle (New York: *PublicAffairs*, 2013), chapter 7.

7. *". . . children most often inherit abnormalities in appetite and weight from their parent . . ."* Pembrey, M. R., Saffery, and L. O. Bygren, "Human transgenerational responses to early-life experience: potential impact on development, health and biomedical research," *Journal of Medical Genetics* 51(9) (2014): 563–72. doi: 10.1136/jmedgenet-2014-102577.

8. *". . . 15–20 percent of all children and teens qualifying [as obese]"* Fryar, C.D., M.D. Carroll, and C. L. Ogden. "Prevalence of Overweight and obesity among children and adolescents: United States, 1963–1965 through 2011–2012." Centers for Disease Control and Prevention. Accessed December 5, 2016. http://www.cdc.gov/nchs/data /hestat/obesity_child_11_12/obesity_child_11_12.htm.

9. *". . . morbid obesity, alone rose from 1.6% to 13.3%: a 700 percent increase."* Finkelstein, E. A., O. A. Khavjou, H. Thompson, J. G. Trogdon, L. Pan, B. Sherry, and W. Dietz. "Obesity and severe obesity forecasts through 2030." *American Journal of Preventive Medicine* 42(6) (2012): 563–570. doi: http://dx.doi.org/10.1016/j.amepre.2011.10.026.

10. *"The US now shares with China the highest obesity rate in the world."* NCD Risk Factor Collaboration. "Trends in adult body-mass index in 200 countries from 1975 to 2014: a pooled analysis of 1698 population-based measurement studies with 19.2 million participants." *The Lancet* 387(10026) (2016): 1377–96. doi: http://dx.doi.org/10.1016 /S0140-6736(16)30054-X.

11. *"In 2000, for the first time in history, the number of people who were over-fed and over-weight in the world exceeded the number of people who were under-fed and under-weight."* NCD Risk Factor Collaboration. "Trends in adult body-mass index in 200 countries from 1975 to 2014: a pooled analysis of 1698 population-based measurement studies with 19.2 million participants." *The Lancet* 387(10026) (2016): 1377–96. doi: http://dx.doi.org /10.1016/S0140-6736(16)30054-X.

12. *". . . study of the alarming consequences of a single 12 week, 1,500 calorie diet."* Keys,

A. J. Brozek, and A. Henschel. *The Biology of Human Starvation*. University of Minnesota Press, January 1950.

13. *Re Biggest Loser:* Fothergill, E. J., Guo, L. Howard, J. C. Kerns, N. D. Knuth, R. Brychta, K. Y. Chen, M. C. Skarulis, M. Walter, P. J. Walker, and K. D. Hall. "Persistent metabolic adaptation 6 years after 'The biggest loser' competition." *Obesity* 24(8) (2016):1612–1619. doi: 10.1002/oby.21538.

14. *". . . eat far fewer calories by their trainers."* Kolata, Gina. "After 'The Biggest Loser,' Their Bodies Fought to Regain Weight." *New York Times*. Published May 2, 2016. Accessed March 10, 2017. https://www.nytimes.com/2016/05/02/health/biggest-loser -weight-loss.html?rref=collection%2Fbyline%2Fgina-kolata.

15. *"These alterations are all known to increase cravings and/or slow metabolism."* Sumithran, P., L. A. Prenderast, E. Delbridge K. Purcell, A. Shulkes, A. Kriketos, and J. Proietto. "Long-term persistence of hormonal adaptations to weight loss." *New England Journal of Medicine* 365 (2011):1597–1604, doi : 10.1056/NEJMoa1105816.

16. *". . . of calories considered adequate for sustaining life is considered by the United Nationals to be 1,800."* "Undernourishment around the world in 2010." Food and Agriculture Organization of the United Nations. http://www.fao.org/docrep/013/i1683e /i1683e02.pdf. Accessed December 14, 2016.

17. *". . . by 2015, only 19 percent of people surveyed were on a diet."* Kell, J. "Lean times for the diet industry." *Fortune*. May 22, 2015. Accessed September 29, 2016. http://fortune .com/2015/05/22/lean-times-for-the-diet-industry/.

18. *"We urge them to work toward getting between 10,000 steps known to promote health . . ."* Bassett, D. R., H. R. Wyatt, H. Thompson, J. C. Peters, and J. O. Hill. "Pedometer-measured physical activity and health behaviors in U.S. adults." *Medicine and Science in Sports and Exercise* 42(10) (2010):1819–25. doi: 10.1249/MSS.0b013e3181dc2e54.

19. *"sixty percent of our current calories are now completely devoid of nutrients."* Steele, E. M., L. G. Baraldi, M. L. da Costa Louzada, J.-C.Moubarac, D. Mozaffarian, and C. A. Monteiro, "Ultra-processed foods and added sugars in the US diet: evidence from a nationally representative cross-sectional study." *BMJ* Open 6(3) (2016). doi:10.1136/ bmjopen-2015-009892.

20. *". . . 25% fewer nutrients than they did before 1970."* David, D., M. Epps, and H. Riordan. "Changes in USDA food composition data for 43 garden crops, 1950 to 1999." *Journal of the American College of Nutrition* 23(6)(2004):669–82.

   Barnaski, M., et al. "Higher antioxidant and lower cadmium concentrations and lower incidence of pesticide residues in organically grown crops: a systematic literature review and meta-analyses." *British Journal of Nutrition* 112(5)(2014):794–811. doi: 10.1017/S0007114514001366

21. *"This means that 75 percent of irreplaceable nutrients can drop below minimal levels on any comparable low-calorie diet."* Ames, BN. "Micronutrient deficiencies. A major cause of DNA damage," *Annuals of NY Academy of Science* 889 (1999):87–106.

22. *"Some of the vitamins, minerals, and fats found to be particularly deficient among those who are most . . ."* Via, M. "The malnutrition of obesity: Micronutrient deficiencies that promote diabetes." *ISRN Endocrinology* (2012): 103472. doi: 10.5402/2012/103472.

23. *"A genetic analysis of young bulls who'd been subject to . . ."* Keogh, K., D. A. Kenney, P. Cormican, A. K. Kelly, and S. M. Waters. "Effect of dietary restriction and subsequent re-alimentation on the transcriptional profile of hepatic tissue in cattle." *BMC Genomics* 17:244 (2016). doi: 10.1186/s12864-016-2578-5.

24. *". . . children exposed through their forebears to under-or over-nutrition are known to have increased risks . . ."* Johansen, B. "Feed your genes: How our genes respond to the

foods we eat." *ScienceDaily*. Norwegian University of Science and Technology (NTNU) (2011), https://www.sciencedaily.com/releases/2011/09/110919073845.htm.

25. *"Studies of women in Scandinavia and Holland . . ."* Pembrey, M., R. Saffery, and L. O. Bygren. "Human transgenerational responses to early-life experience: potential impact on development, health and biomedical research." *Journal of Medical Genetics* 51(9) (2014):563–72. doi: 10.1136/jmedgenet-2014-102577.

26. *"Young boys who gorged after a famine . . ."* Lumey, L. H., M. D. Khalangot, and A. M. Vaiserman. "Association between type 2 diabetes and prenatal exposure to the Ukraine famine of 1932–33: a retrospective cohort study." *The Lancet: Diabetes & Endocrinology* 3(10) (2015):787–94. doi: 10.1016/S2213-8587(15)00279-X.

27. *Re Dr. Kenneth Blum, the neuroscientist:* Blum, K, A. L. Chen, T. J. Chen, P. Rhoades, T. J. Prihoda, B. W. Downs, R. L. Waite, L., Williams, E. R Braverman, D. Braverman, V. Arcuri, M. Kerner, S. H. Blum, and T. Palomo. "LG839: anti-obesity effects and polymorphic gene correlates of reward deficiency syndrome." *Advances in Therapy* 25(9) (2008):894–913. doi: 10.1007/s12325-008-0093-z.

   For more on Dr. Blum, visit The Alliance For Addiction Solutions site at http://www.allianceforaddictionsolutions.org/resources/kenneth-blum-phd/blums-scientific-work-in-addiction-medicine/.

28. *"Positive expression replaced negative expression . . ."* Ornish D., M. J. Magbanua, G. Weidner, V. Weinberg, C. Kemp, C. Green, M. D. Mattie, R. Marlin, J. Simko, K. Shinohara, C. M. Haqq, and P. R. Carroll. "Changes in prostate gene expression in men undergoing an intensive nutrition and lifestyle intervention." *Proceedings of the National Academy of Sciences of the USA* 105(24) (2008): 8369–8374. doi: 10.1073/pnas.0803080105

29. *" . . . adoption of traditional eating habits itte . . ."* *ScienceDaily*. "Feed your genes: How our genes respond to the foods we eat." Norwegian University of Science and Technology. Last modified 20 September 2011. Accessed September 29, 2016. www.sciencedaily.com/releases/2011/09/110919073845.htm.

30. *". . . if sugar returns to the diet . . ."* El-Osta, A., and D. Brasacchio, D. Yao, A. Pocai, P. L. Jones, R. G. Roeder, M. E. Cooper, and M. Brownlee. "Transient high glucose causes persistent epigenetic changes and altered gene expression during subsequent normoglycemia." *Journal of Experimental Medicine*. 205(10 (2008):2409–17. doi: 10.1084/jem.20081188.

31. *Re freakishly blonde and obese mice:* Dolinoy, D.C. "The agouti mouse model: an epigenetic biosensor for nutritional and environmental alterations on the fetal epigenome." *Nutrition Reviews* 66 Suppl 1 (2008):S7–11. doi: 10.1111/j.1753-4887.2008.00056.x.

CHAPTER 5

1. *". . . Richard and Judith Wurtman, found early on that inadequate brain levels . . ."* Wurtman, J. H., and Frusztajer, N. T. *The Serotonin Power Diet: Eat Carbs—Nature's Own Appetite Suppressant—to Stop Emotional Overeating and Halt Antidepressant-Associated Weight Gain* (paperback). New York: Rodale, 2009.

2. *". . . Richard and Judith Wurtman, found early on that inadequate brain levels of the anti-depressant neurotransmitter . . ."* Wurtman, R. J., and J. D. Fernstrom. "Brain serotonin content: increase following ingestion of carbohydrate diet." *Science* 174(4013) (1971):1023–5.

3. *". . . sugar, chocolate, and fat could significantly raise levels of endorphin, our natural opiate."* Fortuna, J. L. "Sweet preference, sugar addiction and the familial history of alcohol dependence: shared neural pathways and genes." *Journal of Psychoactive Drugs*. 422(2)(2010): 147–51. doi: 10.1080/02791072.2010.10400687.

4. "'hard' drug substances, can stimulate and deplete, not only serotonin and endorphin, . . ." Volkow, N. D., and R. D. Baler. "NOW vs LATER brain circuits: implications for obesity and addiction." *Trends in Neuroscience* 38(6) (2015):345–52, doi: 10.1016/j.tins.2015.04.002.

5. "*Dr. Kenneth Blum, . . . describes this concert as "The Reward Cascade."*" Blum, K., E. R. Braverman, J. M. Holder, J. F. Lubar, V. J. Monastra, D. Miller, J. O. Lubar, T. J. Chen, and D. E. Comings. "Reward deficiency syndrome: a biogenetic model for the diagnosis and treatment of impulsive, addictive, and compulsive behaviors." *Journal of Psychoactive Drugs* 32(Suppl) (2000):i-iv, 1–112.

6. "*Individual aminos are also flourishing as ingredients in a broad range of consumer products . . .*" "Research and markets: Global amino acid market 2012–2016: Amino-acid based dietary supplements a key factor causing market growth." *BusinessWire*, March 21, 2013. http://www.businesswire.com/news/home/20130321005806/en/Research-Markets-Global-Amino-Acids-Market-2012-2016. Accessed December 16, 2016.

7. Petrou I., R. Heu, M. Stranick, S. Lavender, L. Zaidel, D. Cummins, R. J. Sullivan, C. Hsueh, and J. K. Gimzewski. "A breakthrough therapy for dentin hypersensitivity: how dental products containing 8% arginine and calcium carbonate work to deliver effective relief of sensitive teeth." *Journal of Clinical Dentristry* 20 (2009):23–31.

8. Sheihet, L, P. Chandr, P. Batheja, D. Devore, J. Kohn, and B. Michniak. "Tyrosine-derived nanospheres for enhance topical skin penetration." *International Journal of Pharmaceutics*. 350(1–2)(2008): 312–9. doi: 10.1016/j.ijpharm.2007.08.022.

9. Dr. Blum has published over 500 papers and several books. I refer you to his page at http://www.allianceforaddictionsolutions.org/ My favorite of his books is *Alcohol and the Addictive Brain*. Out of print now, it is available used and tells the inside story of how the neurochemical causes of addiction were discovered by the International Brotherhood of Neuroscientists in the 1970s and '80s. He continues to research and publish on many neuroscientific topics including innovative applications of amino acid therapy.

10. "*Dr. Blum's cocaine-targeted amino acid formula reduced the number of patients who left treatment . . .*" Blum, K., D. Allison, M. C. Trachtenberg, R. W. Williams, and L. A. Loeblich. "Reduction of both drug hunger and withdrawal against advice rate of cocaine abusers in a 30 day inpatient treatment program by the neuronutrient Tropamine." *Current Therapeutic Research* 43(6) (1988): 1204–1214.

11. "*Those in the control group, who had started out with the same high level of cravings, . . .*" Blum, K., J. G. Cull, T.J.H. Chen, S. Garcia-Swan, J. M. Holder, R. Wood, E. R. Braverman, L. R. Buci, and M. C. Trachtenberg. "Clinical evidence for effectiveness of Phencal in maintaining weight loss in an open-label, controlled, 2-year study." *Current Therapeutic Research* 58(10) (1997).

12. Reference books by nutrient therapy pioneers:
Seven Weeks to Sobriety by Joan Mathews-Larson, Ph.D.
End Your Addiction Now by Charles Gant, M.D.
The Mood Cure by Julia Ross

13. "*Depression, insomnia, and anxiety have been increasing right along without cravings and overeating since the 1970s of course.*" Twenge, J. M. "Time period and birth cohort differences in depressive symptoms in the US, 1982–2013." *Social Indicators Research* 121(2) (2015): 437–454. doi:10.1007/s11205-014-0647-1.

CHAPTER 6

1. *"The primary stress response chemicals, adrenaline and cortisol"* Tran-Nguyen, L. T., J. G. Bellew, K. A. Grote, and J. L. Neisewander. "Serotonin depletion attenuates co-caine seeking but enhances sucrose seeking and the effects of cocaine priming on re-instatement of cocaine seeking in rats." *Psychopharmacology* (Berlin) 157(4) (2001): 340–8. doi: 10.1007/s002130100822.

2. *". . . when fructose dominates, . . . decreased tryptophan result."* Ledochowski, M., B. Widner, C. Murr, B. Sperner-Unterweger, and D. Fuchs. "Fructose malabsorption is associated with decreased plasma tryptophan." *Scandinavian Journal of Gastroenterology* 36(4) (2001): 367–371.

3. *"poultry and cattle can't make adequate amounts of tryptophan."* The Merck Veterinary Manuals. "Acute Bovine Pulmonary Emphysema and Edema (Fog fever, Bovine aty-pical interstitial pneumonia)" Last review March 2015. Accessed September 29, 2016 http://www.merckvetmanual.com/mvm/respiratory_system/respiratory_diseases_of _cattle/acute_bovine_pulmonary_emphysema_and_edema.html.

4. *". . . a recent study, eating corn chips or popcorn (and who doesn't?) can quickly reduce tryptophan levels. . . ."* Fernstrom, J. D., Fernstrom, M. H., Irvine, Z.L.E, Langham, K. A. Marcelino, L. M., and Kaye, W. H. "The ingestion of different dietary proteins by humans induces large changes in the plasma tryptophan ratio, a predictor of brain tryp-tophan uptake and serotonin synthesis." *Clinical Nutrition* (32(6)(2013):1073–6.

5. *"chronic depletion of tryptophan by low-calorie dieting can lead to bulimia."* Smith, K. A., C. G. Fairburn, and P. J. Cowen. "Symptomatic relapse in bulimia nervosa follow-ing acute tryptophan depletion." *Archives of General Psychiatry* 56(2) (1999): 171–176.

   This study has been repeated several times, including by big tryptophan expert Simon Young, who showed similar results.

   Bruce, K. R., H. Steiger, S. N. Young, N. M. Kin, M. Israël, and M. Lévesque. "Im-pact of acute tryptophan depletion on mood and eating-related urges in bulimic and nonbulimic women." *Journal of Psychiatry & Neuroscience* 34(5) (2009): 376–82.

6. *"Too many anti-serotonin drugs (aspartame) . . ."* Sharma, R. P., and Roger A. Cou-lombe, Jr., "Effects of repeated doses of aspartame on serotonin and its metabolite in various regions of the mouse brain." *Food and Chemical Toxicology* 25(8) (1987): 565–8. doi: 10.1016/0278-6915(87)90015-9.

7. *"The brain could be easily tricked to activate more serotonin."* Fernstrom, John D., and Richard J. Wurtman. "Brain serotonin content: Physiological dependence on plasma tryptophan levels. " *Science* 173(3992) (1971):149–152.

8. *"Judith wrote several books and toured the country touting her . . ."* Wurtman, J. J., PhD. and N. T. Frusztajer, M.D. *The Serotonin Power Diet: Eat Carbs—Nature's Own Appe-tite Suppressant—to Stop Emotional Overeating and Halt Antidepressant-Associated Weight Gain.* New York: Rodale, 2009.

9. *"Cravings are temporarily dampened, and positive feelings are generated."* Fernstrom, J. D., and R. J. Wurtman. "Brain serotonin content: Physiological dependence on plasma tryptophan levels." *Science* 173(3992) (1971):149–152.

   "Brain serotonin content: increase following ingestion of carbohydrate diet." *Sci-ence.* 174(4013)(1971):1023–5.

10. *"Diabetics have doubled rates of depression . . ."* Holt, R.I.G., M. de Groot, , and S. H. Golden, "Diabetes and Depression" *Current Diabetes Report* 14(6) (2014):491. doi: 10.1007/s11892-014-0491-3.

11. *"raising tryptophan raised levels of serotonin . . ."* Young, S. N., and S. Gauthier. "Effect of tryptophan administration on tryptophan, 5-hydroxyindoleacetic acid and

indoleacetic acid in human lumbar and cisternal cerebrospinal fluid." *Journal of Neurology, Neurosurgery & Psychiatry* 44(4) (1981): 323–8.

12. *"5-HTP alleviating cravings and mood problems"* Cangiano, C. A. Laviano, M. D. Ben, I. Preziosa, F. Angelico, A. Cascino, and F. Rossi-Fanelli. "Effects of oral 5-hydroxy-tyrptophan on energy intake and macronutrient selection in non-insulin dependent diabetic patients." *International Journal of Obesity* 22(7) (1998): 648–654.

13. *"5-HTP alleviating cravings and mood problems"* Rondanelli, M., A. Opizzi, M. Faliva, M. Bucci, and S. Perna. "Relationship between the absorption of 5-hydroxytryptophan from an integrated diet, by means of Griffonia simplicifolia extract, and the effect on satiety in overweight females after oral spray administration." *Eating & Weight Disorders* 17(1) (2012):e22–8. doi: 10.3275/8165.

14. *". . . in a sleep pattern that gives them less than seven hours a night!"* Jones, Jeffrey, M. "In the U.S., 40% Get Less Than Recommended Amount of Sleep." Gallup.com. http://www.gallup.com/poll/166553/less-recommended-amount-sleep.aspx. Published December 19, 2013. Accessed March 2, 2017.

15. *"The less we sleep, the more biochemical commands"* Szewczyk-Golec, K., A. Woźniak, and R. J. Reiter. "Inter-relationships of the chronobiotic, melatonin, with leptin and adiponectin: implications for obesity." *Journal of Pineal Research* 59(3) (2015):277–91. doi: 10.1111/jpi.12257.

CHAPTER 7

1. *". . . increased risk of death within three years after a single incident."* Khunti, K. "Hypoglycemia predicts CV events in Type 1 and 2 diabetes." *Medscape.* December 22, 2014.

2. *"Low blood sugar is a tragically under-appreciated cause of alcoholism."* Mathews-Larson, J., Ph.D. *Seven Weeks to Sobriety: The Proven Program to Fight Alcoholism Through Nutrition.* New York: Ballentine Books, 1997.

3. *"The almost constant glut of triglycerides contributes to our heart disease"* Abbasi, F., P. Kohli, G. M. Reaven, and J. W. Knowles. "Hypertriglyceridemia: A simple approach to identify insulin resistance and enhanced cardio-metabolic risk in patients with pre-diabetes." *Diabetes Research & Clinical Practice* 120 (2016): 156–161. doi: 10.1016/j.diabres.2016.07.024.

4. *". . . the almost constant glut of triglycerides."* Han, T. S., and M.E.J. Lean. "A clinical perspective of obesity, metabolic syndrome and cardiovascular disease." *JRSM Cardiovascular Disease* 5 (2016): 1–13. doi: 10.1177/2048004016633371.

5. *"Fructose impairs insulin signaling in insulin sensitive cells."* Baena, M., G. Sangüesa, A. Dávalos, M. J. Latasa, A. Sala-Vila, R. M. Sánchez, N. Roglans, J. C. Laguna, and M. Alegret. "Fructose, but not glucose, impairs insulin signaling in the three major insulin-sensitive tissues." *Scientific Reports* 6 (2016): 26149. doi: 10.1038/srep26149.

6. *"This means damage to our hormonal appetite-regulating system"* Rezvani R., and K. Cianflone, J. P. McGahan, L. Berglund, A. A. Bremer, N. L. Keim, S. C. Griffen, P. J. Havel, and K. L. Stanhope. "Effects of sugar-sweetened beverages on plasma acylation stimulating protein, leptin and adiponectin: relationships with metabolic outcomes." *Obesity* 21(12) (2013): 2471–2480. doi: 10.1002/oby.20437.

7. *". . . glutamine supplements also restore insulin response . . ."* Samocha-Bonet, Dorit, et al. "L-glutamine and whole protein restore first-phase insulin response and increase glucagon-like peptide-1 in type 2 diabetes patients." *Nutrients* 7(4) (2015): 2101–2108. doi: 10.3390/nu7042101.

8. Pfeiffer, Carl C., and Eric R. Braverman. *The Healing Nutrients Within*. California: Basic Health Pub., Inc., 2003, p. 166.

9. *"Among diabetics, serum levels of glutamine are on."* Guasch-Ferré, M., A. Hruby, E. Toledo, C. B. Clish, M. A. Martínez-González, J. Salas-Salvadó, and F. B. Hu. "Metabolomics in prediabetes and diabetes: A systematic review and meta-analysis." *Diabetes Care* 39(5) (2016): 833–846. doi: 10.2337/dc15-2251.

10. *"Research has found that glutamine is effective both in people with hypoglycemia . . ."* Li, C., C. Buettger, J. Kwagh, A. Matter, Y. Daikhin, I. B. Nissim, H. W. Collins, M. Yudkoff, C. A. Stanley, and F. M. Matschinsky. "A signaling role of glutamine in insulin secretion." *Journal of Biological Chemistry* 279(14) (2004): 13393–13401. doi: 10.1074/jbc.M311502200.

11. *"It also reduced weight, and insulin levels."* Laviano, A., and A. Molfino, M. T. Lacaria, A. Canelli, S. De Leo, I. Preziosa, F. R. Fanelli. "Glutamine supplementation favors weight loss in nondieting obese female patients. A pilot study." *European Journal of Clinical Nutrition* 68(11) (2014): 1264–1266. doi: 10.1038/ejcn.2014.184.

12. *"L-glutamine also improves the deadly diarrhea associated with HIV"* Leite, R. D., N. L. Lima, C. A. Leite, C. K. Farhat, R. L. Guerrant, and A. A. Lima. "Improvement of intestinal permeability with alanyl-glutamine in HIV patients: a randomized, double blinded, placebo-controlled clinical trial." *Arquivos de Gastroenterologia* 50(1) (2013): 56–63.

13. *"Cancer treatment relies on the use of glutamine."* Martins, H. A., C. C. Sehaber, C. Hermes-Uliana, F. A. Mariani, F. A. Guarnier, G. E. Vicentini, G. D. Bossolani, L. A. Jussani, M. M. Lima, R. B. Bazotte, and J. N. Zanoni. "Supplementation with L-glutamine prevents tumor growth and cancer-Induced cachexia as well as restores cell proliferation of intestinal mucosa of Walker-256 tumor-bearing rats." *AminoAcids* (2016):1–12. DOI: 10.1007/s00726-016-2313-1.

14. *". . . prevent infections, decrease oxidative stress, and improve survival."* Novak, F., D. K. Heyland, A. Avenell, J. W. Drover, and X. Su. "Glutamine supplementation in serious illness: a systematic review of the evidence." *Critical Care Medicine.* 2002; 30(9): 2022–2029.

15. Williams, Roger J. *Prevention of Alcoholism Through Nutrition*. New York: Bantam Books, 1984.

16. *". . . the mineral chromium and the vitamin biotin are both often depleted, especially in obese and diabetic Americans."* Via, M. "The malnutrition of obesity: Micronutrient deficiencies that promote diabetes." *ISRN Endocrinology* (2012): 103472. doi: 10.5402/2012/103472.

17. *"When we have occasionally run out of it (chromium)"* Brownley, K. A., A. von Holle, R. M. Hamer, M. La Via, and C. M. Bulik. "A double-blind, randomized pilot trial of chromium picolinate for binge eating disorder: results of the Binge Eating and Chromium (BEACh) study." *Journal of Psychosomatic Research* 75(1) (2013): 36–42. doi: 10.1016/j.jpsychores.2013.03.092.

18. *"When we have occasionally run out of it (chromium)"* Dakshinamurti, K. "Vitamins and their derivatives in the prevention and treatment of metabolic syndrome diseases (diabetes)." *Canadian Journal of Physiology & Pharmacology* 93(5) (2015): 355–362. doi: 10.1139/cjpp-2014-0479.

19. *"When we have occasionally run out of it (chromium)"* Via, M. "The malnutrition of obesity: Micronutrient deficiencies that promote diabetes." *ISRN Endocrinology* (2012): 103472. doi: 10.5402/2012/103472.

20. *". . . scores of diabetes studies have now confirmed the superiority of a low carbohydrate diet"* Feinman, R. D., W. K. Pogozelski, A Astrup, R. K. Bernstein, E. J. Fine, E. C. Westman, A. Accurso, L. Frassetto, B. A. Gower, S. I. McFarlane, J. V. Nielsen, T. Krarup, L. Saslow, K. S. Roth, M. C. Vernon, J. S. Volek, G. B. Wilshire, A. Dahlqvist, R. Sundberg, A. Childers, K. Morrison, A. H. Manninen, H. M. Dashti, R. J. Wood, J. Wortman, and N. Worm. "Dietary carbohydrate restriction as the first approach in diabetes management: critical review and evidence base." *Nutrition* 31(1) (2015): 1–13. doi: 10.1016/j. nut.2014.06.011.

21. *"This kind of bitter complaining about the 'unwillingness' of diabetics"* Kolata, G. "Diabetes and your diet: The low-carb debate." *New York Times.* http://www.nytimes.com /2016/09/16/health/type-2-diabetes-low-carb-diet.html?_r=0. Published September 15, 2016. Accessed January 6, 2017.

22. *"The amino acid glutamine (no surprise . . ."* Mansour A., M. Mohajer-tehrani, M. Qurbani, R. Heshmat, B. Larijani, S. Hosseini. "Effect of glutamine supplementation on cardiovascular risk factors in patients with type 2 diabetes." *Nutrition.* 31(1) (2015):119–26. doi: 10.1016/j.nut.2014.05.014.

23. *"This resulted in lowered blood glucose . . ."* Mansour A., M. Mohajer-Tehrani, M. Qurbani, R. Heshmat, B. Larijani, S. Hosseini. "Effect of glutamine supplementation on cardiovascular risk factors in patients with type 2 diabetes." *Nutrition.* 31(1)(2015): 119–26. doi: 10.1016/j.nut.2014.05.014.

24. *". . . glutamine has been repeatedly proven safe."* Mansour A., M. Mohajer-Tehrani, M. Qurbani, R. Heshmat, B. Larijani, S. Hosseini. "Effect of glutamine supplementation on cardiovascular risk factors in patients with type 2 diabetes." *Nutrition.* 31(1) (2015): 119–26. doi: 10.1016/j.nut.2014.05.014.

25. *". . . carnosine . . ."* Budzen, Sandra, and Joanna Rymaszewska. "The biological role of carnosine and its possible applications in medicine." *Advances in Clinical and Experimental Medicine* 22(5) (2013): 739–744.

26. *". . . taurine . . ."* Ito, Takashi, and S. W. Schaffer, J. Azuma. "The potential usefulness of taurine on diabetes mellitus and its complications." Amino Acids. 42(5)(2012):1529– 39. doi: 10.1007/s00726-011-0883-5.

27. *". . . the minerals chromium, and zinc . . ."* May, J. M. "Famine from feast: Low red cell vitamin C levels in diabetes." *EBioMedicine* 2(11) (2015): 1586–1587. doi: 10.1016 /j.ebiom.2015.10.023.

28. *". . . the phospholipid choline, and vitamins C, D, B_1 (Thiamin), and biotin."* Oh, Y. S. "Bioactive compounds and their neuroprotective effects in diabetic complications." *Nutrients* 8(8) (2016). doi: 10.3390/nu8080472.

29. *". . . the phospholipid choline, and vitamins C, D, B_1 (Thiamin), and biotin."* Schwab, S., A. Zierer, M. Heier, B. Fischer, C. Huth, J. Baumert, C. Meisinger, A. Peters, and B. Thornad. "Intake of vitamin and mineral supplements and longitudinal association with HbA1c levels in the general non-diabetic Population—Results from the MONICA/KORA S3/F3 Study." *PLoS One* 10(10) (2015). doi: 10.1371/journal.pone.0139244.

    Cazeau, R., H. Huang, J. A. Bauer, and R. P. Hoffman. "Effect of vitamins C and E on endothelial function in type 1 diabetes mellitus." *Journal of Diabetes Research* (2016). doi: 10.1155/2016/3271293.

    Khosravi-Boroujeni, H., and F Ahmed, N. Sarrafzadegan. "Is the association between vitamin D and metabolic syndrome independent of other micronutrients." *International Journal for Vitamin & Nutrition Research* (2016): 1–16. doi: 10.1024/0300-9831/a000277.

30. *". . . the phospholipid choline, and vitamins C, D, B1 (Thiamin), and biotin."* Wolak, N., M. Zawrotniak, M. Gogol, A. Kozik, and M. Rapala-Kozik. "Vitamins B_1, B_2, B_3, and

B_9—occurrence, biosynthesis pathways and functions in human nutrition." *Mini-Reviews in Medicinal Chemistry* (2016).

31. *". . . zinc lowered HA1C percentage significantly . . ."* Al-Maroof, R. A. and Al-Sharbatti, S. S. "Serum zinc levels in diabetic patients and effect of zinc supplementation on glycemic control of type 2." *Saudi Medical Journal* 27(3)(2006): 344–50.

32. *"and the (benefits of) omega-3 fats (DHA and EPA) which both show good reduction in HA1C levels in response to supplementation"* Tortosa-Caparros, E., D. Navas-Carrillo, F. Marin, and E. Orenes-Pinero. "Anti-inflammatory effects of omega 3 and omega 6 polyunsaturated fatty acids in cardiovascular disease and metabolic syndrome." *Critical Reviews in Food Science and Nutrition* (2016). doi: 10.1080/10408398.2015.1126549.

    "and the omega-3 fats (DHA and EPA)" Polus, A., B. Zapala, U. Razny, A. Gielicz, B. Kiec-Wilk, M. Malczewska-Malec, M. Sanak, C. E. Childs, P. C. Calder, and A. Dembinska-Kiec. "Omega-3 fatty acid supplementation influences the whole blood transcriptome in women with obesity, associated with proresolving lipid mediator production." *Biochimica et Biophysica Acta* 1861(11) (2016): 1746–1755. doi: 10.1016/j.bbalip.2016.08.005.

CHAPTER 8

1. *". . . sugar and chocolate-fueled surge to be comparable, in brain-effect, to that elicited by the drug opium."* DiFeliceantonio, A. G., O. S. Mabrouk, R. T. Kennedy, and K. C. Berridge. 2012. "Enkephalin surges in dorsal neostriatum as a signal to eat." *Current Biology* 22(20) (2012): 1918–1924. doi: 10.1016/j.cub.2012.08.014.

2. *". . . we're consuming at least 3 billion pounds of chocolate and spending 31 billion dollars on it every year . . ."* The World Atlas of Chocolate. Simon Fraser University, British Columbia, Canada. Accessed September 28, 2016. https://www.sfu.ca/geog351fall03 /groups-webpages/gp8/consum/consum.html.

3. *". . . you could have inherited her addicted, 'desensitized' opioid system . . ."* Gugusheff J.R., Ong Z.Y., and B.S. Muhlhausler "A maternal 'junk-food' diet reduces sensitivity to the opioid antagonist naloxone in offspring postweaning."B. *FASEB Journal* 2013 Mar;27(3):1275–84. doi: 10.1096/fj.12-217653.

4. *"A recent study on chocolate chip cookies . . ."* Giraudo S. Q., M. K. Grace, C. C. Welch, C. J, Billington, and A. S. Levine. "Naloxone's anorectic effect is dependent upon the relative palatability of food." *Pharmacology, Biochemistry, and Behavior* 46(4)(1993):917–21.

5. *". . . charm is lost when the brain's endorphin reception is sealed off."* Fortuna, J. L. "Sweet preference, sugar addiction and the familial history of alcohol dependence: shared neural pathways and genes." *J Psychoactive Drugs.* 2010 Jun;42(2):147–51. doi: 10.1080/02791072.2010.10400687.

6. *". . . putting a brain device on audience members to identify the images in a potential ad for Cheetos . . ."*. "Neuromarketing: Understanding the why of what we buy." *Frozen Fire* http://frozenfire.com/neuromarketing-understanding-the-why-of-what -we-buy/.

    "NeuroFocus receives Grand Ogilvy Award from the Advertising Research Foundation." *PR Newswire*. Published April 02, 2009. Accessed March 7, 2017. http://www .prnewswire.com/news-releases/neurofocus-receives-grand-ogilvy-award-from-the -advertising-research-foundation-61707317.html.

7. *". . . sugar's effect is so powerful that many studies are comparing it to the impact of 'hard' opiates . . ."* Colantuoni, C., P. Rada, J. McCarthy, C. Patten, N. M. Avena, A. Chadeayne, and B. G. Hoebel. "Evidence that intermittent, excessive sugar intake causes endogenous opioid dependence." *Obesity Research* 10(6)(2002): 478–88.

8. *"Mindfulness can raise endorphin levels and temporarily reduce "reward-driven eating."* Mason A. E., E. S. Epel, K. Aschbacher, R. H. Lustig, M. Acree, J. Kristeller, M. Cohn, M. Dallman, Moran, P. J. B. Pacchetti, B. Laraia, F. M. Hecht, and J. Daubenmier. "Reduced reward-driven eating accounts for the impact of a mindfulness-based diet and exercise intervention on weight loss: Data from the SHINE randomized controlled trial." *Appetite.* 2016 May 1;100:86–93. doi: 10.1016/j.appet.2016.02.009. Epub 2016 Feb 8.

9. *"Eating disorders (binging, purging or starving) are known to trigger endorphin elevations."* Lienarda, Y., and Vamecqa, J. "[The auto-addictive hypothesis of pathological eating disorders]." *Presse Med.* 33(18)(2004): 33–40.

10. *". . . D-phenylalanine had strong endorphin-building power."* Ehrenpreis, S. "Pharmacology of enkephalins inhibitors: animal and human studies." *Acupuncture & Electro-Therapeutics Research,* 10(3)(1985): 203–208(6).

11. Gant, Charles, M.D. and Greg Lewis. *End Your Addiction Now: The Proven Nutritional Supplement Program That Can Set You Free.* New York: Square One, Publishers, 2010, pp. 203–214.

CHAPTER 9

1. *"The World Health Organization calls stress the "health epidemic of the 21st century,"* Wilkinson, R.G. and M. Marmot, ed. *Social Determinants of Health: The Solid Facts.* 2d. Edition." Demark: World Health Organization 2003. pp. 12–13.

2. *"70 percent of those feeling stressed"* Adam, T. C., and E. S. Epel. "Stress, eating and the reward system." *Physiology & Behavior* 91 (2007): 449–58. doi: 10.1016/j.physbeh.2007.04.011

3. *"A study that measured EEG responses to a GABA supplement."* Abdou, A. M., S. Higashiguchi, K. Horie, M. Kim, H. Hatt, and H. Yokogoshi. "Relaxation and immunity enhancement effects of gamma-aminobutyric acid (GABA) administration in humans." *BioFactors* 26(3) (2006):201–8.

4. *"GABA depletion can ignite food cravings and GABA supplementation decreases this drive for food."* Tews, J. K., Q. R. Rogers, J. G. Morris, and A. E. Harper. "Effect of dietary protein and GABA on food intake, growth and tissue amino acids in cats." *Physiology & Behavior* 32(2) (1984):301–8.

   This was reported in the seminal and still best book ever written on amino acid therapy *The Healing Nutrients Within*, by brilliant pioneer Carl C. Pfeiffer, M.D. Since his death, lead author on the new editions has been listed as Eric Braverman, M.D.

5. *"Among the overeaters most triggered by stress are food restrictors."* Wardle, J., A., G. O. Steptoe, and Z. Lipsey. "Stress, dietary restraint and food intake." *Journal of Psychosomatic Research* 48(2) (2000):195–202.

6. *"Sweet foods can shunt GABA out of active function."* Wang, C., K. Kerckhofs, M. Van de Casteele, I. Smolders, D. Pipeleers, and Z. Ling. "Glucose inhibits GABA release by pancreatic beta-cells through an increase in GABA shunt activity." *American Journal of Physiology: Endocrinology & Metabolism* 290(3) (2006):E494–9.

7. *"rumor . . . GABA supplements do not cross blood-brain-barrier . . ."* Boonstra, E., R. deKleijn, L. S. Coizato, A. Alkemade, B. U. Forstmann, and S. Nieuwenhuis. "Neurotransmitters as food supplements: the effects of GABA on brain and behavior." *Frontiers in Psychology* 6(2015): 1520. doi: 10.3389fpsyg.2015.01520.

8. *"low-calorie dieting elevates cortisol levels . . ."* Walter, K. N., E. J. Corwin, J. Ulbrecht, L. M. Demers, J. M. Bennett, C. A. Whetzel, and L. C. Klein. "Elevated thyroid stimulating hormone is associated with elevated cortisol in healthy young men and women." *Thyroid Research* 5(1) (2012):13. doi: 10.1186/1756-6614-5-13.

CHAPTER 10

1. *"sugar can specifically unleash dopamine, setting up a drug-like dependence"* Pepino, M. Y., S. A. Eisenstein, A. N. Bischoff, S. Klein, S. M. Moerlein, J. S. Perlmutter, K. J. Black, and T. Hershey, "Sweet Dopamine: Sucrose preferences relate differentially to striatal D2 receptor binding and age in obesity." *Diabetes* 65(9)(2016):2618–23.doi: 10.2337/ db16-0407.

2. *"Studies have found that they reduce calorie intake . . ."* Ballinger, A. B., and M. L. Clark. "L-phenylalanine releases cholecystokinin (CCK) and is associated with reduced food intake in humans: evidence for a physiological role of CCK in control of eating." *Metabolism* 43(6) (1994):735–8.

3. *"In one study, participants who were given phenylalanine ate 400 calories"* Pohle-Krauza, R. J., J. L. Navia, E. Y. Madore, J. E. Nyrop, and C. L. Pelkman. "Effects of L-phenylalanine on energy intake in overweight and obese women: interactions with dietary restraint status." *Appetite* 51(1) (2008):111–9. doi: 10.1016/j.appet.2008.01.002.

4. *"Many overeaters are low in both serotonin and the Cat called dopamine."* Jimerson, D. C., M. D. Lesem, W. H. Kaye, and T. D. Brewerton. "Low serotonin and dopamine metabolite concentrations in cerebrospinal fluid from bulimic patients with frequent binge episodes." *Archives of General Psychiatry* 49(2) (1992): 132-B.

5. *"The current 'obesogenic' (obesity-promoting) American diets is known to lower dopamine levels."* A. V. Kravitz, T. J. O'Neal, and D. M. Friend. "Do dopaminergic impairments underlie physical inactivity in people with obesity?" *Frontiers in Human Neuroscience* 10:514. doi: 10-3389/fnhum.2016.00514.

6. *"Charles Gant, M.D., who has researched and written about"* Gant, Charles, M.D. and Greg Lewis. *End Your Addiction Now: The Proven Nutrtional Supplement Program That Can Set You Free.* Garden City, NY: Square One Publishers, 2010.

7. Liu, Junxie, M. D. "Association of coffee consumption with all-cause and cardiovascular disease mortality." *Mayo Clinic Proceedings* 88(10) (2013): 1006–74. doi: 10-1016 /j.mayocp.2013.06.020.

    One study author, Carl J. Lavie, MD, describes these findings in his book, *The Obesity Paradox,* which contains many other important surprises as well.

8. *"It reduces the levels of the Cat-fueling amino acids phenylalanine . . ."* Hajnal A., and R. Norgren. "Accumbens dopamine mechanisms in sucrose intake." *Brain Research* 904(1) (2001): 76–84.

9. *"Caffeine can accelerate your progression toward diabetes."* Keijzers, G. B., B. E. De Galan, C. J. Tack, and P. Smits. "Caffeine can decrease insulin sensitivity in humans." *Diabetes Care* 25(2) (2002): 364–369. doi: 10.2337/diacare.25.2.364

10. *". . . are associated with an increased risk of stroke."* Gardener, H., T. Rundek, M. Markert, C. B. Wright, M.S.V. Elkind, and R. L. Sacco. "Diet soft drink consumption is associated with an increased risk of vascular events in the Northern Manhattan study." *Journal of General Internal Medicine* 27(9)(2012):1120–1126. Doi: 10.1007 /s11606-011-1968-2.

11. *"For many of us chocolate is a super-drug."* Greenberg, J. A., and B. Buijsse. "Habitual chocolate consumption may increase body weight in a dose-response manner." *PLoS ONE* 8(8) (2013): e70271. doi:10.1371/journal.pone.0070271.

    Farhat, G. E. Al-Dujaili, S. Drummond, and L. Fyfe. "Dark chocolate low in polyphenols increases BMI in normal weight and overweight adults (121.3)" *FASEB Journal* 28(1) (2014): Supplement 121.3.

12. *". . . unsweetened (dark) chocolate contains three times more caffeine and other stimulants and it, too, is linked with weight gain."* Greenberg, James A., and B. Buijsse.

"Habitual Chocolate Consumption May Increase Body Weight in a Dose-Response Manner." *PLoS ONE* 8(8) (2013): e70271. doi:10.1371/journal.pone.0070271.

13. Farhat, G., E. Al-Dujaili, S. Drummond, and L Fyfe. "Dark chocolate low in polyphenols increases BMI in normal weight and overweight adults (121.3)" *FASEB Journal* 28(1) (2014): Supplement 121.3.

CHAPTER 12

1. *"If, like 70% of diabetics, you have non-alcoholic fatty liver disease . . ."* Jinjuvadia, J., F. Antaki, P. Lohia, and S. Liangpunskul. "The association between nonalcoholic fatty liver fisease and metabolic abnormalities in the United States population." *Journal of Clinical Gastroenterology* (2016).

2. *"If, like 70% of diabetics, you have non-alcoholic fatty liver disease . . ."* Sherriff, J. L. and T. A. O'Sulllivan, C. Properzi, J. L. Oddo, L. A. Adams. "Choline, its potential role in nonalcoholic fatty liver disease, and the case for human and bacterial genes." *Advances in Nutrition* 7(1) (2016): 5–13 doi: 10.3945/an.114.007955.

3. *". . . a methylated multi B-complex for extra Vitamin B-1 and B-6 (in the P5P form), twice a day."* Polizzi, F. C., G. Andican, E. Cetin, S. Civelek, V. Yumuk, and G. Burcak. "Increased DNA-glycation in type 2 diabetic patients: the effect of thiamine and pyridoxine therapy." *Experimental and Clinical Endocrinology & Diabetes* 120(6) (2012): 329–334. doi: 10.1055/s-0031-1298016.

4. *"Also the amino carnosine daily."* Budzen, Sandra, and Joanna Rymaszewska. "The biological role of carnosine and its possible applications in medicine." *Advances in Clinical and Experimental Medicine* 22(5) (2013): 739–744.

5. *"Also the amino carnosine daily."* Stegen, S., B. Stegen, G. Aldini, A. Altomare, L. Cannizzaro, M. Orioli, S. Gerlo, L. Deidicque, M. Ramaekers, P. Hespel, and W. Derave. "Plasma carnosine, but not muscle carnosine, attenuates high-fat diet-induced metabolic stress." *Applied Physiology, Nutrition and Metabolism* 40(9) (2015): 868–876. doi: 10.1139/apnm-2015-0042.

6. *"For those who need an alternative to Metformin (which can cause digestive problems) the herb . . ."* Liu, C., Z. Wang, Y. Song, D. Wu, X. Zheng, P. Li, J. Jin, N. Xu, and L. Li. "Effects of berberine on amelioration of hyperglycemia and oxidative stress in high glucose and high fat diet-induced diabetic hamsters in vivo." *BioMed Research International* 2015 (2015): 313808. doi: 10.1155/2015/313808.

   Zhang, H., J. Wei, R. Xue, J. D. Wu, W. Zhao, Z. Z. Wang, S. K. Wang, Z. X. Zhou, D. Q. Song, Y. M. Wang, H. N. Pan, W. J. Kong, and J. D. Jiang. "Berberine lowers blood glucose in type 2 diabetes mellitus patients through increasing insulin receptor expression." *Metabolism* 59(2)(2010):285–92. doi: 10.1016/j.metabol.2009.07.029.

7. *"Widespread vitamin D deficiency is contributing to the U.S. increase in insulin resistance (even in children under age five) that sets us up for obesity and diabetes."* Talaei, A., M. Mohamadi, and Zahra Adgi. "The effect of vitamin D on insulin resistance in patients with type 2 diabetes." *Diabetology & Metabolic Syndrome* 5(2013):8. doi: 10.1186/1758-5996-5-8.

CHAPTER 13

1. *"Whether you approve of the Homo sapien brain, or not,. . . ."* Wrangham, R., Ph.D. *Catching Fire: How Cooking Made Us Human.* New York: Basic Books, 2010.

2. *". . . a recent study found that egg consumption lowers blood pressure and weight!"* Skórkowska-Telichowska, K., J. Kosińska, M. Chwojnicka, D. Tuchendler, M. Tabin, R.

Tuchendler, Ł. Bobak, T. Trziszka, and A. Szuba. "Positive effects of egg-derived phospholipids in patients with metabolic syndrome." *Advances in Medical Science* 61(1) (2016):169–74. doi: 10.1016/j.advms.2015.12.003.

3. *"Go back to the ten eggs per week we ate before 1970. It certainly wasn't raising blood pressure or weight, or increasing heart disease then!"* C. A. Eunjung. "Eggs are okay again." *Washington Post.* Published January 7, 2016. Accessed January 11, 2017. https://www.washingtonpost.com/news/to-your-health/wp/2016/01/07/cholesterol-new-u-s-dietary-guidelines-remove-warnings-making-eggs-okay-again/?utm_term=.5e6367cbcda8.

4. *"Multiple studies have shown that people on low carbohydrate but unrestricted fat diets lose more weight than those on low-fat diets, even when the calories are equal. Their cholesterol and diabetes markers drop lower too!"* Feinman, R. D., W. K. Pogozelski, A. Astrup, R. K.Bernstein, E. J. Fine, E. C. Westman, A. Accurso, L. Frassetto, B. A. Gower, S. I. McFarlane, J. V. Nielsen, T. Krarup, L. Saslow, K. S. Roth, M. C. Vernon, J. S. Volek, G. B. Wilshire, A. Dahlqvist, R. Sundberg, A. Childers, K. Morrison, A. H. Manninen, H. M. Dashti, R. J. Wood, J. Wortman, and N. Worm. "Dietary carbohydrate restriction as the first approach in diabetes management: critical review and evidence base." *Nutrition* 31(1) (2015): 1–13. doi: 10.1016/j.nut.2014.06.011.

5. *"farmed fish contain some omega-3 fat, but also much more omega-6 fat . . ."* Sprague, M., J. R. Dick, and D. R. Tocher. "Impact of sustainable feeds on omega-3 long-chain fatty acid levels in farmed Atlantic salmon, 2006–2015." *Scientific Reports* 6(2016). doi:10.1038/srep21892.

   Strobel, C., G. Jahreis, and K. Kuhnt. "Survey of n-3 and n-6 polyunsaturated fatty acids in fish and fish products." *Lipids in Health and Disease* 11(2012):144. doi: 10.1186/1476-511X-11-144.

6. *"We can now, once again, derive some DHA and EPA from the fat of land animals, but only if they're traditionally grass fed."* Masterjohn, Christopher. "Fatty Acid Analysis of Grass-fed and Grain-fed Beef Tallow." The Weston A. Price Foundation. Published 21, 2014. Accessed January 11, 2017. http://www.westonaprice.org/know-your-fats/fatty-acid-analysis-of-grass-fed-and-grain-fed-beef-tallow/.

7. *" . . . can derive some DHA and EPA from the fatty meat of land animals, but only if they're grass fed"* Średnicka-Tober, D., et al. "Composition differences between organic and conventional meat: a systematic literature review and meta-analysis." *British Journal of Nutrition* 115(6) (2016):994–1011. doi: 10.1017/S0007114515005073.

8. *"Organic whole milk products have recently been found to contain twice as much omega-3 as nonorganic (or low-fat) versions."* Benbrook, C. M., G. Butler, M. A. Latif, C. Leifert, D. R. Davis. "Organic production enhances milk nutritional quality by shifting fatty acid composition: a U.S. wide, 18-month study." *PLOS ONE* 8(12): e82429. doi: 10.1371/journal.pone.0082429.

9. *"The nutrient content of organic produce in multinational study was 60% higher . . ."* David, D., M. Epps, and H. Riordan. "Changes in USDA food composition data for 43 garden crops, 1950 to 1999."*Journal of the American College of Nutrition* 23(6)(2004):669–82. Barnaski, M., et al. "Higher antioxidant and lower cadmium concentrations and lower incidence of pesticide residues in organically grown crops: a systematic literature review and meta-analyses." *British Journal of Nutrition* 112(5)(2014):794–811. doi: 10.1017/S0007114514001366.

10. *"Modern conventional fruit has been bred to be bigger."* Harvey, C. "Amazing graphics show how much fruits have changed since humans started growing them." *Business*

Insider. Published October 16, 2014. Accessed January 11, 2017. http://www.business insider.com/how-fruits-have-evovled-over-time-2014-10.

11. *"stevia leaves are 10–15 times sweeter, but the extract is 100–300 times sweeter."* Mogra, R., and V. Dashora. "Exploring the use of Stevia rebaudiana as a Sweetener in Comparison with Other Sweeteners." *Journal of Human Ecology* 25(2) (2009): 117–120.

12. *"We need to drink half to one ounce of water for every pound of body weight."* Elkaim, Yuri. "The truth about how much water you should really drink." *US News.* Published September 13, 2013. Accessed January 11, 2017. http://health.usnews.com/health-news /blogs/eat-run/2013/09/13/the-truth-about-how-much-water-you-should-really -drink.

13. *"The AHA urges a 1,500mg (¾ tsp) cap on daily salt."* "Experts criticize new study about salt consumption." *American Heart Association News.* http://news.heart.org /experts-criticize-new-study-about-salt-consumption/. Published May 20, 2016. Accessed January 5, 2017.

14. *"study found that the death rates of heart disease patients on a low sodium diet . . ."* Mente, A. et al. "Associations of urinary sodium excretion with cardiovascular events in individuals with and without hypertension: a pooled analysis of data from four studies." *The Lancet* 388(10043)(2016):465–475. doi: 10.1016/S0140-6736(16)30467-6.

15. Morell, Sally Fallon. "Why Salt is essential to health and happiness." The Weston A. Price Foundation. http://www.westonaprice.org/health-topics/abcs-of-nutrition/the -salt-of-the-earth/ . Published July 4, 2011. Accessed January 5, 2017.

16. *Re Berlin airlift:* Reeves, R. *Daring Young Men: The Heroism and Triumph of the Berlin Airlift.* New York: Simon & Schuster 2011, p. 94.

17. *"association between no breakfast and fatigue, infertility, heart disease, cognitive defects"* So, H. K., E.A.S. Nelson, A. M. Li, G. S. Guidan, J. Yin, O. C. Ng, and R.Y.T. Sung. "Breakfast frequency inversely associated with BMI and body fatness in Hong Kong Chinese children aged 9–18 years." *British Journal of Nutrition* 106(5)(2011):742–51. doi: 10.1017/S0007114511000754.

Brazier, Y., "Good Breakfast Linked to Better Grades." *Medical News Today.* http://www.medicalnewstoday.com/articles/302942.php. Published November 22, 2015. Accessed January 5, 2017.

Wennberg, M. P., Gustafsson, P. WennBerg, and A. Hammarstrom. "Poor breakfast habits in adolescence predict the metabolic syndrome in adulthood." *Public Health Nutrition* 18(1)(2015):122–9. doi: 10.1017/S1368980013003509.

O'Neil, C. E., T. A. Nicklas, and V. L. Fulgoni. "Nutrient intake, diet quality, and weight/adiposity parameters in breakfast patterns compares with no breakfast in adults: national health and nutrition examination survey 2001–2008." *Journal of the Academy of Nutrition and Dietetics* 114(12 Suppl)(2014):S27–43. doi: 10.1016 /j.jand.2014.08.021.

CHAPTER 14

1. *". . . when we began cultivating plants and husbanding animals for food."* Wrangham, Richard, Ph.D. *Catching Fire: How Cooking Made Us Human.* New York: Basic Books, 2010.

This marvelous resource was suggested by local anthropology professor Christina Milner-Rose, PhD. who also summarized the development of human meat eating and brain development in several fascinating interviews with me in 2016.

2. *". . . weight gain, insulin resistance, and metabolic syndrome have often been the result for those . . ."* Hardy, M., J. A. Tye-Din, J. A. Stewart, F. Schmitz, N. L. Dudek, I.

Hanchapola, A. W. Purcell, and R. P. Anderson. "Ingestion of oats and barley in patients with celiac disease mobilizes cross-reactive T cells activated by avenin peptides and immuno-dominant hordein peptides." *Journal of Autoimmunity* 56 (2014):56–65. doi: 10.1016/j.jaut.2014.10.003.

3. *"10 year study found almost 10% of celiacs reacted to oats as well."* M. Y. Hardy, J. A. Tye-Din, J. A. Stewart, F. Schmitz, N. L. Dudek, I. Hanchapola, A. W. Purcell, and R. P. Anderson. "Ingestion of oats and barley in patients with celiac disease mobilizes cross-reactive T cells activated by avenin peptides and immuno-dominant hordein peptides." *Journal of Autoimmunity*, 2014. doi: 10.1016/j.jaut.2014.10.003.

4. *"Type O's, not surprisingly, have the lowest rates of type 2 diabetes."* Fagherazzi, G., Gusto, F. Clavel-Chapelon, B. Balkau, and F. Bonnet. "ABO and Rhesus blood groups and risk of type 2 diabetes: evidence from the large E3N cohort study." *Diabetologia* 58(3) (2014): 519–22. doi: 10.1007/s00125-014-3472-9.

5. *"Since gluten intolerance is known to be a causative factor in diabetes, gluten certainly must go."* Feinman, R. D., W. K. Pogozelski, A. Astrup, R. K. Bernstein, E. J. Fine, E. C. Westman, A. Accurso, L. Frassetto, B. A. Gower, S. I. McFarlane, J. V. Nielsen, T. Krarup, L. Saslow, K. S. Roth, M. C. Vernon, J. S. Volek, G. B. Wilshire, A. Dahlqvist, R. Sundberg, A. Childers, K. Morrison, A. H. Manninen, H. M. Dashti, R. J. Wood, J. Wortman, and N. Worm. "Dietary carbohydrate restriction as the first approach in diabetes management: critical review and evidence base." *Nutrition* 31(1) (2015): 1–13. doi: 10.1016/j.nut.2014.06.011.

6. *". . . diabetics can only rarely reintroduce any of the above higher carbohydrate foods."* Haimoto, Ha., T. Sasakabe, T. Kawamura, H. Umegaki, M. Komeda, and K. Wakai. "Three-graded stratification of carbohydrate restriction by level of baseline hemoglobin A1c for type 2 diabetes patients with a moderate low-carbohydrate diet." *Nutrition & Metabolism* 11(33) (2014). doi: 10.1186/1743-7075-11-33.

7. *". . . adding healthy, undamaged fats seems to be actually life-saving for diabetics . . ."* Busko, Marlene. "High-Fat Diet Best for Diabetes Prevention in Obesity Prone." *Medscape.* Last updated June 29, 2016. Accessed September 29, 2016. www.medscape.com/viewarticle/865525.

8. Yakoob, M. Y., P. Shi, W. C. Willett, K. M. Rexrode, H. Campos, E. J. Orav, F. B. Hu, and D. Mozaffarian. "Circulating Biomarkers of Dairy Fat and Risk of Incident Diabetes Mellitus Among U.S. Men and Women in Two Large Prospective Cohorts." *Circulation.* 2016; CIRCULATIONAHA. 115.018410. https://doi.org/10.1161/CIRCULATIONAHA. 115.018410.

9. *".lean further toward soups, stews, poaching, steaming, and marinating with lemon or vinegar any meats, poultry, or fish before cooking over more direct heat."* Vlassara, H., and J. Uribarri. "Advanced glycation end products (AGE) and diabetes: cause, effect, or both?" *Current Diabetes Report* 14(1)(2014):453. doi: 10.1007/s11892-013-0453-1.

10. Masterjohn, C. "The Trouble With Measuring AGEs—Butter and More." Accessed September 17, 2017. https://chrismasterjohnphd.com/2011/10/06/trouble-with-measuring-ages-butter-and/.

CHAPTER 15

1. *". . . beta-casein cow's milk . . ."* Jianquin, Sun, et. al. "Effects of milk containing only A2 beta casein versus milk containing both A1 and A2 beta casein proteins on gastrointestinal physiology, symptoms of discomfort, and cognitive behavior of people with self-reported intolerance of traditional cow's milk." *Nutritional Journal* 15 (2016): 35. doi: 10.1186/s12937-016-01472.

2. Masterjohn, Christopher. "Milk gone bad: A1 beta-casein and GI distress." *Examine .com Research Digest* 19(1 of 2) (2016): 8–14. http://vb.examinecdn.com/erd/chris masterjohn2.pdf.

CHAPTER 16

1. *"thyroid medication is often the top prescription drug sold in America"* Brown, Troy, RN. WebMD. Published May 8, 2015. Accessed May 9, 2017. http://www.webmd .com/drug-medication/news/20150568/most-prescribed-top-sellings drugs.
2. *"Over 20 million Americans diagnosed with forms of thyroid disease."* American Thyroid Association. "Genual Information/PressRoom." Accessed May 10, 2017. http:// www.thyroid.org/media-main/about-hypothyroidism/.
3. *"More than 13 million Americans undiagnosed."* Ibid.
4. *"One in eight women encounter thyroid disease in . . ."* Ibid.
5. *"Women are 10 to 20 times more likely than men . . ."* Ibid.

Index